PEARLS of WISDOM

Emergency Medicine

ORAL BOARD REVIEW

Sixth Edition

Editors and Chief

William G. Gossman, MD, FAAEM
Chairman, Department of Emergency Medicine
Creighton University School of Medicine
Omaha, Nebraska

Scott H. Plantz, MD, FAAEM
Associate Professor of Emergency Medicine
University of Louisville Emergency Medicine Residency
Louisville, Kentucky

Mc Graw Hill Education

New York Chicago San Francisco Athens London Madrid Mexico City
Milan New Delhi Singapore Sydney Toronto

Emergency Medicine Oral Board Review, Sixth Edition

1 2 3 4 5 6 7 8 9 0 RHR/RHR 20 19 18 17 16 15

ISBN 978-0-07-184362-1
MHID 0-07-184362-0

Notice

Medicine is an ever-changing science. As new research and clinical experience broaden our knowledge, changes in treatment and drug therapy are required. The authors and the publisher of this work have checked with sources believed to be reliable in their efforts to provide information that is complete and generally in accord with the standards accepted at the time of publication. However, in view of the possibility of human error or changes in medical sciences, neither the authors nor the publisher nor any other party who has been involved in the preparation or publication of this work warrants that the information contained herein is in every respect accurate or complete, and they disclaim all responsibility for any errors or omissions or for the results obtained from use of the information contained in this work. Readers are encouraged to confirm the information contained herein with other sources. For example and in particular, readers are advised to check the product information sheet included in the package of each drug they plan to administer to be certain that the information contained in this work is accurate and that changes have not been made in the recommended dose or in the contraindications for administration. This recommendation is of particular importance in connection with new or infrequently used drugs.

This book was set in Adobe Garamond Pro
The editors were Catherine A. Johnson and Christina M. Thomas.
The production supervisor was Rick Ruzycka.
Project management was provided by Amit Kashyap, Aptara, Inc.
RR Donnelley was the printer and binder.

This book is printed on acid-free paper.

Library of Congress Cataloging-in-Publication Data

Emergency medicine oral board review / [edited by] William G. Gossman, Scott H. Plantz. – Sixth edition.
p. ; cm. – (Pearls of wisdom)
Includes bibliographical references.
ISBN 978-0-07-184362-1 (pbk. : alk. paper) – ISBN 0-07-184362-0 (pbk. : alk. paper)
I. Gossman, William G., editor. II. Plantz, Scott H., editor. III. Series: Pearls of wisdom.
[DNLM: 1. Emergency Medicine–Case Reports. 2. Emergency Medicine–Examination Questions. WB 18.2]
RC86.9
616.02'5076–dc23

2015009152

DEDICATION

For my wife, Sherry, who is the most important person in my life and my best friend.

Bill

For my son, Huntly Conway Plantz, thank you for the hug you bring me everyday.

Scott

CONTENTS

CONTRIBUTORS

ASSOCIATE EDITORS

Steve C. Christos, DO, MS, FACEP, FAAEM
Clinical Assistant Professor
Department of Emergency Medicine
Presence Resurrection Medical Center
Chicago, Illinois

Martin Huecker, MD
Assistant Professor and Research Director
Department of Emergency Medicine
University of Louisville
Louisville, Kentucky

Stephen W. Leslie, MD, FACS
Associate Professor of Surgery
Division of Urology
Creighton University School of Medicine
Omaha, Nebraska

Kelly Mullin, PA-C
Creighton University Medical Center
Omaha, Nebraska

Robert Oelhaf, MD, FAAEM
Clinical Instructor and Research Director
Creighton University School of Medicine
Omaha, Nebraska

Hugh Schoff, MD
Assistant Professor
Department of Emergency Medicine
University of Louisville
Louisville, Kentucky

Kathryn Walenz, PA-C
Creighton University Medical Center
Omaha, Nebraska

CONTRIBUTORS TO PREVIOUS EDITIONS

Bobby Abrams, MD, FAAEM

Jonathan Adler, MD, FAAEM

David F. M. Brown, MD

Eduardo Castro, MD

James Corrall, MD

Bikram S. Dhillon, MD

Stephen Emond, MD

Craig Feied, MD, FAAEM

Mitchell J. Goldman, DO, FAAEM, FAAP

Lindsey Harrell, MD

Christine Head, PA-C

Melanie S. Heniff, MD, FAAEM, FAAP

James Holmes, MD

Eddie Hooker, MD, FAAEM

Lance W. Kreplick, MD, FAAEM

Joe Lex, MD, FAAEM

Bernard Lopez, MD, FAAEM

Mary Nan Mallory, MD, FAAEM

David Morgan, MD, FAAEM

Carlo Rosen, MD

David C. Smith, DO

Dana Stearns, MD

Jack "Lester" Stump, MD, FAAEM

Loice Swischer, MD, FAAEM

Stephen H. Thomas, MD

James Unger, MD, FAAEM

Thomas Widell, MD

John Wipfler, MD

Leslie Zun, MD

INTRODUCTION

Congratulations on your purchase of *Emergency Medicine Oral Board Review: Pearls of Wisdom.* Originally designed as a study aid to improve performance on the EM Oral Board Exam, this book is full of useful information. First intended for EM specialists, we have learned that this unique format has also been useful to house officers and medical students in the ED.

The primary intent of *Emergency Medicine Oral Board Review* is to serve as a study aid to improve performance on the EM Oral Board Exam. To achieve this goal, the text is written in three formats: a topic review, a rapid-fire question/answer format, and actual practice cases. Emphasis has been placed on distilling true trivia and key facts that are easily overlooked, quickly forgotten, or needed on the oral board exam.

The ABEM oral exam is an anxiety-provoking exam, and this is understandable. This is a unique type of test that requires you to "imagine" a patient is having stroke, see it in your mind, and talk through the details of diagnosing, managing, and dispositioning the patient. There are few tests like this in medical school or residency. After many years of teaching residents how to take this exam, we have come up with a few key points to decrease your anxiety:

1. You have already proven that you know the material being covered because you passed the written test. The medical knowledge required is far less than that for the written part.
2. The scenarios are contrived and you must learn to "play the game." You can conquer this exam by coming up with a format that can be used to get you through any case, from a 1 day old to a 99 year old.
3. Traits being measure are things like interpersonal skills, patient relationships, and ability to cope with stress while being evaluated. Basically the test attempts to simulate what you do every day at work.
4. Practice, practice, practice. Do every case you can or read through them for an idea of what is being expected of you.

The first third of this book is presented in a straightforward format with essential facts. The second section of the book consists of random pathophysiology, procedure, and treatment pearls with some questions selected from the *Emergency Medicine Written Board Review: Pearls of Wisdom*, sixth edition. The questions are grouped into small clusters by topic presented in no particular order. The Random Pearls section repeats much of the factual information contained in the Pearls Topics and builds on this foundation with greater emphasis on linking information and filling in gaps from the Pearls Topics. The final section of the text, *Sample Cases*, is the most important and contains actual practice cases that should be used with your study partner to gain confidence and experience in attacking boards cases.

Emergency Medicine Oral Board Review has limitations (directly proportional to those of the senior editor/authors!): We have found *many* conflicts among sources of information. Variation between the definition of "apneustic" breathing provided in Tintinalli versus Stedman's causes little consternation. Variations between half-life of paralyzing agents and of naloxone, or between rankings of stability of cervical spine fractures, provided in Tintinalli versus Rosen are of more concern. We have tried to verify in other references the most accurate information. Some texts have internal discrepancies further confounding clarification of information.

Emergency Medicine Oral Board Review risks accuracy by aggressively pruning complex concepts down to the simplest kernel—the dynamic knowledge base and clinical practice of emergency medicine is not like that! For the most part, the information taken as "correct" is that indicated in the resources such as *Emergency Medicine, A Comprehensive Study Guide*, edited by Tintinalli, Krome, and Ruiz, *The Clinical Practice of Emergency Medicine*, edited by Harwood-Nuss, Linden, Luten, Shepherd, and Wolfson, eMedicine Medscape, and UpToDate.

New research and practice occasionally deviates from that which likely represents the “right” answer for test purposes. In such cases, we have selected the information that we believe is most likely to be “correct” for test purposes. This text is designed help you pass and maximize your score on a *test.* Refer to your most current sources of information and mentors for direction for *practice.*

We welcome your comments, suggestions, and criticism. Great effort has been made to verify these topics, questions and answers, and cases. There will be information we have provided that is at variance with your knowledge. Most often this is attributable to the variance between original sources (previously discussed). *Please* make us aware of any errata you find. We hope to make continuous improvements and would greatly appreciate any input with regard to format, organization, content, presentation, or about specific questions.

Study hard and good luck!
Bill and Scott

ORAL BOARDS PREPARATION

"Learning to learn is to know how to navigate in a forest of facts, ideas and theories, a proliferation of constantly and changing items of knowledge. Learning to learn is to know what to ignore but at the same time not rejecting innovation and research."

Raymond Queneau

Oral Boards Preparation

"Two roads diverged in a wood and I took the one less traveled by, And that has made all the difference."
Robert Frost

GENERAL EXAMINATION INFORMATION

1. **Where:**

   The examination is administered twice a year in April and October at the Chicago-O'Hare Marriott. Most graduating residents take the written examination in November of the year they graduate from residency. You will be notified of the results around January, and assigned a position in the spring or fall for your oral examination.

2. **Pass Rate:**

   Residency-trained, first-time examinees have a pass rate of 90% to 93%.

3. **Expenses:**

   Examination fee plus the cost of hotel, food, and travel.

4. **Duration of Examination:**

   The examination will be completed in about 6 hours. The 6-hour block includes 30 minutes for orientation, 2.5 hours of waiting periods, and 3 hours of testing. The orientation will include a 5-minute welcome, a 10-minute case demonstration, a 5-minute description of the rating and scoring, and a 5-minute explanation of the logistics of the examination day.

5. **Detailed Description of the Examination:**

   After the orientation, you will go to an examination area, which is a small group of hotel rooms clustered together on a particular floor. A lounge area will be on one of the floors where you can wait between simulations. A receptionist will be available on each floor to assist and direct you. You will present to your examining room 5 minutes before a simulation is scheduled to begin and wait outside the room. You are not allowed to take anything with you, and paper and pencil for notes will be provided in the room. After the test case is done, you must leave all notes you have made in the room.

6. **Number of Cases Comprising the Examination:**

   There will be five single cases each lasting 15 minutes, and two triple cases each lasting 30 minutes. One of the cases will consist of a field-test case and will not be scored.

7. Time of the Day:

Testing sessions will be either in the morning (6:30 AM–12:30 PM) or afternoon (1:30 PM–7:30 PM). You may request to change the time and the day of the examination. If submitted early, your request is usually granted.

8. Scoring:

Each case is scored individually by assessing the eight component skills described below. Information was taken directly from the *ABEM Examination Information for Candidates* booklet for 2014.

8.1. The 8-point scale contains the following sections.

A. **Data Acquisition:** This assesses your ability to gather a history perform an appropriate physical examination and obtain appropriate tests. This rating addresses the following:
- Elicited in an orderly fashion and timely manner the appropriate data required to correctly diagnose and manage the patient.
- Data collection approach was well integrated into the overall management plan.

B. **Problem Solving:** This assesses your ability to create a differential diagnosis, analyze data accurately to narrow your differential, and draw reasonable conclusions. It addresses the following:
- Approach to the clinical situation was well organized in a manner to collect data, select among reasonable alternative diagnosis while ensuring patient stabilization and anticipating future problems.
- Efficient arrival at an informed and appropriate management plan.

C. **Patient Management:** This assesses your ability to plan and provide therapy in a timely and efficient manner. It addresses the following:
- Treat at the appropriate times throughout the encounter.
- Proper referral of the patient at the appropriate time.
- Patient was properly attended when treating other patients during the encounter.

D. **Resource Utilization:** This section will ascertain your ability to utilize available resources to aid in caring for your patient. You are being tested on your ability to be resourceful (have paramedics find the pill bottles). Do not do a "shotgun" approach to each patient, this will hurt your score. Examples include the following:
- Use economic efficiency when ordering x-rays and laboratory tests. Seldom are a CT and MRI required on the same patient.
- Order diagnostic imaging in children that does not use ionizing radiation when a satisfactory alternative imaging is available.
- Exhibit actions that reflect logic, cost sensitivity, and limit patient discomfort and exposure.

E. **Health-Care Provided (Outcome):** The examiner will ask two questions: (1) Did the patient receive timely and appropriate medical treatment? (2) Did the patient's condition improve by the care provided? This rating is based on actual patient outcome, such as the following:
- The patient received timely and appropriate care with regard to the national standards of care.
- The patient's condition stabilized and maximally improved by the medical interventions provided.

F. **Interpersonal Relations:** You will be evaluated on your ability to interact with patients and family members in a compassionate and informative manner, such as:
- Explain all procedures or painful examination techniques, giving the patient an option.
- Always assume that an unconscious patient can still hear and warn him/her of impending painful maneuvers and procedures.
- Show respect to other medical staff.
- Communication should be clear, concise, and not full of medical language.

G. **Comprehension of Pathophysiology:** This assesses your understanding of the underlying pathophysiology, and the rationale for the clinical procedures that have been ordered. Your comprehension will be assessed during the case management, not at the end with specific questions.

H. **Clinical Competence (Overall):** Overall, how well did you do? The examiner will judge your level of proficiency by accessing your combined cognitive and procedural skills in providing emergency care in this setting.

8.2. The eight performance ratings are scored on an 8-point scale for each oral case.

- **A. Very Acceptable (7, 8):** The examiner does not have significant criticisms of the candidate's ability to diagnose and manage the case.
- **B. Acceptable (5, 6):** All critical actions were addressed and no dangerous actions were undertaken. Several minor inefficiencies or errors where found, but the performance was within the range of acceptable health-care standards.
- **C. Unacceptable (3, 4):** One or more critical actions were not taken and/or one or more dangerous actions were implemented. Several deficiencies in data acquisition and management were observed. Health care was provided in an incomplete, unorganized, and unacceptable manner.
- **D. Very Unacceptable (1, 2):** Gross negligence and/or mismanagement were observed.

8.3. Critical Actions:

Critical actions are few in number (2–5), and describe actions important in properly managing the case. These are predetermined and impossible to know what is or is not a critical action. It is possible to miss one or more critical actions and still pass the examination. The pass/fail decision depends on your performance across all critical actions and cases.

8.4. Pass/Fail Criteria: A candidate passes the examination by fulfilling A or B stated below:

- **A.** The average score calculated from all of the cases is 5.75 or higher.
- **B.** The highest and lowest cases are averaged. If this score and the scores from the remaining four cases are all 5.00 or above, you pass.
- **C.** You fail a case by scoring less than 5.00, performing a dangerous act, or missing a critical action.

9. Examination Procedures:

9.1. Obtain initial vital signs and a brief history. While discussing medical history, communicate with the examiner as you would talk to a real patient.

9.2. Perform a physical examination. Remember you will be in charge. Nothing will be done unless you ask for it.

9.3. Order laboratory studies, x-rays, etc., without "shot gunning."

9.4. Review laboratory studies, x-ray results, etc. Abnormal laboratory values will not be highlighted.

9.5. Based upon all the information gathered, make a diagnosis and take the appropriate actions. The patient will deteriorate or improve depending on your actions.

9.6. The examiner will end the case, ask one or more questions, and then excuse you.

9.7. Feedback will not be provided.

10. Strategies:

10.1. Take your time and approach the examination systematically.

10.2. Ask for general information. For example, "What do I see, hear, and smell as I observe the patient?"

10.3. Develop a system for taking notes and practice it.

10.4. Be direct in verbalizing your actions.

10.5. Listen to the examiner's feedback and cues.

10.6. If certain information cannot be obtained, continue to manage the case.

10.7. Don't verbally interpret x-ray and ECG findings unless asked to do so.

10.8. Know the dosages for commonly used drugs.

10.9. Use consultants as needed.

10.10. Acknowledge that all the examiner's information is correct.

10.11. Normal laboratory values will be provided.

10.12. Look up information, if necessary.

10.13. Never get into a conflict with the examiner, you will lose.

10.14. You are in charge, so take control of the case early.

10.15. If something goes wrong backup and reassess.

10.16. All abnormal vital signs require immediate stabilization.

SUGGESTED OUTLINE OF ATTACK

The following outline provides one method of consistently approaching and treating a simulated patient. This outline includes a "Primary Survey," which may be interrupted for acute interventions and test ordering, a "Secondary Survey," and treatment and disposition. A brief outline is provided below; details of each phase are described in the following sections. It is usually important to cover all of these issues during each case. The editors strongly encourage you to develop your own individualized approach based on the history, physical, and on the treatment approach of your own practice.

Primary Survey

Obtain a complete set of vital signs, which may include bilateral BPs and use of a rectal probe or temperature sensing Foley catheter. Ask, "When I walk in the room, what do I see, hear, and smell?" Introduce yourself to the patient and all family members.

A. **Airway:** Includes C-spine precaution, check for pooled secretions, gag reflex, and tracheal deviation.

B. **Breathing:** Check the rate and depth of respirations, breath sounds, and chest movement.

C. **Circulation:** BP, capillary refill, skin color, and temperature. Perform interventions as determined thus far, that is, restrain, security, intubation, needle thoracostomy, chest tube, etc. Consider interrupting primary survey here to order other interventions or tests.

D. **Disability:** Pupils, GCS, and perform a brief neuro examination (are they moving everything).

E. **Expose:** Undress, perform a swift abbreviated examination, roll patient, check skin, and look for medical alert tags.

F. **Finger and Rectal Examination:** Check for gross blood, occult blood, high riding or "boggy" prostate, and blood at urethral meatus. Insert a Foley as needed.

G. **NG:** Insert and check aspirate.

H. **History:** A complete history requires **AMPLE FRIENDS**.

A	Allergies	**F**	Family medical history, family, friends, and family doctor as the sources of information
M	Meds	**R**	Records, ROS
P	Past medical history	**I**	Immunizations
L	Last meal	**E**	EMS personnel as sources of information
E	Events/environment and chief complaint	**N**	Narcotic and other drugs/substances of abuse
		D	Doctor for admission and consultation
		S	Social history (living environment, etc.)

Consider pausing here at the end of the Primary Survey to re-evaluate vital signs and to order additional tests and treatments.

Secondary Survey

This part is a detailed head-to-toe full body survey looking for any and all potential abnormalities.

General

Skin

HEENT

Neck

Lungs/Heart/Chest

Back

Abdomen

Extremities

Neuro

Vascular

Perineum/Rectum/Vagina/Pelvis

Primary/Secondary Survey Pearls:

- Complete the procedures and order additional tests.
- Evaluate all laboratory and x-ray results.
- Recheck vital signs.
- Be consistent and complete the physical examination.
- Talk to family and inform them of your findings and plan.
- Ask patients and/or family if they have any other information to give.
- Make sure transfers are arranged and consultants are contacted.

THE PRIMARY SURVEY

Obtain a complete set of vital signs, which may include bilateral BPs and use of a rectal probe. Ask, "When I walk in the room, what do I see, hear, and smell?"

1. **Airway:**

   1.1. Assessment: Along with the C-spine,

   A. immobilize C-spine, if indicated
   B. place patient in a cervical collar

   1.2. Management:

   A. Ask patient if he/she can speak and breath: If yes, move on to "breathing," if no, stop and correct the problem.
   B. Open the airway, perform the chin-lift maneuver (use the jaw-thrust maneuver for patients with a possible C-spine injury).
   C. Clear the airway of foreign bodies and see if the patient is pooling secretions.
   D. If above maneuvers do not work, a definitive airway is required (oropharyngeal, nasopharyngeal, orotracheal intubation, or cricothyrotomy).
   E. If intubation is required, preoxygenate with 100% O_2 by using a bag-valve-mask, auscultate the chest, and obtain a postintubation chest x-ray.
   F. Continue to maintain the C-spine in a neutral position.

2. Breathing:

2.1. Assessment:

A. Expose the neck and chest.
B. Determine the rate and depth of respirations.
C. Inspect and palpate the neck and chest for tracheal deviation, for unilateral and bilateral chest movements, and for any signs of injury, such as bruising, crepitance, and tenderness.
D. Auscultate the chest bilaterally.

2.2. Management:

A. Administer a high concentration of oxygen.
B. Treat a tension pneumothorax.
C. Seal an open pneumothorax.
D. Place the patient on a pulse oximeter.

3. Circulation:

3.1. Assessment:

A. Inspect color of the skin and the presence of rash and petechiae.
B. Ascertain pulse rate and regularity.
C. Determine capillary refill.
D. Obtain blood pressure.
E. Find sources of external bleeding.

3.2. Management:

A. Initiate one to two large bore IVs (14–16 gauge) of warm LR or NS, if indicated.
B. Simultaneously obtain appropriate laboratory studies.
C. Apply direct pressure to bleeding sites.
D. Place on a cardiac monitor.

3.3. Order:

IV (bilateral anticubital fossa), O_2, monitor, ABG, ECG, x-ray (C-spine, CXR, and pelvis), and laboratory studies.

3.4. Treatment:

D_{50} or glucose check, naloxone (Narcan), thiamine, and tetanus.

4. Disability—Brief Neurologic Examination:

4.1. Assessment:

A. Determine the level of consciousness by using the GCS.
B. Assess the pupils for size, equality, and reaction.
C. Test the patient's ability to move all extremities.

4.2. Management: Consider using the following coma protocol:

A. Thiamine, 100 mg IV (not indicated in children younger than 10 years).
B. Naloxone (Narcan), 2 mg IV in adults or 0.01 to 0.1 mg/kg in pediatrics.
C. Bedside glucose check or give glucose, 50 to100 mL of $D_{50}W$ for adults patients, 2 to 4 mL/kg of $D_{25}W = 0.5$ to 1.0 g/kg for pediatric patients aging 1 month to 8 years, and 0.5 to 1.0 g/kg of $D_{10}W$ for the neonates.

5. Exposure:

5.1. Completely undress the patient.

5.2. Look for a medic alert tag and check his/her wallet for potential medical information.

5.3. Prevent hypothermia.

6. **Finger and Foley:**
   - **6.1.** Finger in every orifice. Check for contraindications to placement of Foley.
   - **6.2.** After assessment of the pelvic bones, genitalia, and rectum, insert all appropriate catheters.

7. **Gastric:**
   - **7.1.** Check for contraindications to placement of a nasogastric tube (NG).
   - **7.2.** Insert an NG tube as needed.

8. **History:**

   Acquisition of a detailed history will aid in determining a diagnosis as well as in obtaining points in the data acquisition, problem solving, interpersonal relations, and clinical competence sections of the performance criteria. Developing a systematic approach and practicing will help you in collecting the pertinent information in an efficient, complete, and timely manner. The following mnemonic may be useful: **AMPLE FRIENDS.**

A Allergies
M Medications
P Past medical history
L Last meal
E Events/environment related to the injury or illness (History of present illness or HPI)

F Family history, friends, and family doctor (as historians)
R Records.
I Immunizations
E EMTs and paramedics
N Narcotic and other substances of abuse
D Doctor for admission including consultants
S Social history (alcohol, tobacco, and living conditions)

THE SECONDARY SURVEY

1. **General:**
   - **1.1.** Take another look at the patient.
   - **1.2.** Recheck vital signs.

2. **Skin:**
   - **2.1.** Check for lacerations, bruising, abrasions, or any abnormal lesions.
   - **2.2.** Reassess turgor, color, and capillary refill.

3. **Head and Maxillofacial:**
   - **3.1.** Assessment:
     - **A.** Inspect and palpate the entire head and face for lacerations, contusions, and fractures.
     - **B.** Re-evaluate the pupils while examining the eyes for hemorrhage, penetrating injury, jaundice, visual acuity, and the presence of a contact lens.
     - **C.** Recheck level of consciousness.
     - **D.** Evaluate ears and nose for cerebrospinal fluid leakage and check for a septal hematoma.
     - **E.** Inspect the mouth for evidence of trauma.
   - **3.2.** Management:
     - **A.** Maintain an adequate airway.
     - **B.** Control hemorrhage.
     - **C.** Prevent secondary brain injury.

4. Neck:

4.1. Assessment:

A. Open the c-collar and inspect for JVD, tracheal deviation, scars, deformity, or masses.
B. Palpate for tenderness, deformity, swelling, or subcutaneous emphysema.
C. Auscultate for carotid bruits.

4.2. Management:

A. Maintain adequate in-line immobilization and protection of the c-spine.
B. Consider a complete c-spine series or obtain a CT scan.

5. Lungs/Heart/Chest:

5.1. Assessment:

A. Inspect for symmetrical rise and fall, bruising, wounds, hemorrhage, flail segment, and use of accessory muscles. Palpate for tenderness and crepitation.
B. Auscultate the anterior chest wall and posterior bases for bilateral breath sounds and any adventitious sounds.
C. Listen to the heart for murmurs, rubs, gallops, or clicks, and distant or muffled tones.

5.2. Management:

A. Obtain a chest x-ray, if it hasn't already been ordered.
B. Place the patient on a cardiac monitor and ask for a rhythm strip. Perform an ECG, if indicated.
C. Perform a tube thoracostomy, if indicated.
D. Perform a pericardiocentesis, if indicated.

6. Back:

6.1. Assessment:

A. Log-roll the patient while maintaining alignment of the entire spinal column.
B. Palpate, from top to bottom, all areas of the occiput, neck, back, and buttocks.
C. Inspect for deformity, wounds, abrasions, ecchymoses, or tenderness.
D. Auscultate the posterior aspect of the chest if needed.
E. Consider doing the rectal at this time if indicated.

6.2. Management:

Order x-rays and a CT, if indicated.

7. Abdomen:

7.1. Assessment:

A. Inspect the anterior abdomen for signs of blunt and penetrating injury, deformity, gross appearance (distended or flat), surgical scars, and pregnancy.
B. Auscultate for the presence or the absence of bowel sounds.
C. Percuss for dullness or subtle rebound tenderness.
D. Palpate for rebound tenderness, guarding, rigidity, pulsatile mass, or thrill.
E. Compress the pelvis while examining for tenderness, abnormal motion, deformity, or crepitance.
F. Request a fetal heart tone monitor as needed.

7.2. Management:

A. Transfer the patient directly to the operating room, if indicated.
B. Perform a FAST examination. Consider a CT scan.
C. Obtain a pelvic x-ray.

8. Extremities:

8.1. Assessment:

- **A.** Inspect upper and lower extremities for the presence of deformities, an expanding hematoma, open wounds, or abrasions.
- **B.** Palpate for sensation, tenderness, crepitation, abnormal movement, and the presence/absence of pulses.
- **C.** Monitor compartment pressures, if indicated.

8.2. Management:

- **A.** Apply appropriate splinting for fractures as indicated.
- **B.** Relieve pain by prescribing a medication and/or reducing fractures and dislocations.
- **C.** Give tetanus immunization and antibiotics, if indicated.
- **D.** Treat compartment syndrome aggressively.
- **E.** Perform an escharotomy with circumferential burns.
- **F.** Order an angiogram or CT angio, if indicated.
- **G.** Obtain x-rays of suspected fracture sites as indicated. If it hurts after a traumatic event, acquire an x-ray.

9. Neurologic:

9.1. Assessment:

- **A.** Re-evaluate the pupils and the level of consciousness.
- **B.** Determine the GCS.
- **C.** Evaluate the upper and lower extremities for motor and sensory responses.
- **D.** Evaluate the DTRs and note the presence/absence of pathologic reflexes (Babinski and ankle clonus).
- **E.** Check cerebellar function.
- **F.** Evaluate the gait, if possible.
- **G.** Evaluate cranial nerve function.
- **H.** Perform mini-mental status examination as needed.

9.2. Management:

- **A.** Continue to ventilate and oxygenate.
- **B.** Ensure that the patient is adequately immobilized.

10. Vascular:

10.1. Assessment:

- **A.** Evaluate symmetry and the strength of pulses.
- **B.** Re-evaluate for bleeding.

10.2. Management:

- **A.** Apply pressure dressings or tourniquet to the bleeding sites and tie bleeding vessels, when appropriate.
- **B.** Arrange for a surgical consultation as appropriate.

11. Perineum/Rectum/Vagina/Pelvis:

11.1. Perineal Assessment:

- **A.** Inspect the perineum and genitalia for wounds, swelling, urethral bleeding, or for a scrotal hematoma.
- **B.** Inspect the testicles for swelling, pain, nodules, or for the presence of a varicocele.

11.2. Rectal Assessment:

- **A.** Check the anal sphincter tone.
- **B.** Assess the bowel wall integrity examining for the presence of bone fragments, tenderness, or gross blood (hemocult stool from nontraumatized patients).
- **C.** Palpate the prostate noting its position, size, and quality.

11.3. Vaginal Assessment:

A. Check for blood in the vaginal vault.
B. Examine for retained tampons, lacerations, or for the presence of bone fragments.
C. Note for any indications of cervical motion tenderness, abnormal discharge, an enlarged uterus, enlarged ovaries, or for an adnexal mass, and/or tenderness.

11.4. Pelvis:

A. Check for pelvis deformity or laxity.
B. Pelvic rock is no longer encouraged.

11.5. Management:

A. Perform a perineum/rectum/vaginal examination at the end of the primary survey, if a DPL and a Foley catheter are required.
B. Treat injuries and obtain appropriate consultations.

PEARLS

- All problems exist until proven otherwise. All patients with chest pain require a rectal.
- All patients who need thrombolytics actually have a contraindication.
- All children are abused.
- All cardiac patients become hypotensive when given morphine or nitroglycerin.
- All alcoholics have multiple problems.
- All seizure patients dislocate something.
- All pills are somewhere.
- All patients have allergies.
- All overdoses are real and need a psychiatric consult.
- All joints are septic.
- All patients with an altered level of consciousness have fallen and require a c-collar and spine precautions.
- All patients with an abnormal temperature need a rectal probe or temperature sensing Foley catheter.
- All seizure patients are noncompliant with their medication.
- All single encounter patients need to be admitted.
- All burns have CO poisoning.
- All pain that goes away will be replaced by something worse.
- All patients who have an arrhythmia will eventually need to be shocked.
- All patients with "the flu" have CO poisoning, or some other toxin ingestion, or a dangerous infection.
- All children younger than 3 months will need a septic workup.
- All females are pregnant.
- All patients who wake up with D50 will need admission.
- All patients with a pneumothorax need to be quickly needled.
- All trauma and burn patients are at risk for myoglobinuria.
- All females of child-bearing age with abdominal pain have an ectopic pregnancy.
- All children with a head injury have hemophilia.
- All pearls have exceptions.
- All patients with an altered mental status have a serious cause, there not just drunk.
- Always look for the worst possible scenario.
- What can happen will happen.

Abbreviations Used in This Text

ABG/VBG	Arterial blood gas/venous blood gas
ACS	Acute coronary syndrome
Abd	Abdomen
AMI	Acute myocardial infarction
AMS	Altered mental status
ASA	Aspirin
BMP	Basic metabolic panel (Na, K, Cl, CO_2, BUN, Cr)
BNP	B-type natriuretic peptide
CMP	Comprehensive metabolic panel
CMT	Cervical motion tenderness
CRP	C-reactive protein
C&S	Culture and sensitivity
CXR	Chest x-ray
DBP	Diastolic blood pressure
ESR	Erythrocyte sedimentation rate
ETT	Endotracheal tube
FAST	Focused abdominal sonography for trauma
FHT	Fetal heart tones
GERD	Gastoesophageal reflux disease
GC	gonorrhea
Hr	Hour or hours
gm	gram
HPTX	Hemo/pneumothorax
HTN	Hypertension
IBS	Irritable bowel syndrome
IO	Intraosseous
IOP	Intraocular pressure
IVIG	Intravenous immunoglobulin
J	Joules
kg	kilogram
KUB	Kidney, ureter, bladder x-ray
LFT	Liver function tests (total, direct, and indirect bilirubin, AST, ALT, Alkaline phosphatase)
LR	Lactated ringers
MTP	Massive transfusion protocol
mL	milliliter
m/o	Month old
NG/OG	Nasogastric/orogastric
NSAIDs	Nonsteroidal anti-inflammatory drugs
N/V/D	Nausea/vomiting/diarrhea
NS	Normal saline
PID	Pelvic inflammatory disease
PRBCs	packed red blood cells
PTX	Pneumothorax
SBP	Systolic blood pressure
SC or SQ	Subcutaneous
S/S	Signs/symptoms
RSI	Rapid sequence intubation
TBI	Traumatic brain injury
TPTX	Tension pneumothorax
tPA	Tissue plasminogen activator
T&S	Type and screen
UA	Urinalysis
US	Ultrasound
VS	Vital signs
WN/WD	Well nourished/well developed
w/o	Week old
y/o	Year old

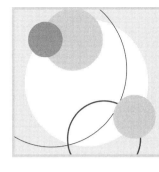

Pearls Topics

"The ultimate measure of a man is not where he stands in moments of comfort and convenience, but where he stands at times of challenge and controversy."
Martin Luther King, Jr.

CARDIOVASCULAR

Cardiac Life Support

1. **Ventricular Fibrillation/Pulseless Ventricular Tachycardia Algorithm (VF/VT):**
   - **1.1.** Access ABCs (Airway, Breathing, Circulation).
   - **1.2.** Perform CPR until a defibrillator is attached
   - **1.3.** FV/VT are present on the monitor
   - **1.4.** Defibrillate: biphasic defibrillator use 120 J; monophasic defibrillator use 360 J
   - **1.5.** Persistent VF/VT
   - **1.6.** Continue CPR for five cycles or about 2 minutes
   - **1.7.** Intubate
   - **1.8.** IV access
   - **1.9.** Administer epinephrine, 1 mg IV push, repeat q 3 to 5 minutes or vasopressin 40 U IV, as a single dose, one time only
   - **1.10.** Defibrillate with 360 J (monophasic) or 200 J (biphasic)
   - **1.11.** Medication sequence includes:
     - **A.** Amiodarone 300 mg IV push, repeat 150 mg IV/IO × 1 (max 2.2 g/24 h).
     - **B.** Lidocaine, 1.0 mg/kg IV push, repeat in 3 to 5 minutes to a maximum dose of 3 mg/kg. Do not give amiodarone if already given.
     - **C.** Consider magnesium sulfate, 1 to 2 g IV/IO in torsades de pointes, suspected hypomagnesemic state, refractory VF, or digoxin toxicity. May repeat in 10 minutes.
     - **D.** Consider procainamide, 20 mg/min in refractory VF to a maximum total dose of 17 mg/kg. Use in arrest is limited by the need for a slow infusion and uncertain efficacy.
     - **E.** Sodium bicarbonate, 1 mEq/kg IV, should be used if the following conditions are present:
       - Pre-existing bicarbonate-responsive acidosis.
       - Tricyclic antidepressant overdose.
       - Long cardiac arrest.
       - Hypoxic lactic acidosis.
       - Spontaneous circulation after long cardiac arrest.
       - Suspicion of hyperkalemic state.
   - **1.12.** Defibrillate. Monophasic unit 360 J for all shocks. Biphasic unit use 120 J. To start then 200 J.

2. Pulseless Electrical Activity Algorithm (PEA):

Pulseless electrical activity includes electromechanical dissociation (EMD), pseudodissociation (EMD), idioventricular rhythms, ventricular escape rhythms, ventricular escape rhythms, bradysystolic rhythms, and postdefibrillation idioventricular rhythms. There is cardiac activity without an associated pulse or blood pressure.

2.1. Continue CPR.

2.2. Intubate.

2.3. IV access.

2.4. Consider possible causes (5 Hs and 5 Ts):

A. Hypovolemia.
B. Hypoxia.
C. Hypothermia.
D. Hypo/hyperkalemia.
E. H+ ion (acidosis).
F. Thrombosis (MI/PE).
G. Tension pneumothorax.
H. Tablets/toxins (drug overdose).
I. Tamponade (pericardial).
J. Trauma.

2.5. Administer epinephrine, 1 mg IV push, and repeat q 3 to 5 minutes.

2.6. Atropine in no longer recommended by the American Heart Association but may be considered. Dose is 1 mg IV/IO q 3 to 5 minutes to a maximum of 3 mg.

2.7. Check rhythm.

3. Tachycardia Algorithm:

3.1. Access ABCs, IV, O_2, pulse oximeter, and monitor. Obtain an ECG and a CXR.

3.2. Unstable tachycardia includes chest pain, SOB, altered mental status (AMS), low BP, Shock, congestive heart failure (CHF), or AMI. When the ventricular rate is >150 bpm, cardiovert or administer medications depending on arrhythmia and blood pressure.

3.3. For stable atrial fibrillation and atrial flutter, consider diltiazem, beta-blockers, verapamil, digoxin, procainamide, quinidine, and anticoagulants.

3.4. For stable PSVT (paroxysmal supraventricular tachycardia), wide-complex tachycardia, and VT, consider the following.

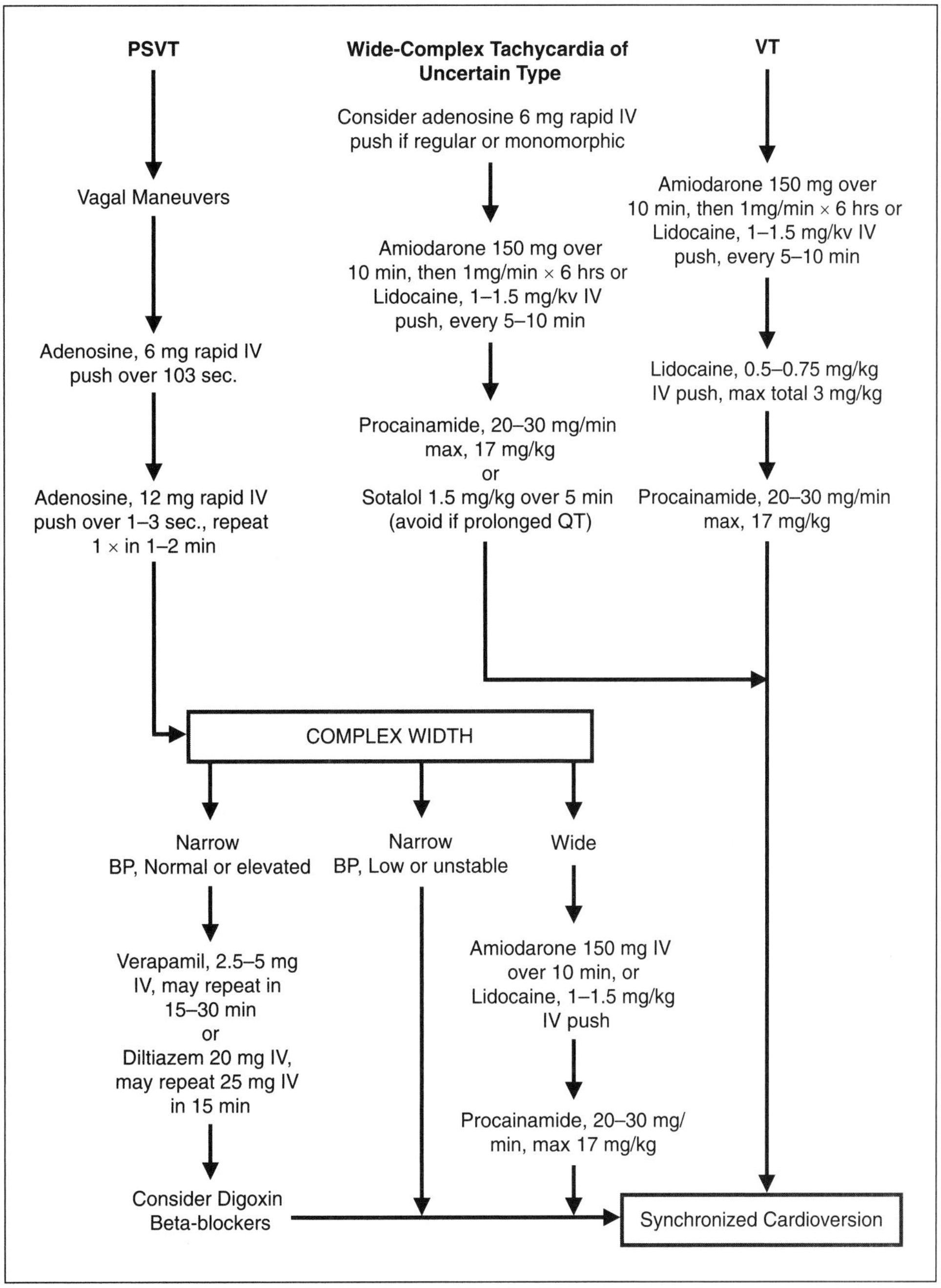

4. **Asystole Algorithm:**
   - **4.1.** Continue CPR.
   - **4.2.** Intubate.
   - **4.3.** IV/IO access.
   - **4.4.** Confirm asystole in more than one lead.
   - **4.5.** Consider possible causes, including the 5 Hs and 5 Ts.

4.6. Consider initiating transcutaneous pacing (no evidence of success).

4.7. Administer epinephrine, 1 mg IV push, and repeat q 3 to 5 minutes.

4.8. Consider giving atropine, 1 mg IV/IO push, and repeat q 3 to 5 minutes to a total of 0.03 to 0.04 mg/kg. Not recommended by the AHA but not considered harmful.

4.9. Consider "termination of efforts."

5. Bradycardia Algorithm:

5.1. Access ABCs

5.2. Start IV/IO, O_2, pulse oximeter, and monitor

5.3. Check vital signs

5.4. Obtain history, perform a physical examination, and order ECG, CXR, and electrolytes

5.5. Bradycardia (<60 bpm)

5.6. Consider serious signs, symptoms, and conditions including:

- **A.** Chest pain.
- **B.** Shortness of breath.
- **C.** Altered mental status.
- **D.** Low BP
- **E.** CHF
- **F.** AMI

5.7. If there are any serious signs/symptoms, perform the following intervention sequence:

- **A.** Administer atropine, 0.5 to 1.0 mg. Doses <0.5 mg IV/IO may cause paradoxical heart rate slowing.
- **B.** Initiate transcutaneous pacing.
- **C.** Administer dopamine, 5 to 20 μg/kg/min.
- **D.** Consider epinephrine 2 to 10 μg/min.
- **E.** Consider isoproterenol 2 to 10 μg/min.

5.8. If no serious signs/symptoms exists, observe the patient in the ICU.

Cardiovascular Cases

1. Post-Resuscitation Care:

1.1. Initial objectives:

- **A.** The goal is to optimize cardiac, pulmonary, and neurologic function.
- **B.** Identify what caused the arrest so that measures can be done to prevent recurrence.
- **C.** Consult cardiology (PCI is of value in selected patients).
- **D.** Consider therapeutic hypothermia. Works best for V-fib arrest but may be of value in non–V-fib arrest. Cool the patient to 89.5° to 93.5°F.
- **E.** Admit to the ICU/CCU.

2. Atrial Fibrillation (AF):

AF is the most common sustained adult tachyarrhythmia and is due to multiple atrial ectopic foci stimulating irregular ventricular responses. The enlarged and poorly contracting left atrium induces the onset of thrombus formation, emboli, and stroke. Etiologies include coronary artery disease, congestive heart failure, cardiomyopathy, thyrotoxicosis, rheumatic heart disease, hypertension, alcohol ingestion, and pulmonary embolism.

2.1. Clinical Evaluation:

- **A. Symptoms:** AF is often chronic in long-standing arteriosclerotic heart disease and may be asymptomatic. In paroxysmal AF, palpitations and skipped beats may be accompanied by weakness and near-syncope.
- **B. Signs:** The rhythm is irregularly irregular with a rate of 80 to 180 bpm. The rate in chronic AF is usually 80 to 120 bpm. Some of the beats may not be transmitted to the peripheral circulation, resulting in a "pulse deficit."
- **C. DDX:** Multifocal atrial tachycardia, PSVT, electrolyte disorder, PE, AMI.
- **D. Workup:** ECG (irregular baseline undulations accompanied by irregular QRS complexes and no clear p waves). CBC, BMP, BNP, LFTs, PT/PTT/INR, D-dimer, cardiac enzymes, ETOH, CXR

2.2. RX:

- **A.** Support ABCs, IV, O_2, pulse oximeter, and monitor.
- **B.** If the rate is less than 120 bpm, usually no immediate treatment is required.
- **C.** Anticoagulation therapy should be considered for AF >48 to 72 hours duration prior to pharmacologic therapy or cardioversion.
- **D.** Rate control is more important acutely. Consider beta-blockers, such as esmolol, metoprolol, propranolol, or calcium channel blockers (diltiazem or verapamil). However, these two classes of drugs are negative inotropic agents and can cause hypotension. May consider amiodarone, procainamide, and vernakalant as alternative therapy.
- **E.** Unstable patients with chest pain, dyspnea, hypotension, congestive heart failure, or cardiac ischemia, require immediate cardioversion after sedation. Start with 200 J monophasic or 120 to 200 J biphasic synchronized energy. If initial dose fails then increase the dose.
- **F.** Consult cardiology.
- **G. Disposition:** Admit to telemetry or CCU.

3. Atrial Flutter:

Atrial flutter occurs when there is an ectopic focus originating from a small area in the atrium. Causes include coronary artery disease, COPD, CHF, PE, thyrotoxicosis, sympathomimetic substances, and rheumatic heart disease.

3.1. Clinical Evaluation:

- **A. Symptoms:** Heart palpitations, with or without symptoms (fatigue, angina, poor exercise tolerance, dyspnea, and syncope).
- **B. Signs:** Cardiac rate is typically about 150 bpm (2:1 block) and the rhythm is usually regular. Rates of 75 bpm occur with 4:1 block. Rate and rhythm may be irregular, alternating between a 2:1 and a 4:1 block.
- **C. Workup:** ECG ("Sawtooth" flutter waves with an atrial rate between 250 and 4,000 bpm. AV block is usually present, commonly 2:1, but 4:1 and alternating blocks are not uncommon. If the ECG has a constant ventricular rate of 150 bpm, it is atrial flutter). CBC, BMP, BNP, LFTs, PT/PTT/INR, D-dimer, cardiac enzymes, CXR.

3.2. RX:

- **A.** Support ABCs, IV, O_2, pulse oximeter, and monitor.
- **B.** β-Blockers or calcium channel blockers should be used to control the rate (refer to the "Atrial Fibrillation" section).
- **C.** Unstable patients can usually be converted with 50 to 100 J (monophasic or biphasic) of synchronized energy, increased as needed.
- **D. Disposition:** Admit to the telemetry or to the CCU.

4. First-Degree AV Heart Block:

Decreased conduction through the right atrium or AV node. Usually an incidental finding in an asymptomatic patient. Etiologies include AMI, sarcoid, amyloidosis, endocarditis/myocarditis, hypothermia, hyperkalemia, and various antiarrhythmic drugs.

4.1. Clinical Evaluation:

- **A. Symptoms:** Usually asymptomatic but may present with syncope.
- **B. Signs:** No specific findings noted.
- **C. Workup:** ECG (PR interval >2 seconds, constant from beat to beat and a P/QRS ratio of 1:1). CBC, BMP, BNP, LFTs, PT/PTT/INR, D-dimer, cardiac enzymes, CXR.

4.2. RX:

- **A.** Support ABCs, IV, O_2, pulse oximeter, and monitor.
- **B.** Administer atropine, 0.5 to 1.0 mg for adults and 0.01 to 0.02 mg/kg for peds, IV q 3 to 5 minutes to a total of 3 mg for the adult patient, and 0.04 mg/kg for the pediatric patient.
- **C. Disposition**: Rarely requires admission, close follow-up acceptable.

5. Second-Degree AV Heart Block Type I:

A type I second-degree AV block is usually due to a conduction disturbance in the AV node. Usually it does not progress to complete heart block. Etiologies include endocarditis/myocarditis, inferior MI, collagen vascular diseases, electrolyte disorders, and medications.

5.1. Clinical Evaluation:

- **A. Symptoms:** Usually asymptomatic unless ventricular rate drops very low.
- **B. Signs:** Regularly irregular heart rate.
- **C. Workup:** ECG (progressive PR prolongation until a QRS complex is dropped. Normal p wave and QRS complex). CBC, BMP, BNP, LFTs, PT/PTT/INR, cardiac enzymes, BNP, D-dimer, CXR.

5.2. RX:

- **A.** Support ABCs, IV, O_2, pulse oximeter, and monitor.
- **B.** Administer atropine, 0.5 to 1.0 mg for adults and 0.01 to 0.02 mg/kg for peds, IV q 3 to 5 minutes to a total of 3 mg for the adult patient, and 0.04 mg/kg for the pediatric patient.
- **C.** Initiate transcutaneous pacing.
- **D.** Administer isoproterenol, 2 to 10 μg/min for adults and 0.05 to 2 μg/kg/min for the pediatric patient.
- **E.** Disposition: Admit all symptomatic patients and those with cardiac ischemia or infarction. If discharging, close follow-up with cardiology.

6. Second-Degree AV Heart Block Type II:

A type II second-degree AV block is usually infranodal and associated with cardiac disease and a high incidence of progression to complete heart block. Etiologies include medications, endocarditis/myocarditis, anterior MI, collagen vascular diseases, and electrolyte disorders.

6.1. Clinical Evaluation:

- **A. Symptoms:** Usually asymptomatic but may have syncope, palpitations, and angina.
- **B. Signs:** Bradycardia.
- **C. Workup:** ECG (constant PR interval with a sudden dropped beat. The QRS complex is usually wide. If two or more p waves are seen between QRS complexes, there is a higher chance of progression to a third-degree block). CBC, BMP, BNP, PT/PTT/INR, cardiac enzymes, CXR.

6.2. RX:

A. Support ABCs, IV, O_2, pulse oximeter, and monitor.
B. If patient is symptomatic, atropine is contraindicated due to increasing sinus rate and precipitating a third-degree block.
C. Initiate transcutaneous pacing.
D. **Disposition**: Admit all patients and consult cardiology.

7. Third-Degree AV Heart Block:

A third-degree AV block implies significant conduction system damage resulting in no conduction through the AV node. A complete dissociation between the atrium and ventricle exits leading to ventricular escape beats. There is an increased risk of sudden death and asystole. Etiologies include endocarditis/myocarditis, AMI, collagen vascular diseases, electrolyte disorders, and medications.

7.1. Clinical Evaluation:

A. **Symptoms:** Usually symptomatic with fatigue, chest pain, syncope, confusion Stokes/Adams attacks, dyspnea and poor exercise tolerance.
B. **Signs:** Bradycardia, signs of CHF, mental status changes, acute MI.
C. **Workup:** ECG (rate of <60 beats per minutes with more p waves than QRS complexes. There is no association between the p waves and QRS and both are regular). CBC, BMP, BNP, LFTs, PT/PTT/INR, D-dimer, CXR, cardiac enzymes, consider Lyme titer, Chagas titer, enterovirus PCR, or adenovirus PCR if indicated.

7.2. RX:

A. Support ABCs, IV, O_2, pulse oximeter, and monitor.
B. Transcutaneous pacing is the treatment of choice.
C. Hemodynamically unstable patients may be treated with atropine. Give with caution. If the block is in the bundle of HIS, you get an increased atrial rate, and a greater degree of block, slowing ventricular rate. Care should be taken in patients with a suspected acute myocardial infarction (cause ventricular arrhythmias).
D. **Disposition:** Admit all patients and consult cardiology.

8. Paroxysmal Supraventricular Tachycardia (PSVT):

Paroxysmal supraventricular tachycardia is characterized by a sudden increase in heart rate, that is, usually 160 to 200 bpm. This condition is induced by the impulse re-entering the AV node. It arises in patients with accessory tracts that bypass part of the normal conducting system, such as in Wolff–Parkinson–White syndrome and Lown–Ganong–Levine syndrome. PSVT usually occurs in healthy individuals but can be caused by hyperthyroidism, mitral valve prolapse, stimulants, alcohol abuse, pericarditis, AMI, pneumonia, COPD, and rheumatic heart disease.

8.1. Clinical Evaluation:

A. **Symptoms:** Palpitations, weakness, dizziness, fatigue, dyspnea, or faintness.
B. **Signs:** The heart rate is between 120 and 280 bpm, with an average rate of 160 to 200 bpm, and the rate is regular.
C. **DDX:** Digitalis toxicity, aflutter with 2:1 block, and VT.
D. **Workup:** ECG (narrow-complex QRS without p waves). CBC, BMP, BNP, LFTs, PT/PTT/INR, D-dimer, cardiac enzymes, CXR

8.2. RX:

A. Support ABCs, IV, O_2, pulse oximeter, and monitor.
B. Attempt appropriate vagal maneuvers, such as carotid message, and valsalva maneuver.
C. Adenosine 6 mg IV fast, repeat at 12 mg IV if no response.
D. Calcium channel blockers or beta-blockers.
E. If unstable cardiovert at 50 to 100 J (monophasic and biphasic).
F. **Disposition:** Admit patients with a new identifiable significant cause, unstable presentation, or severe underlying disease. Consult cardiology.

9. Premature Ventricular Contractions (PVCs):

Premature ventricular contractions are caused by one or more ectopic foci in the ventricle. They can be caused by ischemia, infarction, electrolyte abnormalities, digoxin toxicity, sympathomimetic drugs, and mechanical irritation (central line). It is the most common arrhythmia seen after an AMI. There is an increased risk of precipitating V-tach if the PVC occurs during ventricular repolarization (R on T phenomenon). The cardiac monitor shows a wide QRS with no p wave and a deflection opposite to the normal QRS. The beat occurs earlier than expected and there is a compensatory pause before the next normal beat.

9.1. Clinical Evaluation:

- **A. Symptoms:** PVCs are common in the normal patient, but they are significant in a patient with active cardiac ischemia.
- **B. Signs:** The rhythm is irregularly irregular or regularly irregular, if in bigeminy or trigeminy.
- **C. Workup:** CBC, BMP, BNP, LFTs, PT/PTT/INR, D-dimer, cardiac enzymes, CXR.

9.2. RX:

- **A.** Treatment is usually not necessary unless PVCs are frequent (approximately >6/min), multifocal, or in runs. In the setting of myocardial ischemia or infarction with these criteria, administer lidocaine, 1 mg/kg IV bolus, and start 2 to 3 mg/min IV drip, beta-blockers, or amiodarone.
- **B.** Consider magnesium sulfate in the setting of a myocardial infarction.
- **C. Disposition:** Admit to the ICU, if the patient is experiencing ischemia, infarction, or runs of V-tach.

10. Abdominal Aortic Aneurysm (AAA):

This is an abnormal dilation of the abdominal aorta with 90% due to atherosclerosis. Most patients with an AAA are asymptomatic and most (98%) are located infrarenal. Risk of rupture increases with diameter >5.5 cm, current smoking, high blood pressure, aortic expansion rate >0.5 cm/year, female, and symptomatic. Only 30% of ruptured aneurysms have a known history of AAA.

10.1. Clinical Evaluation:

- **A. Symptoms:** Symptoms begin with a leaking or a rapidly expanding aneurysm. The typical patient is an older male with severe, constant, low abdominal, and/or back pain, which is not relieved by position. Pain may be present in the lower back, scrotum, or perineum.
- **B. Signs:** Patients with a leak or rupture will have hypotension, tachycardia, possible unequal or diminished pulses, abdominal tenderness, and a pulsatile abdominal mass.
- **C. DDX:**
  Shock present: Hemorrhagic pancreatitis, perforated viscus, and mesenteric infarction.
  Shock not present: Renal colic, diverticulitis, lumbar disk disease/compression fracture, small bowel obstruction, appendicitis, and peritonitis.
- **D. Workup:** CBC, BMP, PT/PTT/INR, T&C 10 units of PRBCs (consider MTP), UA, ECG. An ED ultrasound can detect an aneurysm but may not identify if it is leaking. A CT of the abdomen/pelvis with IV contrast is diagnostic but should only be used in the stable patient.

10.2. RX:

- **A.** Support ABCs, two large bore IVs, O_2, pulse oximeter, and monitor.
- **B.** Maintain SBP 90 to 100 with IV fluids or blood.
- **C.** Order an MTP with platelets and FFP.
- **D.** Rush the unstable patient, to the OR for immediate surgery.
- **E.** Admit the more "stable" patient to the ICU and continue evaluation for possible surgery.

11. Aortic Dissection:

The main cause of an aortic dissection is necrosis of the tunica media from atherosclerosis and uncontrolled hypertension. The dissection starts with an intimal tear and blood flows between the layers forming a false lumen distally and often proximally. As the dissection worsens it may involve branch vessels, the aortic valve, and pericardial space. Mortality is 2% per hour for the first 2 days.

- **A.** Stanford Type A (DeBakey I and II): Involves the ascending aorta and is usually best managed with surgery. The mortality rate of the untreated is approximately 60%. With treatment, the rate decreases to approximately 30%.
- **B.** Stanford Type B (DeBakey III): Involves the descending aorta only. Medical management is the treatment of choice unless unstable. The mortality rate with medical treatment is approximately 10%.

11.1. Clinical Evaluation:

- **A. Symptoms:** A typical patient is an older hypertensive male with a sudden onset of severe chest pain (90%), "tearing" quality, and radiation to the back.
- **B. Signs:** Rales, diastolic murmur of aortic insufficiency, differences in left and right or upper, and lower extremity blood pressures and pulses. Abdominal tenderness and/or pulsatile mass and neurologic deficits are caused by compromised arterial supply. Neurological findings are present, if the carotid arteries are involved.
- **C. DDX:** New-onset angina, variant (Prinzmetal's) angina, MI, pericarditis, pneumonia, pulmonary embolus, pneumothorax, biliary disorders, and GI disorders, gastritis, pancreatitis, peptic ulcer, and esophagitis.
- **D. Workup:** ECG, CBC, BMP, PT/PTT/INR, D-dimer, UA, cardiac enzymes, T&C 6 to 8 units of PRBCs (consider MTP). CXR (mediastinal widening, prominent ascending aorta, enlargement of the aortic knob, pleural effusion). CT angiography of the chest is the test of choice. If the patient is stable, consider transesophageal echocardiography, if it is available in the ED.

11.2. RX:

- **A.** Support ABCs, IV, O_2, pulse oximeter, and monitor.
- **B.** Consult thoracic surgery immediately or arrange transfer if unavailable.
- **C.** Pain management.
- **D.** Control hypertension and tachycardia.
  - To decrease the force of a contraction, use a beta-blockers, esmolol (Brevibloc), 50 μg/kg IV over 1 minute, then infuse at 50 μg/kg/min, **or** propranolol, 1 mg/min to total of 10 mg or labetalol, 5 to 20 mg IV bolus, then 20 to 40 mg every 10 to 15 minutes.
  - Start nitroprusside (Nipride), 1 μg/kg/min IV, and lower systolic pressure to 100 to 120 mm Hg. Observe for organ perfusion and neurologic status. Do not overshoot BP.
- **E. Disposition:** Transfer the patient to the ICU or to surgery.

12. Acute Coronary Syndrome (ACS):

Acute coronary syndrome refers to a spectrum of disease including unstable angina (UA), ST-segment elevation myocardial infarction (STEMI), and non-STEMI. There is a decrease or blockage of blood flow from a thrombus in an atherosclerotic coronary artery. If compromised blood flow is persistent, myocardial heart muscle necrosis occurs.

12.1. Clinical Evaluation:

- **A. Symptoms:** Chest pain is substernal, severe, steady, "squeezing," "heavy," "tight," or "pressure like," often radiating to left jaw or shoulder. Associated symptoms include nausea, vomiting, dyspnea, diaphoresis, palpitations, and weakness.
- **B. Signs:** Cold, clammy skin, pallor, variable heart rate and rhythm, +/– murmur.
- **C. DDX:** Stable angina, variant (Prinzmetal's) angina, aortic dissection, pericarditis, pneumonia, pulmonary embolus, pneumothorax, chest wall pain, biliary disorders, gastritis, dyspepsia, peptic ulcer, esophagitis, and esophageal spasm.

D. Workup: Obtain an ECG within 10 minutes of arrival. Elevations in leads, II, III, and aVF (inferior wall); V1 to V3 (anteroseptal); I, aVL, and V4 to V6 (lateral); and V1 to V6 (anterolateral). ST depression in leads, V1 to V3 (posterior). Nonspecific ST and T-wave abnormalities in an NSTEMI. ST depression consider ischemia of unstable angina.

Order cardiac enzymes (elevated in 70% of cases of STEMI and NSTEMI), CBC, BMP, BNP, PT/PTT/INR, D-dimer, CXR.

12.2. RX:

STEMI: Full-thickness myocardial necrosis with a high morbidity and mortality.

A. Support ABCs, IV, O_2, pulse oximeter, and monitor.
B. Aspirin 325 mg po, Clopidogrel 300 mg po, in patients who cannot take aspirin.
C. Give nitroglycerin (NTG) 0.4 mg SL × 3 q 5 minutes apart while starting IVs. Give an NTG IV drip at 10 to 20 μg/min and titrate to pain and SBP. Contraindicated in an inferior MI, right ventricular MI, and recent phosphodiesterase inhibitor (sildenafil) use.
D. Consider morphine 2 to 4 mg IV q 10 minutes (if pain is refractory to NTG), until pain is gone.
E. Consult cardiology, immediately.
F. Percutaneous coronary intervention (PCI) is the preferred reperfusion strategy if available within 90 minutes.
G. Thrombolytic therapy protocol given within 30 minutes of arrival.
- **Precise indications:** Choice of agent and dosing regimen for thrombolysis depends on local practice and current research. Therapy should be given within 30 minutes of ED presentation in patients diagnosed with an STEMI unable to receive PCI within 90 minutes.
- **Absolute contraindications:** Active GI bleeding, intracranial aneurysm, AVM or tumor, history of hemorrhagic CVA, CVA within 1 year, suspected aortic dissection, and pericarditis.
- **Relative contraindications:** Time to therapy >24 hours, prolonged CPR (>10 minutes), uncontrolled HTN (BP >180/110 mm Hg), recent internal bleeding, pregnancy, current anticoagulant use, active peptic ulcer disease, trauma, or surgery within the last 2 to 3 weeks, and a history of CVA (>1 year).
- **Suggested guidelines:**
  Alteplase: >65 kg: 15 mg initial IV bolus, 50 mg infused over the next 30 minutes, 35 mg infused over the next 60 minutes (max dose 100 mg).
  Streptokinase: 1.5 million units infused over 60 minutes. No heparin is required.
  Reteplase (r-PA, retavase, reptilase): Derivative of rt-PA that is effective as rt-PA and may work more quickly. Infuse 10 units IV over 2 minutes followed by a repeat dose in 30 minutes. Heparin must be used to prevent reclosure.
  Tenecteplase (TNKase): <60 kg: 30 mg IV over 5 seconds. >60 to 69 kg: 35 mg IV over 5 seconds. 70 to 79 kg: 40 mg over 5 seconds. 80 to 89 kg: 45 mg IV over 5 seconds. >90 kg: 50 mg IV over 5 seconds.

H. Consider a beta-blockade if tachycardic or hypertensive. It is not mandatory to give in the ED. May use metoprolol, 5 mg IV q 5 minutes × 3 doses.
I. Start unfractionated heparin at 60 to 70 U/kg bolus followed by a 12 to 15 U/kg/h IV drip. May also use low–molecular-weight heparin.
J. Disposition: Admit to the cath lab or CCU.

NSTEMI: Subendocardial necrosis that is less extensive than an STEMI. If high-risk patient: (elevated cardiac enzymes, TIMI score >4, ECG changes), do the following:

A. Support ABCs, IV, O_2, pulse oximeter, and monitor.
B. Aspirin 325 mg po, Clopidogrel 300 mg po, in patients who cannot take aspirin.
C. Give NTG 0.4 mg SL × 3 q 5 minutes apart while starting IVs. Give an NTG IV drip at 10 to 20 μg/min and titrate to pain and SBP. Contraindicated in an inferior MI, right ventricular MI, and recent phosphodiesterase inhibitor (sildenafil) use.

D. Consider morphine 2 to 4 mg IV q 10 minutes (if pain is refractory to NTG), until pain is gone.
E. Consult cardiology immediately.
F. PCI is strongly recommended.
G. Thrombolytic therapy is contraindicated.
H. Consider a beta-blockade if tachycardic or hypertensive. It is not mandatory to give in the ED. May use metoprolol, 5 mg IV q 5 minutes × 3 doses.
I. Start unfractionated heparin at 60 to 70 U/kg bolus followed by a 12 to 15 U/kg/h IV drip. May also use low–molecular-weight heparin.
J. **Disposition:** Admit to the cath lab or CCU.

NSTEMI: If medium to low risk, do the following:

A. Support ABCs, IV, O_2, pulse oximeter, and monitor.
B. Aspirin 325 mg po, Clopidogrel 300 mg po, in patients who cannot take aspirin.
C. Give NTG 0.4 mg SL × 3 q 5 minutes apart while starting IVs. Give an NTG IV drip at 10 to 20 μg/min and titrate to pain and SBP. Contraindicated in an inferior MI, right ventricular MI, and recent phosphodiesterase inhibitor (sildenafil) use.
D. Consider morphine 2 to 4 mg IV q 10 minutes (if pain is refractory to NTG), until pain is gone.
E. Consult cardiology.
F. PCI not recommended.
G. **Thrombolytic therapy is contraindicated.**
H. Consider a beta-blockade if tachycardic or hypertensive. It is not mandatory to give in the ED. May use metoprolol, 5 mg IV q 5 minutes × 3 doses.
I. Consider starting unfractionated heparin at 60 to 70 U/kg bolus followed by a 12 to 15 U/kg/h IV drip. May also use low–molecular-weight heparin.
J. **Disposition:** Admit to a telemetry floor or CCU.

Unstable Angina: An ACS where there is no detectable release of enzymes and biomarker[illegible] necrosis.

A. Support ABCs, IV, O_2, pulse oximeter, and monitor.
B. Aspirin 325 mg po, Clopidogrel 300 mg po, in patients who cannot take aspirin.
C. Give NTG 0.4 mg SL × 3 q 5 minutes apart while starting IVs. Give an NTG IV drip at 10 to 20 μg/min and titrate to pain and SBP. Contraindicated in an inferior MI, right ventricular MI, and recent phosphodiesterase inhibitor (sildenafil) use.
D. Consider morphine 2 to 4 mg IV q 10 minutes (if pain is refractory to NTG), until pain is gone.
E. Consult cardiology.
F. PCI not recommended.
G. **Thrombolytic therapy is contraindicated.**
H. Consider a beta-blockade if tachycardic or hypertensive. It is not mandatory to give in the ED. May use metoprolol, 5 mg IV q 5 minutes × 3 doses.
I. Start unfractionated heparin at 60 to 70 U/kg bolus followed by a 12 to 15 U/kg/h IV drip. May also use low–molecular-weight heparin.
J. **Disposition:** Admit to a telemetry floor or CCU.

13. Hypertensive Emergencies:

Hypertension urgency is defined as a sustained elevated blood pressure (SBP >180 mm Hg or DBP >90 mm Hg) in an asymptomatic patient. A hypertensive emergency is uncontrolled hypertension causing end-organ dysfunction. There is no evidence that any specific antihypertensive agent or class is superior to any other in treating a hypertensive emergency.

13.1. Clinical Evaluation:

A. **Symptoms:** Headache, nausea, vomiting, visual disturbances, chest pain, shortness of breath, orthopnea, confusion, stupor, coma, and abdominal pain.

B. **Signs:** Neurologic deficits, seizures, fundal abnormalities, rales, pulmonary edema, hemorrhage, thrombosis, embolus, acute renal failure, dyspnea, and murmurs.

C. **DDX:** Acute myocardial infarction, congestive heart failure, thoracic aortic dissection, coarctation of aorta, renovascular disease, and primary aldosteronism.

D. **Workup:** CBC, BMP, U/A, cardiac enzymes, BNP, CXR, ECG, CT head if neuro findings or severe headache.

13.2. RX:

A. Support ABCs, IV, O_2, pulse oximeter, and monitor.

B. Antihypertensive agents:
- Labetalol, 20 mg IV, repeat q 15 minutes (max. dose 300 mg),
- Nitroprusside infusion, 0.5 to 10 µg/kg/min IV (avoid in pregnancy),
- Hydralazine bolus, 5 to 15 mg (preferred in pregnancy), or,
- Nitroglycerin infusion, start at 10 to 20 µg/min titrating to BP,
- Esmolol load 500 µg/kg over 1 minute, then infuse 50 to 200 µg/kg/min,
- Enalapril 1.25 to 5 mg IV q 6 hours,
- Phentolamine 1 to 5 mg IV boluses for catecholamine crises.

C. Specific disease state recommendations:
- For hypertensive encephalopathy, use nicardipine, esmolol, or labetalol. The goal is to reduce the MAP by 25% over 8 hours.
- For CNS events, use nitroprusside, NTG, or labetalol.
- For myocardial ischemia, use NTG infusion or beta-blockers.
- For CHF, use nitroprusside or NTG.
- For eclampsia/preeclampsia, use hydralazine or labetalol.
- For interactions between MAO inhibitors and foods or drugs, use phentolamine or labetalol.
- For antihypertensive withdrawal, use labetalol or nitroprusside.
- For renal failure, use NTG or labetalol.
- For cocaine toxicity, use a benzodiazepine as the first agent.

D. **Disposition:** Send the patient home if uncomplicated hypertension. Admit the patient if the BP is difficult to control and there is evidence of end-organ damage.

14. Congestive Heart Failure (CHF):

CHF is a clinical syndrome secondary to the inability of the ventricle to effectively eject blood or fill with blood. Systolic dysfunction is impaired ejection of blood from the ventricle while diastolic dysfunction is abnormal left ventricular filling.

14.1. Clinical Evaluation:

A. **Symptoms:** Dyspnea, PND, orthopnea, nocturia, edema, chest pain, fatigue, and cough.

B. **Signs:** Respiratory distress, tachycardia, tachypnea, hypotension, JVD, hepatojugular reflex, rales, murmurs, pulsatile liver, S3 (ventricular gallop), S4 (atrial gallop), or cyanosis.

C. **DDX:** Constrictive pericarditis, cardiac tamponade, myocardial infarction, COPD, pneumonia, renal failure, cirrhosis, anemia, or pulmonary embolism.

D. **Workup:** ABG, CBC, BMP, cardiac enzymes, BNP (proBNP), LFTs, UA, CXR, ECG.

14.2. RX:

A. Support ABCs, IV, O_2, pulse oximeter, and monitor.

B. CPAP or BiPAP may help avoid intubation.

C. Keep patient in a sitting position, if possible.

D. Insert a Foley catheter for monitoring I/Os, IVs, and TKO.

E. Anticipate BP drop as patient's failure improves.

F. Consider administrating the following medications:
- Furosemide, 40 to 80 mg IV or 2x the previous dose.
- NTG 10 to 20 µg/min IV, titrated to effect and BP. This reduces preload, afterload, and cardiac workload.

- Consider an ACE inhibitor (captopril 25 mg po or SL or Enalapril 1.5 mg IV) for afterload reduction.
- Morphine 2 to 4 mg IV to reduce the catecholamine response, preload reduction, and provide analgesia.
- Dobutamine, 2.5 to 10 μg/kg/min. Increases cardiac output and cause vasodilatation.
- Dopamine, 5 to 20 μg/kg/min. Increases inotropy and chronotropy.
- Milrinone increases inotropy, chronotropy, and lusitropy. Potent venous and arterial dilatory without causing tachycardia.
- Treat bronchospasms with albuterol, 2.5 mg in NaCl Nebs q 30 to 60 minutes.
- For hypertension, consider nitroprusside, 0.5 to10 μg/kg/min IV.

G. **Disposition:** Admit the patient to the ICU, if there is an evidence of pulmonary edema with respiratory distress or cardiac ischemia or infarction. The patient may be admitted to telemetry if stable after ED managements. All patients with new-onset CHF or pulmonary edema require admission.

15. Pulmonary Embolism:

Pulmonary embolism most commonly occurs when the venous thrombi in the deep venous system dislodge and enter the pulmonary arterial circulation. Risk factors include prolonged bed rest, elderly, CHF, carcinoma, CVA, pregnancy, oral contraceptives, postoperative, leg trauma, previous DVT/PE, and obesity. Risk stratify with Wells or PERC if starting empiric anticoagulation.

15.1. Clinical Evaluation:

A. **Symptoms:** Patients present with anxiety, pleuritic chest pain, dyspnea (most common symptom), agitation, hemoptysis, and syncope.

B. **Signs:** Examination reveals tachycardia, tachypnea, low-grade fever, hypotension, rales, rub, decreased breath sounds, hypoxia, and possible signs of a DVT.

C. **DDX:** Myocardial infarction, angina, pneumonia, pleural effusion, pneumothorax, musculoskeletal chest pain, pleurisy, and pericarditis.

D. **Workup:** CBC, BMP, BNP, PT/PTT/INR, cardiac enzymes, D-dimer (good for low-risk patients and if normal, can exclude DVT/PE/dissection).

- CXR: Usually normal but may show nonspecific abnormalities like an elevated hemidiaphragm, infiltrate or small pleural effusion. Westermark sign and Hampton hump are rare findings.
- ECG: S1Q3T3 pattern, incomplete RBBB, nonspecific ST-T wave changes, and tachycardia (most common abnormality).
- V-Q scan: Positive, if multiple segmental or lobar perfusion defects with normal ventilation. A normal scan excludes a pulmonary embolism. Normal ventilation with decreased perfusion is suggestive of a pulmonary embolism. Low and intermediate probability scans often require further testing for confirmation. High probability requires immediate anticoagulation.
- Lower extremity Doppler ultrasound: If a diagnosis is suspected but not confirmed by a V-Q scan or CT, consider a venous Doppler study of the lower extremities. This is an appropriate first test for a pregnant female with signs and symptoms of a PE. If the test is positive then no pulmonary imaging (except a CXR) is needed.
- Pulmonary angiogram: "Gold standard" test for the diagnosis of PE. Intraluminal filling defects and/or arterial cutoffs suggest a PE. This test has been replaced by VQ and CT angiography.
- High-resolution CT angiography chest: This has become the screening test of choice due to its safety, speed, availability, and excellent specificity for diagnosing PE and other pulmonary pathology. Good for detecting emboli in large pulmonary vessels but misses peripheral clots in small vessels. Less radiation to fetus than a VQ scan.
- Echocardiogram: Right ventricular dysfunction. Valuable in unstable patients who cannot leave the ED.

15.2. RX:

- **A.** Manage ABCs, IV, O_2, pulse oximeter, and monitor.
- **B.** Treat pain as needed.
- **C.** IV fluid bolus if hypotensive.
- **D.** Treat with unfractionated heparin, 80 U/kg bolus, followed by an IV infusion at 18 U/kg/h. May use low–molecular-weight heparin (enoxaparin, tinzaparin, or fondaparinux).
- **E.** Use thrombolysis in a patient with hypotension requiring vasopressors and with angiographically documented PE. May be considered empirically for a patient in extremis.
- **F.** t-PA, 100 mg over 2 hours **or** streptokinase.
- **G.** STAT thoracic surgery consult for consideration of embolectomy.
- **H.** **Disposition:** Admit all patients with a PE.

16. Arterial Embolism:

Thrombi or atheromatous material embolize and occlude a peripheral vessel causing a true vascular emergency. Ninety percent originate from the heart and are due to atrial fibrillation, mitral/aortic valve disease, CHF, cardiomyopathies, and endocarditis. Femoral (40%) and iliac (20%) arteries are the most commonly involved.

16.1. Clinical Evaluation:

- **A.** **Symptoms:** Sudden onset of pain, pallor, paralysis, paresthesias, and coolness.
- **B.** **Signs:** Pulselessness, necrosis of skin, abscess of hair, sensorimotor deficit, prolonged capillary refill, and an abnormal Doppler signal (absent flow, monophasic flow, abnormal ABI)
- **C.** **DDX:** DVT, cellulitis, osteomyelitis, and septic joint.
- **D.** **Workup:** CBC, BMP, T&C, PT/PTT/INR, cardiac enzymes, ECG, CXR, CT angiography.

16.2. RX:

- **A.** Support ABCs, IV, O_2, pulse oximeter, and monitor.
- **B.** Treat pain.
- **C.** Start heparin 60 U/kg IV bolus then 12 U/kg infusion, or low–molecular-weight heparin (Enoxaparin) 1 mg/kg sq.
- **D.** Consult vascular surgery.
- **E.** Aspirin 325 mg po.
- **F.** **Disposition:** Admit to ICU after postoperative embolectomy.

17. Deep Vein Thrombosis (DVT):

A deep vein thrombosis is the development of single or multiple clots within the deep veins of the pelvis or extremities. The most important concern is embolization, most commonly to the lung, which results in a life-threatening pulmonary embolism. Isolated calf DVT is a low risk for embolization, although up to 20% may propagate proximally. Risk factors include recent travel, sedentary/debilitated state, cancer, surgery, pregnancy, BCP use, previous DVT/PE, and tobacco use.

17.1. Clinical Evaluation:

- **A.** **Symptoms:** Calf pain, unilateral leg swelling, warmth, erythema.
- **B.** **Signs:** Unilateral leg swelling, palpable cords, calf firmness, warmth, tenderness, Homan's sign.
- **C.** **DDX:** Cellulitis, lymphangitis, ruptured Baker's cyst, muscle strain, edema from other causes (CHF and pregnancy).
- **D.** **Workup:** CBC, BMP, D-dimer, PTT/PT/INR, ECG. The type of tests ordered is based on suspected location.
  - Duplex ultrasound (US with color flow Doppler) is noninvasive and particularly useful at detecting popliteal and femoral thrombi.
  - Contrast venography is the gold standard test but has fallen out of favor because invasive and duplex US is just as specific and sensitive.
  - MRI is highly sensitive and useful for iliac vein, and vena cava evaluation.

17.2. RX:

A. Support ABCs, IV, O_2, pulse oximeter, and monitor prn.
B. Give heparin 80 U/kg IV bolus, followed by an 18 U/kg/h IV drip or enoxaparin (Lovenox) 1.0 mg/kg sc.
C. **Disposition:** Admit and treat a proximal DVT patient. Consider outpatient treatment for stable patients, without severe disease or comorbidities, who have adequate follow-up.

18. Syncope:

Syncope is a sudden transient loss of consciousness characterized by unresponsiveness, loss of postural tone, and spontaneous recovery. Near-syncope or presyncope is the feeling of faintness. The etiologies are similar for both conditions. Most causes of syncope are benign, but assume a life-threatening etiology until proven otherwise.

- Reflex-mediated syncope (40% of cases). This is neutrally mediated and due to excessive afferent discharge from mechanoreceptors. A reflex-mediated increase in parasympathetic tone causes vasodilation, bradycardia, and hypotension. Examples include vasovagal syncope, situational syncope, and carotid sinus hypersensitivity.
- Orthostatic hypotension syncope (5%). This occurs from intravascular volume depletion. Examples include GI bleed, vomiting, diarrhea, diuretic use, and anemia.
- Neurologic syncope (10% of cases). Examples include first-time seizure, atonic and temporal lobe seizures, TIAs, and migraines.
- Cardiovascular syncope (5% of cases). These are divided into two categories based on an organic cause or an arrhythmia. Organic causes include aortic stenosis, PE, pulmonary hypertension, AMI, cardiac tamponade, aortic dissection, and cardiomyopathy. Arrhythmias of concern are second-/third-degree blocks, sick sinus syndrome, V-tach, torsades, PSVT, pacemaker malfunction, and prolonged QT syndromes. If there is a cardiac cause for syncope, the 1-year mortality is 30% if undiagnosed or treated.
- Idiopathic (40% of cases). The diagnosis is unknown after initial workup. Disposition is based on the presence of significant risk factors for death or disability.

18.1. Clinical Evaluation:

A. **Symptoms:** Determine events immediately preceding the episode, including associated symptoms, that is, chest pain, palpitations, prodrome, dyspnea, or headache. The patient usually has a history of cardiac, pulmonary, or endocrine disease, and/or a prior history of syncope or seizure disorder. Talk with all witnesses and family members.
B. **Signs:** Evaluate vital signs and check for orthostatic hypotension. Pinpoint or dilated pupils may suggest toxidrome. Carotid bruits suggest cerebral ischemia. Evaluate neurologic status, including mental status, sensory, motor, reflexes, and cerebellar signs. Look for a tongue laceration or bowel and bladder incontinence. Consider hemocculting stools.
C. **DDX:** Refer to above.
D. **Workup:** Glucose, CBC, BMP, T&C, PT/PTT/INR, cardiac enzymes, drug screen, ETOH, ECG, CXR, CT head if a neurologic cause is suspected.

18.2. RX:

A. Support ABCs, IV, O_2, pulse oximeter, and monitor.
B. **Disposition:** Patients with syncope, resulting from seizure, vasovagal episode, corrected hypovolemia, and hypoglycemia, who improve in ED and who have no complications can usually be safely discharged. Admit patients, especially the elderly, with conditions caused by an arrhythmia, valvular disease, cerebrovascular accident, subarachnoid hemorrhage, pulmonary embolism, aortic dissection, or myocardial infarction, as well as those individuals with undetermined causes to a monitored bed.

DERMATOLOGY

1. Henoch–Schönlein Purpura (HSP):

Henoch–Schönlein purpura is an acute IgA–mediated disorder characterized by a vasculitis of the small vessels in the GI tract, skin, joints, kidneys, and rarely lungs and CNS.

1.1. Clinical Evaluation:

A. Symptoms: The onset is gradual to abrupt, with a prodrome of headache, fever, and anorexia. Over time, the patient develops a rash (especially to the legs), abdominal pain, vomiting, joint pain, edema, and possible bloody stools. HSP is most common in children aged 4 to 11 years with a recent history of upper respiratory or GI infection.

B. Signs: Palpable purpura begins on gravity-dependent areas of the legs and buttocks and the extensor surface of the arms. Diffuse abdominal pain and arthritis may be evident on examination. Edema may be present on the face and ears.

C. DDX: Acute abdomen, drug reaction, glomerulonephritis, bacterial endocarditis, meningococcal infection, Rocky Mountain spotted fever (RMSF), Kawasaki disease, septic shock, child abuse, mononucleosis, and ITP.

D. Workup: CBC, BMP, UA, PT/PTT/INR, lipase, hemoccult stool. Consider ESR, CRP, abdominal x-ray, and a CXR.

1.2. RX:

A. Resolves in 1 to 4 months. No treatment has been found to shorten the duration or degree of HSP.

B. Anti-inflammatory agents may be used for fever and arthritis.

C. Treat with corticosteroids, such as prednisone 1 to 2 mg/kg/d, for angioedema and severe GI symptoms. Steroids do not help alleviate the lesions.

D. Plasmapheresis may be effective in delaying progression of kidney disease.

E. Disposition: Outpatient therapy is appropriate unless complications occur such as renal failure, secondary infection of vasculitis lesions, or intestinal tract perforations or intussusception.

2. Thrombotic Thrombocytopenic Purpura (TTP):

TTP is a consumptive thrombocytopenia that is characterized by fever, mental status changes, renal insufficiency, severe thrombocytopenia, and a microangiopathic hemolytic anemia. The mortality rate is 80% if left untreated.

2.1. Clinical Evaluation:

A. Symptoms: Fever, fatigue, altered mental status, and headache.

B. Signs: Flat, nonpalpable purpura in areas of pressure, petechiae <3 mm, and ecchymosis >3 mm. Fluctuating neurologic symptoms may occur, including stroke, seizures, and altered mental states. Hematuria, proteinuria, jaundice, or pallor may be present. Purpura may involve the mucous membranes and optic fundi.

C. DDX: Drug reaction, meningococcal infection, septic shock, and ITP.

D. Workup: CBC (platelet count vital), PT/PTT/INR, type and cross, BMP, UA, blood smear (fragmented RBCs), reticulocyte count, LFTs, D-dimer, fibrinogen. CT head if stroke is suspected.

2.2. RX:

A. Give methylprednisolone 1 mg/kg/d IV.

B. Plasmapheresis coupled with FFP infusion is emergently required.

C. Anticoagulation, aspirin, and dipyridamole are controversial and fallen out of favor.

D. Consult dermatology.

E. Platelet transfusion should be avoided unless life-threatening bleeding is present.

F. Disposition: ICU admission is required for all of these patients.

3. Idiopathic Thrombocytopenic Purpura (ITP):

ITP is a decrease in the circulating number of platelets due to a defective IgG immunoglobulin binding to normal platelets. This complex is phagocytized by macrophages predominately in the spleen. The acute form occurs in children, 2 to 6 y/o, usually following a viral prodrome. The chronic form of the disease is seen in adults 20 to 50 y/o. The latter condition presents with no prodrome, easy bruising, prolonged menses, and mucosal bleeding. The hallmark of ITP is isolated thrombocytopenia without other blood dyscrasias.

3.1. Clinical Evaluation:

A. **Symptoms:** Bruising, gingival bleeding, menometrorrhagia, menorrhagia, recurrent epistaxis, and neurologic symptoms secondary to intracerebral bleeding.
B. **Signs:** Petechiae and purpura. Nonpalpable spleen (absence of an enlarged spleen is an essential diagnostic criteria). Neurologic deficits secondary to intracerebral bleeding. Hemoccult positive stools.
C. **DDX:** Lupus, myelodysplastic syndromes, lymphoma, TTP, drug reaction, bacterial endocarditis, meningococcal infection, and septic shock.
D. **Workup:** PT/PTT/INR, CBC (platelet count), BMP, LFTs, ANA, blood smear.

3.2. RX:

A. Treat acute ITP with prednisone, 4 to 8 mg/kg/d for 7 to 10 days and then taper.
B. Patient should be considered for a splenectomy but less frequently done due to the use of rituximab.
C. Administer IV gamma globulin (IgG), 1 to 2 g/kg single dose.
D. Aspirin is contraindicated.
E. Avoid gamma globulin, if the patient has IgA deficiency.
F. Obtain a hematology consult.
G. Other therapies include vincristine, vinblastine, danazol, plasmapheresis, azathioprine, cyclophosphamide, and interferon.
H. **Disposition:** Consider outpatient management unless the individual has a platelet count <20,000. Admit patients with active bleeding.

4. Staphylococcal Scalded Skin Syndrome (SSSS):

A superficial blistering syndrome caused by *Staphylococcus aureus* species that produces epidermolytic toxins A&B. The toxin is spread hematogenously from a local source causing damage at distant sites. SSSS differs from TEN by the fact it causes intraepidermal separation where TEN involves sloughing of the entire epidermis from the dermis. It most commonly affects children/infants <5 y/o. Self-limiting disorder with a 3% mortality in children and a 30% mortality in adults (very rare). Symptoms usually resolve within 5 to 7 days.

4.1. Clinical Evaluation:

A. **Symptoms:** Prodrome of fever, malaise, sore throat, irritability, and skin tenderness. A faint erythematous rash is seen with blistering and sloughing occurring 24 to 48 hours later.
B. **Signs:** The macular rash is red, tender, and in the flexor creases. Mucous membranes are spared and the Nikolsky sign is positive. Perioral crusting, facial edema, and signs of dehydration are seen.
C. **DDX:** TEN/SJS, drug reactions, Kawasaki disease, meningococcal or possibly gram-negative sepsis, RMSF, and streptococcal scarlet fever.
D. **Workup:** CBC, BUN, blood culture, Strep screen, wound culture, ESR, and CRP. Consider a CXR if pneumonia is considered.

4.2. RX:

A. Support ABCs, IV, pulse oximeter, and monitor.
B. Administer, nafcillin, 50 to 100 mg/kg/d IV, with or without clindamycin (toxin synthesis inhibitor). Use Cefazolin if penicillin allergic.
C. Manage fluids and electrolytes.
D. Pain control.
E. Avoid steroids.
F. Disposition: Admit.

5. Toxic Epidermal Necrosis/Steven–Johnson Syndrome (TEN/SJS):

TEN results from an immune cytotoxic reaction that destroys keratinocytes. It is life threatening and characterized by wide spread erythema, necrosis, and bullous detachment of the epidermis and mucous membranes. SJS/TEN is most commonly caused by drugs such as sulfonamides, barbiturates, phenytoin, phenylbutazone, or penicillin. Rare causes include a graft-versus-host reaction (after a bone marrow transplant) or administration of blood products.

- SJS and TEN are a disease continuum distinguished by severity, based upon the percentage of body surface involved with skin detachment. SJS is the less severe form, with skin detachment of <10% and two or more mucous membrane sites involved. TEN involves detachment of >30% of the body surface area along with mucous membrane involvement. SJS was once considered a severe form of erythema multiforme (major) but is now considered a different entity with different, distinct causes.
- Erythema multiforme minor is characterized by target lesions that are raised papules distributed acrally.
- Erythema multiforme major is exactly like EM minor except for two or more mucous membranes involved, and epidermal detachment of <10% total body surface.

5.1. Clinical Evaluation:

A. Symptoms: Affects adults primarily. Flulike prodrome of malaise, rash, fever, myalgias rhinitis, headache, and anorexia. Skin becomes red, hot with blisters and sloughing of skin.
B. Signs: Skin becomes red, hot with blisters, and sloughing of skin. Mucous membranes are involved and the entire thickness of the epidermis separates from the dermis. Nikolsky sign is positive.
C. DDX: SSSS, drug reactions, Kawasaki disease, meningococcal or possibly gram-negative sepsis, RMSF, and streptococcal scarlet fever.
D. Workup: CBC, BMP, ESR, CRP, PT/PTT/INR, skin biopsy.

5.2. RX:

A. Support ABCs, IV, O_2, pulse oximeter, and monitor.
B. Remove offending agent.
C. Manage fluids and electrolytes similar to that used for burn treatments.
D. Keep the patient warm.
E. Pain control.
F. Consult a dermatologist and an ophthalmologist for eye involvement.
G. Corticosteroids, plasmapheresis, cyclosporine, and tumor necrosis factor-alpha inhibitors are controversial.
H. Disposition: Admit to burn unit.

6. Erythema Multiforme:

Erythema multiforme is an acute, self-limited type IV hypersensitivity reaction involving the skin and mucous membranes. Exposure to drugs (50% of cases), herpes, hepatitis, influenza, fungal infections, collagen vascular disease, and various viral infections are the most common etiologies. Rash will resolve in 7 to 10 days.

6.1. Clinical Evaluation:

A. Symptoms: Acute, rapidly progressive rash with minor constitutional symptoms.
B. Signs: Red raised rash with central clearing (target lesions). Found on palms, soles of the feet, dorsum of the hand, face and extensor surfaces. Twenty-five percent will have mucous membrane involvement with a negative Nikolsky sign.
C. DDX: Toxic epidermal necrolysis, urticaria, necrotizing vasculitis, drug reaction, contact dermatitis, viral exanthems, RMSF, meningococcemia, and syphilis.
D. Workup: CBC, BMP, LFTs, calcium, PT/PTT/INR, ESR, CRP, consider HSV testing.

6.2. RX:

A. Support ABCs, IV O_2, pulse oximeter, and monitor as indicated.
B. Discontinue offending agent.
C. Treat pain.
D. For severe cases, use 80-mg prednisone q day (controversial).
E. Consult an ophthalmologist for corneal lesions.
F. Disposition: Admit severe cases to the hospital.

7. Toxic Shock Syndrome (TSS):

Toxic shock syndrome is a toxin-mediated multisystem shock state from an immune reaction to super antigens. *S. aureus* (endotoxin toxic shock syndrome-1 [TSST-1]) infection is the most common followed by *Streptococcus pyogenes* exotoxin A/B. Toxic shock criteria for *Staph* are (1) fever, (2) hypotension, (3) rash, (4) ≥3 organ systems involved. Criteria for *Strep* are (1) isolation of *Group A Strep*, (2) hypotension, (3) ≥organ systems involved. Mortality <3% for *Staph* but 30% to 70% for *Strep*. The syndrome is linked to nasal packing, superabsorbent tampons, Post-partum, DM, HIV, chronic cardio/pulmonary disease, and influenza infection.

7.1. Clinical Evaluation:

- **A. Symptoms:** Fever >38.9°C (102.2°F), rash, headache, arthralgia, vomiting, watery diarrhea, pain at infection site, and syncope.
- **B. Signs:** Diffused, blanching, macular erythroderma rash, hypotension, petechial, mental status changes, dysrhythmias, pharyngitis, conjunctivitis, vaginitis, renal, and hepatic or hematologic dysfunction. Full-thickness desquamation involves the hands and feet in 1 to 2 weeks. Hair and nail loss occur 1 to 2 months later.
- **C. DDX:** Kawasaki disease, RMSF, scarlet fever, TEN/SJS, drug reactions, SSSS, and meningococcal sepsis.
- **D. Workup:** CBC, cultures (blood, wound), BMP, LFTs, calcium, PT/PTT/INR, UA, rapid strep, RMSF serology, ANA, ECG, CXR.

7.2. RX:

- **A.** Support the ABCs, IV, O_2, pulse oximeter, and monitor.
- **B.** Start IV with nafcillin, vancomycin, cefazolin, or clindamycin.
- **C.** Initiate drainage of staphylococcal infection and remove any foreign bodies (FBs).
- **D.** Complications include coagulopathy, respiratory depression, and myocardial depression.
- **E. Disposition:** Admit all patients to the ICU. Consider consulting ID, surgery, and possible cardiology.

8. Scarlet Fever:

This is due to an erythrogenic toxin producing group A beta-hemolytic *Streptococcus* infection of the pharynx, cellulitic or surgical wounds, or uterus. The exotoxin causes skin inflammation, edema, renal damage, myocarditis, and sepsis.

8.1. Clinical Evaluation:

- **A. Symptoms:** Fever 40°C (104°F), sore throat, myalgias, nausea/vomiting, and malaise followed by a rash in 12 to 24 hours.
- **B. Signs:** Bright red mucous membranes, flushed face, and circumoral pallor (Forchheimer spots). Skin rash is a papular eruptions on an erythematous base, diffuse, with a rough texture ("sandpaper"). Pastia lines in inguinal folds and axilla are common Pharynx is injected, petechiae on palate (red strawberry tongue), and desquamation occurs 5 days to 6 weeks later.
- **C. DDX:** Measles, rubella, infectious mononucleosis, roseola, syphilis, Toxic shock syndrome, SSSS, TEN/SJS, Kawasaki disease, and drug hypersensitivity.
- **D. Workup:** Rapid strep, throat culture, antistreptolysin-O titer, CBC, BMP, ESR, CRP, UA, ECG, CXR, and wound/blood culture if indicated.

8.2. RX:

- **A.** Support the ABSc, IV, O_2, pulse oximeter, and monitor.
- **B.** NS bolus of 20 mL/kg bolus.
- **C.** Treat with penicillin. Alternative treatment include erythromycin or a first-generation cephalosporin.
- **D.** Diphenhydramine and/or antihistamines for itching.
- **E. Disposition:** Discharge with close follow-up, unless there are severe secondary complications.

9. Meningococcemia:

Neisseria meningitidis is a gram-negative diplococcus that is transmitted by airborne droplets to the nasopharynx where it becomes colonized. The infection enters the bloodstream and spreads to multiple sites (meninges, joints) leading to shock and death within hours of presentation. If fulminant infection is present, the mortality rate is 50% to 70% within 48 hours.

9.1. Clinical Evaluation:

A. Symptoms: Fever, headache, malaise, myalgias, cough, lethargy, and arthralgias.
B. Signs: Petechial rash beginning on the trunk and legs. Lesions become palpable purpura, confluent, and widely disbursed. Altered mental status, meningeal signs, tachycardia, tachypnea, hypotension, cyanosis, arthritis, and pulmonary edema are other findings.
C. DDX: Sepsis, RMSF, Henoch–Schönlein, gonococcemia, endocarditis, hemolytic uremic syndrome, TTP, and influenza.
D. Workup: CXR, CBC, PT/PTT/INR (prolonged), BMP, ABG/VBG, lactate, blood cultures (70–80% positive), CT head, LP (elevated pressure, positive culture and Gram stain, rapid PCR positive).
E. Special Consideration: Do CT before LP for the following: Immunocompromised state, history of CNS disease (stroke, mass lesion, focal infection), new-onset seizure, focal neuro deficit, abnormal level of consciousness and papilledema. **Give antibiotics before going to CT scanner.**

9.2. RX:

A. Support ABCs, IV, O_2, pulse oximeter, and monitor.
B. NS IV bolus, consider inotropic agents (norepinephrine, dopamine).
C. Ceftriaxone or Cefotaxime is the drug of choice until cultures are available. Empiric treatment with vancomycin is recommended by many sources.
D. Manage complications like seizures DIC, coma, septic arthritis, and thrombocytopenia.
E. Do not use steroids.
F. Disposition: Admit to the ICU. Prescribe prophylactic treatment for all close contacts.

10. Lyme Disease:

The spirochete *Borrelia burgdorferi* is transmitted by the deer tick Ixodes scapularis and pacificus. This is a multiseptemic disorder with three clinical stages and is accounts for 95% of all vector borne illnesses in the United States.

10.1. Clinical Evaluation:

A. Symptoms:
- Stage 1: In 1 to 30 days after the tick bite. Rash, malaise, myalgias, fatigue lethargy, headache, and fever are seen.
- Stage 2: Early disseminated Lyme disease develops 4 to 10 weeks after the tick bite. Fever, malaise, and one or more organ systems (CNC, CV, musculoskeletal) are involved.
- Stage 3: Late (chronic) disease occurs months to years after exposure. Arthritis (knees most common), neuro deficits (Bell's palsy) cognitive problems and skin changes are seen.

B. Signs: Initially, a small red papule forms which expands to a large lesion (>15 cm) consisting of a bright red outer border, with central clearing. The lesions are not painful or pruritic and the palms and soles are spared. Regional lymphadenopathy, meningeal signs, focal neurologic deficits, altered mental status, conjunctivitis, papilledema, and joint swelling are common.
C. DDX: Meningitis, babesiosis, Ehrlichiosis, fibromyalgia, septic arthritis, hepatitis, erythema multiforme, meningitis, myocarditis, and Guillain–Barré syndrome.
D. Workup: CBC, BMP, PT/PTT/INR, LFTs, ECG, ECHO, EIA, or ELISA serologic tests (Western blot if positive or equivocal), cultures, LP (pleocytosis).

10.2. RX:

- **A.** Support ABCs, IV, O_2, pulse oximeter, and monitor.
- **B.** Doxycycline 100 mg bid or amoxicillin 50 mg/kg/d tid for 14 to 21 days.
- **C.** Use ceftriaxone 75 to 100 mg/kg/d (2 g max), IV for Lyme meningitis, arthritis, or carditis.
- **D.** **Disposition:** Most patients can be treated as an outpatient, but those with neurologic or cardiac complications require admission.

11. Rocky Mountain Spotted Fever (RMSF):

RMSF is the most common fatal tick disease in the United States (mortality rate of 3% if treated). *Rickettsia rickettsii* is transmitted by the female ticks *Dermacentor variabilis* (dog tick) and *Dermacentor andersoni* (wood tick). The infection causes a small vessel vasculitis with an inflammatory cascades leading to multiorgan damage. Common disorders include meningitis, pulmonary edema, liver necrosis, GI injury, and a myocarditis.

11.1. Clinical Evaluation:

- **A.** **Symptoms:** Abrupt high fever, headache, nausea, vomiting, diarrhea, myalgias, abdominal pain, mental status changes, and a rash.
- **B.** **Signs:** Periorbital edema, relative bradycardia, hypotension, ataxia, vertigo, muscle tenderness, meningeal signs, and an enlarged spleen. The rash is red macules that blanch on wrists and ankles. The macules spread from the wrist and ankles to the trunk and face and become petechial lesions on the palms and soles.
- **C.** **DDX:** Drug eruptions, Lyme disease, Ehrlichiosis, babesiosis, dengue fever, meningococcemia, syphilis, TTP, mononucleosis, rubeola, roseola, enteroviruses, erythema infectiosum, drug eruptions, and anaphylactoid purpura.
- **D.** **Workup:** CBC, BMP, LFTs, PT/PTT/INR, ECG, CXR, LP (increased protein and a monocytosis), blood culture (low yield). Confirmation tests are acute and convalescent titers.

11.2. RX:

- **A.** Support ABCs, IV, O_2, pulse oximeter, and monitor.
- **B.** The treatment of choice is doxycycline 100 mg po/IV bid × 7 to 14 days. Prophylactic treatment for 7 to 14 days after tick removal. Alternative treatment is chloramphenicol 50 to 100 mg/kg/d divided qid IV.
- **C.** IV fluids and PRBCs if anemic.
- **D.** Consult renal for acute renal failure.
- **E.** **Disposition:** Admit all patients to the ICU. Report to the public health department.

12. Anaphylaxis/Urticaria:

Anaphylaxis is a life-threatening allergic reaction that occurs in sensitized persons causing the release of histamine, prostaglandins, and kallikrein from mast cells and basophils. Mediators illicit, massive vasodilation, and capillary leakage that results in hypotension, urticaria, and angioedema. Most common antigens are penicillin and bee/wasp stings.

12.1. Clinical Evaluation:

- **A.** **Symptoms:** Pruritus, rash, chest tightness, flushed skin, throat tightness, dizziness, N/V/D, syncope, abdominal pain.
- **B.** **Signs:** Tachycardia, tachycardia, arrhythmia, hypotension, angioedema, stridor, wheezing, urticaria.
- **C.** **DDX:** Angioedema, asthma, PE, scombroid poisoning, alcohol-induced flush, carcinoid syndrome.
- **D.** **Workup:** CBC, ABG, CXR.

12.2. RX:

- **A.** Support ABCs, IV, O_2, pulse oximeter, and monitor.
- **B.** For severe cases, give:
  - Methylprednisolone (Solu-Medrol), 60 to 125 mg IV push (peds, 1 mg/kg).
  - Consider H_2 blocker (ranitidine 50 mg IV).

- Epinephrine (1:1000 solution), 0.3 cc IM/sq (peds, 0.001 mg/kg). In life-threatening situations, give epinephrine 0.1 to 0.25 mg of 1:10,000 solution IV. May give SL and via ETT.
- NS bolus for hypotension.
- Albuterol via MDI or nebulizer.
- Diphenhydramine 25 to 50 mg IV/IM.

C. Consider glucagon 1 mg IV/IM/sq for refractory cases.
D. For persistent hypotension, treat with dopamine infusion.
E. **Disposition:** Admit all unstable patients to the ICU. If patient responds rapidly and completely, observe in ED for 3 hours then discharge with close follow-up.

ENDOCRINE

1. Alcoholic Ketoacidosis:

Alcoholic ketoacidosis is defined as anion gap acidosis with high levels of ketoacids that are secondary to increased mobilization of free fatty acids (ketone formation), decreased insulin production, and increased glucagon production. The combination of poor nutrition plus volume depletion from vomiting further worsens the ketosis and the patient's condition. This is seen in chronic alcoholics with a history of binge drinking, with abrupt cessation, and decreased food intake.

1.1. Clinical Evaluation:

A. **Symptoms:** Abdominal pain, N/V, anorexia, diarrhea, weakness, and muscle pain. Patients often present 1 to 2 days after the last alcohol use.
B. **Signs:** Tachycardia, ketotic breath, dehydration, tachypnea (Kussmaul's respiration), hypothermia, hypotension, altered mental status, and various abdominal findings.
C. **DDX:** Pancreatitis, peptic ulcer disease, gastritis, hypoglycemia, DKA, toxic alcohol ingestion, sepsis.
D. **Workup:** CBC, BMP, calcium/phosphate, serum ketone and lactate level, ABG/VBG, LFTs, hemoccult stool, lipase, UA, ETOH, CXR, ECG.

1.2. RX:

A. Support the ABCs, IV, O_2, pulse oximeter, and monitor.
B. Administer thiamine, 100 mg IV/IM/po, and feed the patient.
C. Replace fluid loses by using D_5NS or NS.
D. Consider treatment with sodium bicarbonate when pH is <7.10.
E. Treat alcohol withdrawal if it exists.
F. Treat pain and use antiemetics if indicated.
G. Insulin is not indicated and may precipitate hypoglycemia.
H. **Disposition:** Admit the patient to a floor or unit depending on his/her stability.

2. Adrenal Crisis (Addisonian Crisis):

Addisonian crisis is a life-threatening condition that occurs in patients with or without chronic adrenal insufficiency. This condition is precipitated by abrupt withdrawal of steroids, acute infection, sepsis, adrenal hemorrhage, acute trauma, AMI, hypothermia, surgery, and burns.

2.1. Clinical Evaluation:

A. **Symptoms:** Weakness, lethargy, confusion, anorexia, N/V/D, and abdominal pain.
B. **Signs:** Hypotension or orthostatic, tachycardia, hyperthermia, hyperpigmentation, disorientation, confusion, or unconsciousness.
C. **DDX:** Myocardial infarction, heart failure, hypovolemia, sepsis, pulmonary embolism, DKA, and shock.
D. **Workup:** CBC, BMP, calcium/phosphorus, cardiac enzymes, D-dimer, BNP, ECG, CXR, cortisol and ACTH levels, CT scan prn.

2.2. RX:

- **A.** Support ABCs, IV, O_2, pulse oximeter, and monitor.
- **B.** NS bolus 1 to 2 L followed by D_5NS 2 to 3 L over the next 8 hours.
- **C.** Check glucose (or give 1 amp D_{50}) (consider giving thiamine before glucose).
- **D.** Naloxone 2 mg IV for altered mental status or COMA.
- **E.** Simultaneous treatment and confirmation of adrenal insufficiency may be achieved.
- **F.** Consider giving cosyntropin (synthetic ACTH), 0.25 mg IV.
- **G.** Dexamethasone (Decadron), 4 mg (10 mg for shock) or hydrocortisone 100 mg IV.
- **H.** Avoid treatment of hyperkalemia with insulin (will resolve with IV fluids and glucocorticoid replacement).
- **I.** **Disposition:** Admit the patient to the ICU.

3. Diabetic Ketoacidosis (DKA):

DKA is a life-threatening complication of diabetes characterized by hyperglycemia, ketonemia, and acidosis. This occurs due to an insulin deficiency followed by a metabolic derangement (ketosis, hyperglycemia, acidosis, dehydration) that makes the patient unable to deal with a significant stressor (AMI, infection, trauma, stroke). Death occurs due to hyperkalemia-induced arrhythmias and cardiovascular collapse.

3.1. Clinical Evaluation:

- **A.** **Symptoms:** N/V, abdominal pain, fruity breath, myalgias, headache, lethargy.
- **B.** **Signs:** Dehydration, hypotension, tachypnea (Kussmaul's breathing), tachycardia, abdominal tenderness, altered mental status.
- **C.** **DDX:** Hyperosmolar hyperglycemic state, alcoholic ketoacidosis, lactic acidosis, pancreatitis, starvation, sepsis, salicylate toxicity.
- **D.** **Workup:** CBC, BMP, lactate, cardiac enzymes, BNP, ABG/VBG, calcium/phosphorus, serum ketones, lipase, UA, ECG, CXR, cultures prn as appropriate. Recheck K^+ and glucose q 1 to 2 hours after treatment is started.

3.2. RX:

- **A.** Support airway, IV, O_2, pulse oximeter, and monitor.
- **B.** Bolus NS IV at 2 L/h for first 1 to 2 hours.
- **C.** Insulin adheres to IV tubing so bolus 10 units of regular insulin through the tubing to cause adherence without altering the delivery concentration of the remainder of the insulin drip.
- **D.** Bolus 0.1 U/kg IV of regular insulin. You may give a 0.1 unit/kg IM/SQ injection of regular insulin instead of an initial IV bolus.
- **E.** Start a 0.1 U/kg/h IV drip of regular insulin. When the glucose drops below 250 mg/dL, change the IV fluid to D_5 half NS.
- **F.** Administer sodium bicarbonate, if the pH is <6.9.
- **G.** Consider potassium and phosphate replacement once the patient produces urine.
- **H.** **Disposition:** Admit to the ICU.

4. Hyperosmolar Hyperglycemic State (HHS):

HHS was previously called hyperosmolar hyperglycemic nonketotic coma but this was changed since only 20% present in a coma. HHS is seen in type 2 diabetes and is characterized by hyperglycemia, hyperosmolarity, and severe dehydration without ketoacidosis. The glucose level, degree of dehydration, and mortality (10–20%) are greater than in those with DKA.

4.1. Clinical Evaluation:

- **A.** **Symptoms:** Polyuria, polydipsia, altered mental status, lethargy, coma frequently weight loss.
- **B.** **Signs:** Dehydration, postural hypotension, tachycardia, tachypnea, caused by cardiovascular collapse. Neurologic findings include seizures, change in mental status, focal deficits, aphasia, nystagmus, tremors, and hyperreflexia.

- **C. DDX:** DKA, AMI, hepatic failure, sepsis, dehydration, uremia, CVA.
- **D. Workup:** Glucose (average value >800 mg/dL), CBC, BMP, U/A, ABG, CXR, ECG, blood and urine culture, lipase, BNP, LFTs, cardiac enzymes, PT/PTT/INR, serum osmolality. Calculate serum osmolarity = 2(Na) + glucose/18 + BUN/2.8.

4.2. RX:

- **A.** Support ABCs, IV, O_2, pulse oximeter, and monitor.
- **B.** Initiate fluid resuscitation with 1 to 2 L NS for the first hour followed by 1 L/h over the next few hours.
- **C.** Replace potassium unless the patient is hyperkalemic or is in renal failure.
- **D.** Hyperglycemia will decrease with fluid resuscitation; however, consider a low dosage of insulin for patients who are hyperkalemic, acidotic, or in renal failure. Administer regular insulin, 0.1/kg/h, until glucose levels drop to 250 mg/dL.
- **E. Disposition:** Admit the patient to the ICU.

5. Hypothyroidism and Myxedema Coma:

Hypothyroidism is a clinical condition resulting from decreased circulating levels of free thyroid hormone. Myxedema coma is severe hypothyroidism. It commonly occurs in elderly females with hypothyroidism in conjunction with a precipitating event, such as hypothermia, shock, hypoglycemia, AMI, CVA, and sepsis. The mortality rate is as high as 50% with treatment.

5.1. Clinical Evaluation:

- **A. Symptoms:** Lethargy, obtundation, hypothermia, weakness, cold intolerance, constipation, muscle cramps, arthralgias, paresthesias, weight gain, menorrhagia, depression, and hoarseness.
- **B. Signs:** Dry skin, dull facial expressions, husky voice, bradycardia, hypothermia, hypotension, periorbital edema, swelling of the hands and feet, reduced and brittle body and scalp hair, delayed relaxation of DTRs (Cheyney reflexes), macroglossia, anemia, hyponatremia, and enlarged heart.
- **C. DDX:** Nephrotic syndrome, dehydration, chronic nephritis, depression, neurasthenia, CHF, amyloidosis, dementia, and sepsis.
- **D. Workup:** CBC, BMP, PT/PTT/INR, cardiac enzymes, BNP, thyroid function tests (TSH & free T_4), UA, ABG (hypercarbia), ECG (low voltage), CXR, CT head (prn neurologic symptoms).

5.2. RX:

- **A.** Intubate and ventilate, IV, pulse oximeter, and monitor.
- **B.** IV fluid bolus.
- **C.** Initiate passive rewarming for hypothermia.
- **D.** For thyroid replacement, use thyroxine, 400 to 500 μg slow IV.
- **E.** Give hydrocortisone, 100–300 mg IV. (Adrenal insufficiency is often a concomitant finding).
- **F.** Treat precipitating cause. Antibiotics for underlying infection.
- **G. Disposition:** Admit to the ICU.

6. Thyroid Storm:

Thyroid storm is a life-threatening hypermetabolic state induced by excessive release of thyroid hormone. It is caused by undiagnosed or undertreated thyrotoxic Graves' disease or a toxic multinodular goiter exaggerated by a stressful event (infection, trauma, vascular AMI, CVA, pregnancy, DKA).

6.1. Clinical Evaluation:

- **A. Symptoms:** Severe weakness, weight loss, heat intolerance, anxiety, profuse sweating, palpitations, dyspnea, N/V/D, increased appetite, tremor, and emotional lability.
- **B. Signs:** Temp >38.7°C (101.7°F), hypertension, wide-pulse pressure, tachycardia, tachypnea, coma, hyperreflexia, atrial fibrillation, SVT, ophthalmopathy, and a goiter.
- **C. DDX:** Heat stroke, neuroleptic malignant syndrome, withdrawal syndromes, psychosis, pheochromocytoma, anxiety disorder, and congestive heart failure.

D. **Workup:** CBC, BMP, BNP, cardiac enzymes, LFTs, calcium/phosphorus, UA, urine drug screen (as needed), thyroid studies (TSH, T_4, T_3), CXR, ECG.

6.2. RX:

A. Support ABCs, IV, O_2, pulse oximeter, and monitor.
B. Block effects with propranolol, 1 to 2 mg IV q 15 minutes, until the desired effect is achieved.
C. Block release with potassium iodide, 3 to 5 gtt po/ng q 8 hours, or NaI 1 g slow IV q 8 to 12 hours (start 1 hour after PTU administration).
D. Block synthesis with PTU, 900 to 1,200 mg po/ng load.
E. Treat hyperthermia with acetaminophen and a cooling blanket.
F. Treat CHF, cardiac arrhythmias, and electrolyte abnormalities.
G. Give hydrocortisone, 100 to 500 mg/d IV (decrease conversion of T_4 to T_3 and prevent adrenal insufficiency).
H. **Disposition:** Admit to the ICU.

7. Wernicke–Korsakoff Syndrome:

Wernicke–Korsakoff syndrome is a potentially fatal disorder caused by a thiamine deficiency (Vitamin B1), predominately seen in chronic alcoholics. Wernicke's encephalopathy has one or more findings of a triad of global confusion, ataxia, and ophthalmoplegia. Korsakoff's psychosis consists of irreversible memory deficit marked by amnestic apathy and confabulation. The mortality rate is between 10% and 15% with 25% requiring long-term supervised care. Infection is the most common cause of death (75%).

7.1. Clinical Evaluation:

A. **Symptoms:** Wernicke's triad: Ataxia, opthalmoplegia, encephalopathy. Korsakoff's: Defects in learning and memory, retrograde/anterograde amnesia, confabulation.
B. **Signs:** Nystagmus (vertical and horizontal), ophthalmoplegia, anisocoria, disorientation, ataxia. Abnormal mental status, hypotension, hypothermia, and tachycardia/bradycardia.
C. **DDX:** Alcohol intoxication/withdrawal, sepsis, seizure, subdural hematoma, intracranial trauma, encephalopathy, CNS infection, CVA, tumor, demyelinating disease, and hypothermia.
D. **Workup:** CBC, BMP, BNP, ETOH, Lipase, PT/PTT/INR, Mg/Ca/P, urine drug screen, lactate, ABG/VBG, ammonia, ECG, CXR, CT head.

7.2. RX:

A. Support ABCs, IV, O_2, pulse oximeter, and monitor.
B. Administer 100 mg of thiamine IV.
C. Monitor cardiac responses and vital signs.
D. Perform serial neuro examinations.
E. Give multivitamin, magnesium, and nutrition.
F. Treat alcohol withdrawal.
G. **Disposition:** Admit patient with a neurology consult.

ENVIRONMENTAL

1. Bee, Wasp, and Ant Stings (Hymenoptera):

Hymenoptera stings originate from bees, wasps, hornets, yellow jackets, and ants. Stings may result in local inflammatory reactions, immediate and delayed hypersensitivity reactions, atypical reactions, and direct systemic toxicity.

1.1. Clinical Evaluation:

A. **Symptoms:** Pruritus, pain, slight erythema, and edema at the sting site.
B. **Signs:**
- Local reaction: Redness and edema is apparent at sting site. Stinger or venom sac may be present.
- Toxic reaction: Ten or more stings may result in vomiting, diarrhea, light headedness, syncope, headache, fever, muscle spasms, and edema.

- Anaphylactic reaction: Generalized urticaria, facial flushing, itching eyes, dry cough, chest or throat constriction, wheezing, dyspnea, cyanosis, abdominal cramps, diarrhea, nausea and vomiting, vertigo, fever, chills, pharyngeal stridor, shock, loss of consciousness, involuntary bowel and bladder action, and bloody frothy sputum. Reaction may be fatal.

1.2. RX:

A. Support ABCs, IV, O_2, pulse oximeter, and monitor.
B. For a local reaction, remove stinger, if present, but do not squeeze. Wash the affected area with soap and water to minimize the risk of infection. Apply ice to the site and elevate the limb to delay absorption and limit edema.
C. For a mild reaction, give prednisone 1 to 2 mg/kg po q day for 3 to 5 days and diphenhydramine (Benadryl), 25 to 50 mg po q 6 to 8 hours.
D. Treat pain as needed
E. For a severe systemic reaction, give epinephrine 1:1,000 0.3 to 0.5 mL sq for an adult, **or** 0.01 mL/kg sq for a child (do not exceed 0.3 mL). A second injection (10–15 minutes) may be given if the reaction continues.
- Diphenhydramine, 25 to 50 mg IM/IV.
- Albuterol, nebulized 2.5 mg for bronchospasm.
- Intubate if impending airway compromise.
- Bolus NS if hypotension develops.
- Persistent hypotension requires dopamine 5 μg/kg/min, titrated to effect.
- Solumedrol, 90 to 120 mg IV.

F. **Disposition:** If treatment requires epinephrine, the patient should be monitored in the ED for several hours to ensure that the symptoms do not intensify. Admit all severe reaction cases for 24 to 48 hours.

2. Black Widow Spider Envenomation:

Latrodectus mactans/hesperus/variolus females are characterized by a globular abdomen, leg spans of 2.5 cm, and a red hourglass design on the ventral surface of the abdomen. These spiders are poisonous, producing a neurotoxin that causes neurologic and autonomic symptoms.

2.1. Clinical Evaluation:

A. **Symptoms:** A brief, sharp pain is noted. Over the next 30 to 60 minutes, pain is deep, burning, and aching, which begins near the bite location and spreads to the back, neck, chest, abdomen, or flanks. N/V, headache, chest tightness, hypertension, salivation, and anxiety, may occur.
B. **Signs:** Two minor puncture wounds are present. No necrosis or significant swelling is apparent. A halo lesion consisting of a circular area of pallor surrounded by a ring of erythema may be exhibited. Rigid and tender abdominal muscles, diaphoresis, hypertension, tachycardia, ptosis, and periorbital ecchymosis/lacrimation/facial muscle spasm (Latrodectus facies)
C. **DDX:** Almost any illness that causes pain must be considered. Therefore, eliminate the possibility of myocardial infarction and acute abdomen.
D. **Workup:** ECG, CXR, CBC, BMP, UA, CPK, myoglobin.

2.2. RX:

A. Support ABCs, IV, O_2, pulse oximeter, and monitor.
B. Wash wound and apply ice.
C. Give tetanus prophylaxis.
D. Relieve pain with narcotics and benzodiazepines.
E. Indications for antivenin (1 vial IV) are severe pain or dangerous hypertension. Antivenin is contraindicated in patients allergic to horse serum. In addition, it is not recommended for patients taking beta-blocking agents. Perform a skin test before administration of antivenin. Consult poison control before giving.
F. Use of calcium and methocarbamol is of no value.

G. **Disposition:** Patients with mild to moderate symptoms who are controlled by oral analgesics may be discharged. If treated with antivenin, shows no complications, and is asymptomatic, he/she may go home after 8 to 10 hours of observation. Admit pregnant patients, symptomatic children, elderly, and those requiring parenteral narcotics.

3. Cat Bites:

Cat bites tend to be puncture wounds with infection rates of 25% to 50%. Long, narrow teeth often produce wounds that are at high risk for producing tenosynovitis. Typical organisms include *S. aureus, Streptococcus* species, *Klebsiella, Enterobacter* species, anaerobes, *Pasteurella multocida,* and small gram-negative rods. If infection occurs in <24 hours then *Pasteurella* is the most common organism. If infection occurs after 24 hours then consider *Streptococcus* species.

3.1. Clinical Evaluation:

A. **Symptoms:** Headache, fever, malaise, tender regional lymphadenopathy, and pain at the site.
B. **Signs:** Lymphadenopathy, possible rash, red, swollen wound, and signs of tenosynovitis.
C. **DDX:** Other animal bite, cellulitis, osteomyelitis, and puncture wound.
D. **Workup:** CBC, possible wound culture, x-ray for FB.

3.2. RX:

A. Copiously irrigate the affected area.
B. Debride devitalized tissue.
C. Normal hosts with relatively clean lacerations, especially of the face, can be safely sutured if the bite is treated within a few hours of injury. Hand bites should not be closed. Do not close puncture wounds.
D. Determine immunization status of the cat. Consider rabies prophylaxis if unsure.
E. Augmentin, 875 mg bid for 10 to 14 days. For moderate to severe infection use ceftriaxone or ampicillin/sulbactam.
F. Give tetanus prophylaxis.
G. Cat scratch disease resolves spontaneously in 1 to 2 months. Antibiotics are not effective for this disorder.
H. **Disposition:** Admit patients who are septic, immunocompromised, or have signs of infection of joints, or deep structures. All patients who are discharged should be re-examined in 24 to 48 hours.

4. Dog Bites:

Dog bites usually present as crush-type lacerations with devitalized adjacent tissue. Approximately 10% of all dog-bite wounds become infected with a much higher rate involving full-thickness bites. The organisms that are typically contracted are the same as those cited for cat bites. Pit Bull Terriers and Rottweilers cause the most deaths. Capnocytophaga infection in splenectomized patients may causes sepsis.

4.1. Clinical Evaluation:

A. **Symptoms:** Pain to wound, fever, redness, FB, nerve/tendon injury.
B. **Signs:** Wound infection, septic arthritis, and osteomyelitis.
C. **DDX:** Other animal bite, cellulitis, osteomyelitis, fracture, and puncture wound.
D. **Workup:** CBC, possible wound culture, x-ray for fracture.

4.2. RX:

A. ABCs if severely mauled.
B. Irrigate wound, debride devitalized tissue.
C. Tetanus prophylaxis.
D. Close most lacerations with the exception of the hand with a potential for joint or tendon involvement. Do not close puncture wounds.
E. Assess immunization status of the dog and give rabies prophylaxis if unsure.

F. Prophylactic antibiotics rarely indicated unless immunocompromised, asplenic, hand wounds, DM, and facial wounds. Treat with Augmentin 875 mg po bid for 3 to 5 days.
G. For moderate to severe infections use ampicillin/sulbactam, or clindamycin + ciprofloxacin IV for 10 to 14 days.
H. Surgery consult for severe infection or injury.
I. **Disposition:** Patient can usually be discharged. However, if there are signs of serious infection the patient must be admitted, particularly if there is any hand involvement.

5. Human Bites:

A human bite may result in a dangerous wound, especially when distal extremities are involved. Aerobic and anaerobic bacteria from mouth become embedded in the wound potentially leading to tenosynovitis, septic arthritis, or osteomyelitis, if untreated. The infection rate is >45%.

5.1. Clinical Evaluation:

A. **Symptoms:** Wound over the knuckles, ears, nose, tongue, nipples, fingertips, or penis. Pain, fever, swelling at wound site, and pruritus.
B. **Signs:** Erythema, swelling, warmth, purulence, pain (out of proportion to findings), lymphangitis, and adenopathy.
C. **DDX:** Animal bite, trauma, cellulitis, and FB.
D. **Workup:** CBC. Consider a blood and wound culture. X-ray all hand wounds and wounds that overlies bones and joints.

5.2. RX:

A. Copiously irrigate the wound and debride.
B. Tetanus prophylaxis.
C. Close facial wounds, if there is no infection and uninfected wounds <12 hours old. Wounds of the hands with tendon injury or joint space involvement should be referred to a surgeon.
D. Treat fractures as open fractures.
E. Immobilize affected body part.
F. If patient is sent home, Augmentin 875 mg po bid for 5 to 7 days or clindamycin + ciprofloxacin.
G. Infected wound or high-risk patient, us ampicillin/sulbactam 3 g IV or cefoxitin 1 to 2 g IV, or a carbapenem.
H. **Disposition:** If patient is sent home, ensure that the wound is rechecked in 24 hours. Patients with signs of soft tissue infection, lymphangitis, adenopathy, symptoms of systemic infection (fever, chills, rigors), receive IV antibiotics in the ED and are admitted. In addition, admit individuals who are immunocompromised, asplenic, DM, and have closed fist injuries.

6. Cold Injuries:

Cold injuries are divided into three categories: (1) Hypothermia, (2) frostbite, (3) nonfreezing injuries.

- Hypothermia: Covered in Section 7.
- Frostbite: Freezing of tissue causing injury and death to tissue. Tissue destruction is due to cold-induced cell death, inflammation, and tissue necrosis.
- Nonfreezing injuries:
  - Trench foot: Tissue damage due to prolonged exposure to a cold and wet environment.
  - Pernio/Chilblains: Inflammatory disorder characterized by pruritic/painful erythematous extremity lesions. It is due to an abnormal vascular response to cold/wet exposure.

6.1. Clinical Evaluation:

A. **Signs:** Skin is pale, waxy white or mottled blue, solid to firm on palpation, numb or painful (burning, stinging).

B. **Symptoms:** Skin necrosis, blisters, diminished pulses.
C. **DDX:** Hypothermia, trench foot, pernio/chilblains.
D. **Workup:** CBC, BMP, ETOH, UA, CPK, myoglobin, PT/PTT/INR, lactate, LFTs, ECG, CXR, and CT as needed.

6.2. RX:

A. Support ABCs and assess for other injuries or illnesses.
B. Ensure that the patient or EMS does not rewarm if there is any chance that refreezing may occur.
C. Remove all wet nonadherent apparel and place patient under a warm blanket.
D. Avoid massaging or rubbing tissue.
E. Tetanus prophylaxis.
F. Rapidly thaw frostbitten part in a 104°F (40°C) water bath for 30 minutes.
G. Treat pain with morphine.
H. Remove clear blisters and apply aloe vera, but leave hemorrhagic blisters intact.
I. Apply aloe vera to damaged tissue and separate damaged digits with gauze after rewarming.
J. Treat pain with ibuprofen, 400 mg po before rewarming (improves tissue salvage).
K. **Disposition:** Admit all patients except very mild cases. A surgical consultation should be obtained. If patient is discharged, re-examine within 24 hours.

7. **Hypothermia:**

An accidental decrease in the core temperature of <95F° (35°C). Several mechanisms contribute to the cause of hypothermia, including conduction (loss of heat by direct contact), convection (body to air loss), radiation (loss to air), and evaporation (sweating) temperature loss.

- Primary accidental hypothermia: This is due to an environmental exposure in a patient with no significant medical conditions. Alcohol use, mental illness, elderly, homeless, hikers, and hunters are the group at risk.
- Secondary accidental hypothermia: This is due to increased heat loss (burns), decreased heat production (elderly, thyroid disease, malnourished), and impaired thermoregulation (CNS diseases, toxic ingestion, medication).

7.1. Clinical Evaluation:

A. Signs/Symptoms: Correlate with the degree of hypothermia.
   - Mild 90° to 95°F (3235°C): Shivering, apathy, lethargy, fatigue, ataxia, slurred speech, tachycardia, tachypnea, and mild altered mental status.
   - Moderate 86° to 90°F (30–32°C): Shivering decreases, dysarthria, bradycardia, delirium, mydriasis, dysrhythmias, Osborn J waves on ECG, and slowing of reflexes.
   - Severe <86°F (<32°C): COMA, acid–base disturbances, hypotension, fixed dilated pupils, cold skin, and asystole or V-tach.

B. **DDX:** CVA, drug overdose, endocrine disorder.
C. **Workup:** CBC, BMP, PT/PTT/INR, UA, ABG/VBG, myoglobin, CPK, calcium, magnesium, phosphate, lactate, LFTs, thyroid studies, cardiac enzymes, ETOH, urine drug screen.

7.2. RX:

A. Support ABCs, IV, O_2, pulse oximeter, and monitor.
B. Monitor temperature continuously with a rectal probe or temperature sensing Foley catheter.
C. Remove wet nonadherent clothing and cover with warm blankets or mechanical warmer.
D. Warm IV fluids to 113°F (45°C).
E. Actively rewarm neonates and adults with moderate and severe hypothermia by providing warm IV fluids and humidified O_2 heated to 107.6° to 113°F (42–45°C).
F. Actively rewarm severe hypothermia by gastric and bladder infusion (113°F), peritoneal lavage with 113°F (45°C) fluid, warming the blood by hemodialysis (femorofemoral cardiopulmonary bypass pump), and by doing pleuromediastinal lavage via thoracostomy tubes.
G. Correct underlying metabolic abnormalities.

H. Consider steroids or thyroid hormone, if patient is unresponsive to aggressive warming or has an underlying endocrine disorder.
I. Treat dysrhythmias per ACLS guidelines.
J. **Disposition:** Observe a patient with mild hypothermia until asymptomatic and normothermic. Individuals who are very young, very old, or those with underlying pathology should be admitted. Admit patients with moderate to severe hypothermia to the ICU.

8. Heat Illnesses:

Heat illness is as continuum of illnesses due to the body's inability to use normal regulatory mechanisms to cope with heat stress.

- Heat cramps: Painful contractions of large muscles groups during or after strenuous exercise. It is due to the replacement of water without replenishment of adequate salt and electrolytes.
- Heat exhaustion: A syndrome of volume depletion due to heat stress. The mental status is normal and the prognosis is excellent if rehydrated.
- Heat stroke: A condition where thermoregulatory mechanisms cannot overcome heat accumulation. There are two forms, (1) classic (nonexertional): usually occurs in infants, elderly and debilitated. (2) Exertional: usually occurs in younger people involved in strenuous activity. Mortality is 10% if treated early and 80% if treated late.

8.1. Clinical Evaluation:

A. Signs/Symptoms:
- Heat cramps: Muscle cramps, diaphoresis, fatigue.
- Heat exhaustion: Elevated temperature <104°F (40°C), dizziness, headache, N/V, diaphoresis, lightheadedness, and anxiety.
- Heatstroke: Temperature >104°F (40°C), anhydrosis, tachypnea, tachycardia, altered mental status, wide-pulse pressure, ataxia, tremors, tachypnea, confusion, coma, and seizures.

B. **DDX:** Meningitis, thyroid disease, drug intoxication, neuroleptic malignant syndrome, salicylate toxicity, cocaine toxicity, sepsis, DKA.
C. **Workup:** CBC, BMP, CPK, myoglobin, PT/PTT/INR, ABG/VBG, LFTs, UA, calcium, magnesium, phosphorous, lactate, uric acid, and consider an ECG and CXR.

8.2. RX:

A. Support ABCs, IV, O_2, pulse oximeter, and monitor.
B. NS bolus 1 to 2 L.
C. Remove from thermal heat stress and remove clothing.
D. Insert a temperature sensing Foley catheter or rectal probe.
E. Search for other injuries or illnesses.
F. Rapidly cool the patient by cool mist and fan or a mechanical cooling devise. The goal is to decrease the temperature to 100°F (37.7°C) within 1 hour.
G. Correct acid–base, electrolyte, and coagulation abnormalities.
H. Consider alkaline diuresis, 2 amp $NaHCO_3$ in 1 L of D_5W run at 250 mL/h, if rhabdomyolysis is present (no evidence that it is superior to using NS alone).
I. Treat shivering benzodiazepines.
J. Treat seizures with benzodiazepines (phenytoin is ineffective). Intubate if in status epilepticus.
K. **Disposition:** Admit heat exhausted patient to the floor. Admit all patients with heatstroke to the ICU.

9. Electrical Injuries:

Electrical injuries encompass low-voltage (600 V), hig-voltage (>600 V), and lightning injuries (>1,000,000 V). Important historical information includes electrical source, low versus high voltage, duration of exposure, and AC versus DC. AC causes muscle tetany which prevents the victim from letting go, while DC (high-voltage, lightning), throws you from the source. Low-voltage AC current is more likely to cause V-fib and is the most common cause of death. DC and high-voltage AC cause asystole, but circulation may spontaneously return.

9.1. Clinical Evaluation:

- **A. Symptoms:** Nausea, vomiting, paresthesias, headache, hearing impairment, amnesia, and pain.
- **B. Signs:** Pallor, ileus, burns, skeletal fractures, joint dislocations (especially posterior shoulder), spinal compression fractures. Altered mental status, irritability, compartment syndrome, seizures, and coma. Small entrance wounds are commonly found on hands and upper extremities and may demonstrate charring, depression, edema, and inflammatory changes. Large exit wounds may be multiple and have an explosive appearance.
- **C. Workup:** CBC, BMP, CPK, myoglobin, cardiac enzymes, UA, PT/PTT/INR, LFTs, calcium, myoglobin, CXR, plane x-rays, CT head, and cervical spine.

9.2. RX:

- **A.** Support ABCs with C-spine immobilization, IV, O_2, pulse oximeter, and monitor.
- **B.** Use standard ACLS and advanced trauma life support protocols as indicated.
- **C.** Insert a Foley catheter.
- **D.** Tetanus prophylaxis.
- **E.** Treat rhabdomyolysis with aggressive fluid resuscitation, mannitol, and diuretics to enhance urinary output. Give sodium bicarbonate 2 amp in 1 L of D_5W at 250 mL/h, to alkalinize the urine and enhance myoglobin excretion.
- **F.** Pain medication.
- **G.** Consult surgery for a potential escharotomy.
- **H. Disposition:** Admit all patients exposed to >1,000 V to a monitored bed or ICU. Admit high-voltage burns, cardiac or neurological dysfunction, acidosis, rhabdomyolysis, or myoglobinuria. Consider burn unit transfer once stabilized.

10. High-Altitude Illness:

Symptoms associated with high-altitude illness can begin at elevations >8,000 ft. Rapid altitude gain and pre-existing cardiopulmonary disease result in a higher incidence of symptoms. There are a spectrum of syndromes ranging from mild acute mountain sickness (AMS), accompanied by headache and insomnia, to high-altitude pulmonary edema (HAPE), and high-altitude cerebral edema (HACE). Death may occur if descent does not occur. Acetazolamide and dexamethazone are useful in prevention.

- AMS: Symptoms start 6 to 10 hours after ascent and resolves in 1 to 3 days without treatment.
- HAPE: Occurs 48 hours at high altitudes of at least 8,000 ft. This is the most common seen in a young, fit climbers, and it accounts for most high-altitude deaths.
- HACE: Occurs after 4 days and is due to increased blood–brain barrier permeability. It is associated with HAPE and death occurs in 1 to 2 days if descent does not occur.

10.1. Clinical Evaluation:

- **A. Signs/Symptoms:**
  - AMS: Dizziness, fatigue, N/V, dyspnea, headache, insomnia, edema, and decreased urine output.
  - HAPE: Cough, exertional dyspnea, fatigue, tachycardia, tachypnea, orthopnea, crackles, mental status changes, and cyanosis.
  - HACE: AMS, muscle weakness, ataxia, bladder dysfunction, papilledema, CN palsy, retinal hemorrhage, seizures, and herniation.
- **B. DDX:** Migraine headache, dehydration, meningitis, hypoglycemia, DKA, electrolyte abnormality, CVA, asthma, exacerbation of COPD, pneumonia, and acute psychosis.
- **C. Workup:** CBC, BMP, LFTs, PT/PTT/INR, UA, ETOH, cardiac enzymes, ABG, CXR, ECG, CT head as needed.

10.2. RX:

- **A.** Support ABCs, IV, O_2, pulse oximeter, and monitor.
- **B.** If AMS is mild, stop ascent or descend about 1,600 ft. Give acetazolamide 125 to 250 mg po.
- **C.** Severe AMS, HAPE, HACE, requires immediate descent.
- **D.** HAPE: BIPAP or CPAP, albuterol, nifedipine 10 to 20 mg po/sl, dexamethasone 8 to 10 mg po/IV/IM. Consider hyperbaric therapy (Gamow bag) on scene.
- **E.** HACE: Keep warm and dry, dexamethasone, acetazolamide, Lasix, and hyperbaric therapy on scene.
- **F.** Acetazolamide and dexamethasone pretreatment can prevent AMS. Nifedipine can prevent HAPE.
- **G.** **Disposition:** A patient who has mild to moderate AMS may be discharged if asymptomatic after 6 to 12 hours. Those with cardiopulmonary or cerebrovascular disease, severe AMS, HAPE, HACE, or complications, such as ECG changes, should be admitted.

11. Submersion Injuries:

Drowning is the process of experiencing respiratory impairment from submersion/immersion in liquid. Drowning outcomes should be classified as: death, morbidity, and no morbidity. The primary organ affected is the lung and hypoxemia is the primary cause of organ damage and subsequent death. Always assume a head or C-spine injury until proven otherwise.

11.1. Clinical Evaluation:

- **A.** **Symptoms:** A history of coughing, choking, dyspnea, or vomiting after submersion.
- **B.** **Signs:** Awake or lethargic or combative or comatose, hypothermic, tachycardia, tachypnea, hypertensive, rhonchi, rales, wheezing, or in cardiac arrest.
- **C.** **DDX:** Head and/or spinal trauma, drug or chemical intoxication, cardiac arrest, stroke, hypothermia.
- **D.** **Workup:** CBC, BMP, BNP, ABG, ETOH, LFTs, UA, PT/PTT/INR, cardiac enzymes. CXR, CT head/C-spine as needed, and an alcohol and drug screen.

11.2. RX:

- **A.** Early resuscitation is the most important factor influencing morbidity and mortality.
- **B.** Provide ACLS, advanced trauma life support.
- **C.** Consider BiPAP/CPAP in alert, cooperative patients.
- **D.** If intubate, ventilate with PEEP.
- **E.** Administer bronchodilators prn, such as albuterol, 2.5 mg/nb.
- **F.** Treat hypotension with NS IV, and prevent hypothermia.
- **G.** Treat bronchospasm with albuterol.
- **H.** Treat agitation and seizures with benzodiazepines.
- **I.** **Disposition:** Asymptomatic patients, or those who become so after 6 hours of observation, with normal findings may be sent home. All discharged patients require follow-up in 24 to 48 hours. Admit all others. The level of care for admits, floor versus ICU, depends on severity and progression of clinical and laboratory findings.

12. High-Pressure Injection Injuries:

High-pressure injection injuries appear innocuously, but can have devastating consequences if treatment is delayed or inadequate. Consultation with a hand or plastic surgeon is always warranted. The index finger is the most commonly injured extremity.

12.1. Clinical Evaluation:

- **A.** **Symptoms:** Pain, numbness, swelling.
- **B.** **Signs:** Extremity or body part is initially pain-free, followed by an acute inflammatory process that causes swelling and intense pain. Usually, a small pinhole entrance wound is present and a drop of injectate can be expressed from the wound. Pallor, pulselessness, and paresthesia may also be present.
- **C.** **DDX:** Envenomation by reptiles, insects, arachnids, tenosynovitis, and FB.
- **D.** **Workup:** Doppler of the palmar arch, labs prn, and x-rays as needed.

12.2. RX:

A. Place hand in a soft, bulky dressing without undue compression. Splint in neutral position and elevate injured area.
B. Administer broad-spectrum antibiotics.
C. Give tetanus.
D. Do not start an IV in the affected arm.
E. Consult a hand or plastic surgeon.
F. **Disposition:** Admit the patient for surgical exploration.

GASTROINTESTINAL

1. Acute Abdominal Pain:

The causes of abdominal pain are unknown (42% of cases), gastroenteritis (31%), gastritis, peptic ulcer disease, gallbladder disease, diarrhea, and pancreatitis. Visceral abdominal pain from the autonomic fibers is crampy, intermittent, and colicky. Somatic abdominal pain resulting from pain fibers in parietal peritoneum is constant, sharp, and localized. Abdominal pain lasting longer than 6 hours, or present in the elderly and immunocompromised requires a surgical consult.

1.1. Clinical Evaluation:

A. **Symptoms:** Location, onset, duration, quality, severity of pain should be noted. N/V/D, urinary complaints, vaginal discharge, or bleeding, previous painful episodes, drugs/alcohol use, and menstrual history.
B. **Signs:** Vital signs, temperature. Listen for diminished breath sounds, rales, rhonchi, and wheezing. Auscultate for bowel sounds and look for distention, stigmata of liver disease, and old scars. Palpate all four quadrants for guarding, rebound, pulsatile mass, hernia, point tenderness, Murphy's sign, and Rovsing's. Examine the back for CVA tenderness, bruising, and musculoskeletal pain. Check for hernias and do a rectal for masses, tenderness, and blood. In males, examine for tenderness, a mass, hernia, and an abnormal painful testicle. In females perform a pelvic examination checking for vaginal discharge or bleeding, cervical motion tenderness, adnexal fullness, and focal tenderness.
C. **DDX:** Common emergencies requiring immediate surgical intervention are perforated viscus, ruptured abdominal aortic aneurysm, acute appendicitis, bowel ischemia, ectopic pregnancy, and strangulated hernia.

- Common etiologies for tenderness according to abdominal regions are:
  - □ **RUQ:** Hepatitis, cholecystitis, cholangitis hepatomegaly, perforated ulcer, pancreatitis, retrocecal appendicitis, and angina.
  - □ **LUQ:** Gastritis, peptic ulcer disease (PUD), gastritis, AMI, pneumonia, PE, and pancreatitis.
  - □ **EPIGASTRIC:** PUD, pancreatitis, AMI, gastritis, DKA, gastroparesis, and cancer.
  - □ **RLQ:** Appendicitis, PID, Meckel's, AAA, ovarian cyst/torsion, tubo-ovarian abscess (TOA), orchitis, prostatitis, PID, endometriosis, ureteral calculi, mesenteric adenitis, hernia, and an ectopic pregnancy.
  - □ **LLQ:** Diverticulitis, PID, AAA, TOA, uterine fibroids, menses, ovarian cyst/torsion, PID, ureteral calculus, testicular pathology, mesenteric adenitis, hernia, endometriosis, and an ectopic pregnancy.
  - □ **SUPRAPUBIC:** Cystitis, hernia, PID, pregnancy, menses, prostatitis, and ovarian/testicular torsion.
  - □ **DIFFUSE/OR ANY QUADRANT:** AAA, pancreatitis, DKA, bowel obstruction, ureteral calculus, perforation/peritonitis, irritable bowel syndrome, gastroenteritis, sickle cell crisis, pneumonia, mesenteric ischemia, and inflammatory bowel disease.
  - □ **Back/FLANK:** Ureteral calculus, pancreatitis, pyelonephritis, gallstones, AAA, and musculoskeletal.

D. **Workup:** CBC, BMP, LFTs, lipase, ETOH, pregnancy test, UA, lactate, calcium, magnesium, phosphorus, cardiac enzymes, BNP, ECG, CT abd/pelvis, abdominal x-ray, CXR, US if indicated.

1.2. RX (refer also to specific cause):

A. Support ABCs, IV, O_2, pulse oximeter, and monitor prn. Insert an NG tube for obstruction or bleeding cases.
B. NPO.
C. Treat pain and vomiting.
D. Obtain appropriate consultation with surgery or obstetrics.
E. **Disposition:** Admit all patients except those with the mildest problems.

2. Appendicitis:

Appendicitis usually arises as an outcome of hyperplasia of the lymphatic tissue or a fecalith causing a luminal obstruction. Mucus accumulates, intraluminal pressure increases, and an obstruction of lymphatic drainage occurs resulting in severe pain. Peak incidence of appendicitis is in the second and third decades.

2.1. Clinical Evaluation:

A. **Symptoms:** Periumbilical pain migrating to the RLQ. Low-grade fever, anorexia, N/V, and constipation or diarrhea.
B. **Signs:** Temperature rarely >100°F without perforation, pain to palpation at McBurney's point, rebound, guarding, psoas sign, obturator sign, and Rovsing's sign.
C. **DDX:** Mesenteric adenitis, PID, torsed ovarian cyst, mittelschmerz, gastroenteritis, diverticulitis, perforated ulcer, cholecystitis, ectopic pregnancy, kidney stone, bowel obstruction, pyelonephritis, endometriosis, and mesenteric infarction.
D. **Workup:** CBC, BMP, LFTs, PT/PTT/INR, lipase, UA, abdominal x-ray, and beta-HCG, US of the RLQ, CT abd/pelvis.

2.2. RX:

A. Support ABCs, IV, O_2, pulse oximeter, and monitor prn.
B. NPO.
C. IV fluid bolus of NS.
D. If decision to operate or suspected perforation is determined start antibiotics. Ampicillin, mefoxin, metronidazole, aztreonam, or carbapenem.
E. Workup for appendicitis in pregnant patient (1) US, (2) MRI.
F. **Disposition:** If the diagnosis is definite, obtain a surgical consultation and transfer the patient to surgery. If the diagnosis is unclear, admit the patient for observation or have them return within 8 hours for recheck.

3. Cholecystitis:

Prolonged blockage of the cystic duct (95% by gallstone(s)) causes distention, inflammation, and possible infection. Acalculous disease (no stone) is seen in debilitated patients, burn victims, those on TPN and those who have sustained serious trauma have been burned or involved in other trauma. Pain <6 hours in duration is usually a stone trying to pass or lodged in the cystic duct (cholelithiasis). Pain lasting longer than 6 hours usually indicates inflammation is present.

- Acute cholangitis: Bacterial infection of the biliary tree due to obstruction and stasis. Presents with RUQ pain, jaundice, and fever (Charcot's triad), or the previous triad plus shock and altered mental status (Reynold's pentad).

3.1. Clinical Evaluation:

A. **Symptoms:** Sudden onset of RUQ pain, colicky, radiating to the back, N/V, and possible fever.
B. **Signs:** Low-grade fevers, RUQ pain to palpation (Murphy's sign), mild icterus, and possible rebound and guarding.
C. **DDX:** Appendicitis, perforated ulcer, pancreatitis, hepatitis, pneumonia, gastritis PUD, and an AMI.
D. **Workup:** CBC, BMP, LFTs, PT/PTT/INR, lipase, UA, US RUQ (stones, sludge, pericholecystic fluid, thickened gallbladder wall (>3 mm), ultrasonographic Murphy's), radionuclide scan (hepato-iminodiacetic acid [HIDA]), if the ultrasound is normal.

3.2. RX:

- **A.** Support ABCs, IV, O_2, pulse oximeter, and monitor prn.
- **B.** Pain control, antiemetic, NPO, NG if ileus is present.
- **C.** IV hydration with NS.
- **D.** Start broad-spectrum antibiotics ampicillin/sulbactam, or zosyn, or third-generation cephalosporin + metronidazole, or carbapenem.
- **E.** Surgical consult.
- **F.** May require a GI consult for ERCP.
- **G.** **Disposition:** A patient with a resolved uncomplicated biliary colic may be sent home with follow-up for elective surgery. Patients with acute cholecystitis should be admitted. Patients with fever, leukocytosis, peritoneal signs, and appear toxic require immediate surgery with possible ERCP.

4. Hepatic Encephalopathy:

This is due to excessive accumulation of nitrogenous waste products due to liver failure. The damaged liver is unable to break ammonia down and portal blood bringing ammonia is shunted away. There are several conditions that may precipitate an episode: GI bleed, dehydration, hypovolemia, renal failure, hypoxia, hypokalemia, acidosis, increased protein intake, narcotics, benzodiazepines, uremia, and medication noncompliance.

4.1. Clinical Evaluation:

- **A.** **Symptoms:** Malaise, lethargy, weight loss, insomnia, personality changes, confusion, coma, pruritus, weakness, muscle wasting, anorexia, N/V/D, and fever.
- **B.** **Signs:** Asterixis, spider angiomas, palmar erythema, hyperpigmentation, jaundice, edema, muscle wasting, ascites, hepatosplenomegaly, rectal bleeding, and cognitive defects.
- **C.** **DDX:** Hepatitis, hypoglycemia, hyponatremia, sepsis, alcohol intoxication, trauma, anemia.
- **D.** **Workup:** CBC, BMP, BNP, lactate, LFTs, PT/PTT/INR, lipase, ammonia, ETOH, UA, urine drug screen, toxic alcohols, hemoccult stools, T&S, CXR, CT head as needed.

4.2. RX:

- **A.** Support ABCs, IV, O_2, pulse oximeter, glucose check, and monitor.
- **B.** Correct fluid and electrolyte abnormalities.
- **C.** Give thiamine, 100 mg IV.
- **D.** For bleeding esophageal varices, use two large bore IVs, give NS and PRBCs, insert an NG tube, give octreotide 50 mcg IV bolus, followed by a 25–50 mcg/hr infusion, consider tamponade with a Sengstaken–Blakemore tube. Consult GI stat. Consider tranexamic acid for severe bleeding.
- **E.** If bleeding is occurring and the patient is coagulopathic, consider vitamin K, FFP, and/or prothrombin-complex concentrate.
- **F.** For hepatic encephalopathy, give lactulose 30 g po/pr/NG.
- **G.** For spontaneous bacterial peritonitis, administer a third-generation cephalosporin or Unasyn 3 g IV. Use caution when administering aminoglycosides caused by a high risk for nephrotoxicity.
- **H.** **Disposition:** Admit all patients except those exhibiting the mildest symptoms. Admit patients with complications to the ICU. Obtain a surgical consultation for bleeding varices.

5. Diverticulitis:

Diverticulitis is an inflammation of the diverticula. This is a herniation of mucosa/submucosa through the muscular layer of the colon (usually sigmoid) near the vasculature. Complications include perforation, bleeding (40% of lower GI bleeding), obstruction, and abscess and fistula formation.

5.1. Clinical Evaluation:

- **A.** **Symptoms:** LLQ pain is intermittent, crampy, nonradiating, and worsens after eating. Altered bowel habits, anorexia, N/V, fever, previous attacks, and hematochezia.

B. **Signs:** Fever, tachycardia, LLQ tenderness, mass, and possible peritonitis.
C. **DDX:** Irritable bowel syndrome, inflammatory bowel disease, colon/rectal cancer, appendicitis (rare), sigmoid volvulus, tubo-ovarian abscess, ischemic colitis, and angiodysplasia (bleeding).
D. **Workup:** CBC, BMP, lipase, lactate, LFTs, PT/PTT/INR, UA, hemoccult tool, abdominal series, CT abd/pelvis.

5.2. RX:

A. Support ABCs, IV, pulse oximeter, and monitor prn.
B. Bolus NS for dehydration.
C. Treat pain and vomiting.
D. For mild diverticulitis, treat with amoxicillin/clavulanate or second-generation cephalosporin or metronidazole + ciprofloxicin po.
E. For severe diverticulitis, treat with amoxicillin/clavulanate or zosyn or metronidazole + ciprofloxacin IV.
F. For massive GI bleeding refer to the "GI Bleeding" section.
G. Surgical consult for complicated disease (abscess, perforation, bleeding).
H. **Disposition:** For mild stable diverticulitis, discharge on antibiotics with a surgical follow-up. Admit complicated toxic-appearing patients.

6. Upper Gastrointestinal Bleeding (UGI Bleeding):

UGI bleeding is defined as bleeding proximal to the ligament of Treitz. Causes include PUD (55%), esophageal varices (15%), AV malformations (5%), Mallory–Weiss tears (5%) tumors (3%), and idiopathic (10%). UGI bleeding may be occult, overt, or massive. Use of ASA, NSAIDs, anticoagulants, an ETOH must be noted.

6.1. Clinical Evaluation:

A. **Symptoms:** Hematemesis or coffee-ground emesis, melena (70%) with or without abdominal pain, weakness, pallor, syncope, diaphoresis, dyspnea, and chest pain.
B. **Signs:** Hypotension, tachycardia, orthostasis, jaundice, ascites, bruising, AMS, hepatomegaly, hemoccult + stools.
C. **DDX:** PUD, esophagitis, angiodysplasia, esophageal varices, cancer, Mallory–Weiss tear, aortoenteric fistula, and erosive gastritis.
D. **Workup:** CBC, BMP, lactate, LFTs, PT/PTT/INR, T&C 4 to 6 units as needed, ETOH, UA, and hemoccult stool.

6.2. RX:

A. Support ABCs, IV, O_2, pulse oximeter, and monitor prn.
B. Intubate for severe bleeding or altered mental status.
C. Insert an NG tube, saline lavage to diagnose continued UGI bleeding.
D. If unstable, start two large bore IVs, bolus 2 L of NS or LR, and give PRBCs if still unstable.
E. GI consult for emergent endoscopy.
F. Vitamin K, FFP, and/or prothrombin-complex concentrate for patients with a coagulopathy.
G. Consider octreotide IV (safer than vasopressin).
H. Consider IV erythromycin. Helps empty stomach of blood before endoscopy.
I. Consider a proton pump inhibitor (pantoprazole, omeprazole) or an H_2 blocker (ranitidine, famotidine).
J. If uncontrolled variceal bleeding, use a Linton–Nachlas tube to tamponade the affected area. Sengstaken–Blakemore tube may be used but it is associated with higher complication rate.
K. **Disposition:** Admit all unstable cases to the ICU and obtain an immediate surgical and/or GI consult.

7. Lower Gastrointestinal Bleeding (LGI Bleeding):

LGI bleeding is defined as bleeding distal to the ligament of Treitz and is less common than a UGI bleed. Causes include diverticulosis (most common), tumors, Meckel's diverticulum, angiodysplasia, IBD, infectious and ischemic colitis, hemorrhoids and polyps. Bleeding will spontaneously stop in 80% to 85% of cases.

7.1. Clinical Evaluation:

A. Symptoms: Hematochezia or melena with or without abdominal pain, weakness, pallor, syncope, diaphoresis, dyspnea, and chest pain.
B. Signs: Hypotension, tachycardia, orthostasis, jaundice, ascites, bruising, AMS, hepatomegaly, hemoccult + stools.
C. DDX: Diverticulosis, cancer, massive UGI bleed, Meckel's diverticulum, angiodysplasia, IBD, infectious and ischemic colitis, hemorrhoids, polyps, aortoenteric fistula.
D. Workup: CBC, BMP, lactate, LFTs, PT/PTT/INR, T&C 4 to 6 units as needed, ETOH, UA, and hemoccult stool.

7.2. RX:

A. Support ABCs, IV, O_2, pulse oximeter, and monitor prn.
B. Angiography can localize site of bleeding and allow for direct embolization or vasopressin infusion. Tagged RBC scan can detect bleeding but poor at localizing site.
C. Consider NG tube with saline lavage to exclude UGI bleeding.
D. Consider anoscopy to differentiate bleeding from more proximal sites.
E. If unstable, start two large bore IVs, bolus 2 L of NS or LR, and give PRBCs if still unstable.
F. Colonoscopy is the test of choice, but not possible if bleeding is continuous.
G. Vitamin K, FFP, and/or prothrombin-complex concentrate for patients with a coagulopathy.
H. Disposition: Low-risk patients who have a negative workup and stable vital signs may be discharged with close follow-up. Admit all unstable cases to the ICU and obtain an immediate surgical and/or GI consult.

8. Inflammatory Bowel Disease:

Category	Regional Enteritis	Ulcerative Colitis
Name	Crohn's disease Regional enteritis Terminal ileitis Granulomatous ileocolitis	Ulcerative colitis
Area	Oral-to-anus Segmental (skip areas) Most common area is ileum	95% rectosigmoid Contiguous (no skip areas)
Demographics	12–30 y 55–60 y Common in Europeans Jews 10–15% have family history	10–20 y 20–30 y 15 × greater risk with first-degree relative
Bowel	ALL LAYERS Thick bowel wall Narrow lumen Creeping fat—mesenteric fat over bowel wall "Cobblestone" mucosal appearance Fissures Fistulas Abscesses	Mucosa and Submucosa Mucosal ulceration Epithelial necrosis Mild—Mucosa is fine, granular, and friable Severe—Spongy, red, oozing ulcerations Crypt abscesses Toxic megacolon
Clinical	Fever, chronic diarrhea without gross blood, RLQ pain, fistula-fissure-abscess	Bloody diarrhea, abdominal pain, ± N/V, fever. If Toxic Megacolon-toxic appearance ± mass
Treatment	Antidiarrheal meds	NO antidiarrheal meds

Most emergency visits are for complications of an already diagnosed disease, including hemorrhage, intestinal obstruction, bowel perforation, and toxic megacolon.

8.1. Clinical Evaluation:

- **A. Symptoms/Signs:** Refer to previous chart.
- **B. DDX:** Bacterial diarrhea (Shigella or Campylobacter, amebiasis), HIV infection, ischemic colitis, gastroenteritis, appendicitis, intestinal obstruction, mesenteric ischemia, lactose intolerance, irritable bowel syndrome, perforation, diverticulitis.
- **C. Workup:** CBC, BMP, PT/PTT/INR, lactate, lipase, ESR, CRP, hemoccult stool, type and cross, UA, LFTs, stool for ova/parasites, CXR, abdominal series, or CT abd/pelvis as needed.

8.2. RX:

- **A.** Support ABCs, IV, O_2, pulse oximeter, and monitor prn.
- **B.** Correct volume and electrolyte abnormalities.
- **C.** First-line therapy for Crohn's is 5-aminosalicylic acid (mesalamine) po and antibiotics (metronidazole + ciprofloxacin) with prednisone added for symptom flares.
- **D.** Mild to moderate ulcerative colitis is treated with 5-aminosalicylic acid (mesalamine) and corticosteroids po/IV/+ rectal. Sever ulcerative colitis is treated with corticosteroids po/IV/+ rectal, and anti-TNF medication.
- **E.** Toxic megacolon: Colon dilation >6 cm on x-ray, fever, diarrhea, shock, and dehydration. Treat aggressively with IV fluids, hydrocortisone IV, broad-spectrum antibiotics and a surgical consult.
- **F. Disposition:** Admit patients with moderate to severe disease, significant pain, and inadequate follow-up.

9. Small Bowel Obstruction (SBO):

The most common cause of mechanical obstruction of the small bowel is adhesions associated with previous surgery, followed by hernia, and carcinoma. Large bowel obstruction usually results from fecal impaction or carcinoma. Obstruction may be partial or complete and occur at one or two points. Adynamic or paralytic ileus, is decreased intestinal motility in the absence of a mechanical barrier.

9.1. Clinical Evaluation:

- **A. Symptoms:** Crampy poorly localized abdominal pains, N/V, distention, and constipation or diarrhea.
- **B. Signs:** Pain to palpation, diminished and/or high-pitched bowel sounds, distention, tympanitic abdomen, rebound, and guarding.
- **C. DDX:** Trauma, postoperative, peritonitis, electrolyte abnormality, medication, cancer, hernia, DKA, constipation, gallstone ileus, FB.
- **D. Workup:** CBC, BMP, lipase, LFTs, UA, CXR, abdominal series, CT abd/pelvis as needed (highly accurate in delineating partial vs. complete obstruction, level of obstruction, cause of obstruction, and type of obstruction).

9.2. RX:

- **A.** Support ABCs, IV, O_2, pulse oximeter, and monitor prn.
- **B.** Treat pain and vomiting.
- **C.** Insert an NG tube to decompress the small bowel and stomach.
- **D.** NPO and IV rehydration.
- **E.** Give broad-spectrum antibiotics for complicated obstructions (perforation), and if going to the OR.
- **F. Disposition:** Admit and obtain a surgical consult.

10. Pancreatitis:

Aberrant activation of enzymes in the pancreatic ducts resulting in the autodigestion of portions of the pancreas. The most common cause of pancreatitis is alcohol use (80%) with cholelithiasis coming in second. Other causes include trauma, medication (azathioprine, sulfa, valproic acid), hyperlipidemia, hypercalcemia, infection, cystic fibrosis, scorpion bites. Ranson's criteria for predicting severity of the condition on admission are age >55, WBC >16,000, glucose >200, LDH >350, AST >250.

10.1. Clinical Evaluation:

A. Symptoms: Constant, severe, epigastric pain, radiating to the back, N/V, tachypnea, diarrhea, and possible jaundice.
B. Signs: Fever, tachycardia, abdominal distention, pain, guarding, decreased bowel sounds. Hemorrhagic pancreatitis causes periumbilical ecchymosis (Cullen's sign) and/or flank ecchymosis (Grey Turner's sign).
C. DDX: Acute cholecystitis, PUD, alcoholic gastritis, perforated viscus, and bowel infarction, bowel obstruction, perforated peptic ulcer, mesenteric thrombosis, ruptured aortic aneurysm, ruptured ectopic pregnancy, and advanced renal insufficiency.
D. Workup: CBC, BMP, LFTs, lipase, calcium, magnesium, ETOH, UA, CXR, consider a CT or ultrasound to evaluate for an abscess or pseudocyst.

10.2. RX:

A. Support ABCs, IV, O_2, pulse oximeter, and monitor prn.
B. NPO and IV NS hydration.
C. Administer narcotic pain medication and treat vomiting.
D. Give broad-spectrum antibiotics (carbapenems) for severe necrotizing pancreatitis.
E. Consult GI for ERCP, if due to a gallstone.
F. Disposition:
- Admit patient to general floor for pain control, vomiting and other complications.
- Consider ICU for serious disease (Ranson's >2, acute organ failure, significant comorbidities).
- Obtain a surgical consultation, if the patient is hemorrhagic or other complications are present.

11. Peptic Ulcer Disease (PUD):

PUD is a disruption of the balance between the gastric acid secretion and gastroduodenal mucosal defense. The term PUD encompasses both gastric and duodenal ulcers. Common offending agents are ASA, NSAIDS, ETOH, tobacco, stress, shock, steroids, and *Helicobacter pylori.*

11.1. Clinical Evaluation:

A. Symptoms:
- PUD: Epigastric pain after eating, worse with movement. Early satiety, belching, bloating, fatigue, dysphagia, hematemesis, weight loss, worsening pain after eating.
- Duodenal ulcer: Epigastric pain 2 to 3 hours after a meal, pain awakens patient at night, N/V hours after a meal, and food brings rapid relief of pain.

B. Signs: Epigastric pain to palpation, normal or abnormal vital signs, rebound, guarding may be present.
C. DDX: Gastritis, gastroenteritis, biliary tract disease, esophagitis, pancreatitis, AMI, angina, GERD, IBS, and pneumonia.
D. Workup: CBC, BMP, LFTs, ETOH, lipase, PT/PTT/INR, T&C, hemoccult stool, ECG, upright CXR and/or flat and upright abdominal films to detect free air.

11.2. RX:

A. Support ABCs, IV, O_2, pulse oximeter, and monitor prn.
B. For uncomplicated cases, relieve pain with antacids, such as Maalox or Mylanta 30 mL po.
C. Consider IV PPI or H_2 blockers.
D. For "bleeding" cases, start O_2 and an IV of isotonic solution (LR or NS). Insert an NG tube and perform a nasogastric lavage with saline (refer also to the "Gastrointestinal Bleeding–Treatment" section).
E. For a perforation consult surgery, insert an NG tube, start two large bore IVs, insert a Foley catheter, and start broad-spectrum antibiotics.
F. Disposition:
- Uncomplicated: Discharge to home with an H_2 receptor blocker, and an antacid. May also use a proton pump inhibitor (lansoprazole [Prevacid], omeprazole [Prilosec]).

- Admit for intractable pain, signs of bleeding, coagulopathy, elderly, hematemesis/hematochezia, and comorbid disease:
- Continued bleeding or perforation: Obtain an immediate surgical consultation and prepare the patient for the OR.

GYNECOLOGY/OBSTETRICS

1. **Ovarian Torsion:**

Ovarian torsion is the twisting of an ovary leading to decreased blood flow. The most common causes are a mass or large cyst on the ovary or fallopian tube.

1.1. Clinical Evaluation:

A. Symptoms: Sudden onset, sharp, intermittent, and unilateral pain, N/V, low-grade fever, dysuria.
B. Signs: Cervical motion and adnexal tenderness, peritoneal signs, adnexal fullness.
C. DDX: Ectopic pregnancy, appendicitis, PID, renal colic, ovarian cyst.
D. Workup: CBC, pregnancy test (urine or blood), US.

1.2. RX:

A. Support ABCs, IV, O_2, pulse oximeter, and monitor prn.
B. Consult gynecology for a stat laparotomy.
C. Disposition: Admit the patient for surgery.

2. **Pelvic Inflammatory Disease (PID):**

PID is an ascending infection from the lower genital tract makes up a spectrum of disease from endometritis, to salpingitis, to TOA. *Neisseria gonorrhoeae* and *Chlamydia trachomatis* are the most common cause.

- TOA: PID complicated by abscess formation. Septic, unilateral adnexal tenderness, and fullness.
- Fitz–Hugh–Curtis syndrome: Perihepatitis which is caused by PID, with chlamydia being the most common cause. Presents with systemic illness, RUQ pain, and elevated LFTs.

2.1. Clinical Evaluation:

A. Symptoms: Pelvic pain, fever, dysuria, N/V, and abnormal vaginal discharge/bleeding, malaise.
B. Signs: Fever, pelvic tenderness, cervical motion tenderness, adnexal tenderness, red, friable cervix, purulent and RUQ pain (Fitz–Hugh–Curtis syndrome).
C. DDX: Ectopic pregnancy, appendicitis, ovarian cyst, ovarian torsion, cystitis, and pyelonephritis.
D. Workup: CBC, BMP, ESR, CRP, HCG, DNA probe for chlamydia/gonorrhea, RPR, HIV, U/A, pregnancy test. Consider a US for severe tenderness or lack of response to antibiotics in 48 to 72 hours.

2.2. RX:

A. Support ABCs, IV, O_2, pulse oximeter, and monitor prn.
B. Treat pain and vomiting if present.
C. For outpatient treatment of PID use ceftriaxone 250 mg IM, and doxycycline, 100 mg po bid for 14 days.
D. For outpatient treatment of cervicitis use ceftriaxone 250 mg IM, and azithromycin 1 g po.
E. For inpatient treatment use cefoxitin, 2 g IV or cefotetan 2 g IV plus doxycycline 100 mg IV.
F. An alternate inpatient regimen, administer clindamycin, 900 mg IV, plus gentamycin, 2 mg/kg IV loading dose, followed by 1.5 mg/kg q 8 hours IV.
G. Complications include infertility, abscess, dyspareunia, chronic pelvic pain, and increased risk of ectopic pregnancy.
H. Disposition: Admit all but the mildest cases of PID. Admit patients with the following conditions and treat with antibiotics: Tubo-ovarian abscess or pyosalpinx, Fitz–Hugh–Curtis syndrome, fever >100.4°, pregnant, unable to tolerate po, IUD present, peritonitis, uncertain diagnosis, failure on outpatient antibiotics for 48 hours, and nulligravida.

3. Sexual Assault:

Rape is carnal knowledge of a female/male, forcible and nonconsensual. The victim is threatened and in fear of bodily harm. Sexual assault can range from fondling of genitals to oral, anal, or vaginal penetration with objects, or any part of the assailant's body. Fifty percent of victims know their attacker but only one in four rapes are reported. Facial and extremity trauma are more common than genital trauma. Child molestation is an illegal act performed on or with a child with lewd intent. Children are usually younger than 11 years and the assailant is typically known to them. Risks of pregnancy (1%), gonorrhea (5–12%), and other STDs should be assessed.

3.1. Clinical Evaluation:

- **A. Symptoms:** Pertinent details include time, date, place of the attack, description of the assailant, penetration area, ejaculation, threats, weapons, and alcohol/drug use. Ask, "did the victim shower, douche, brush teeth, go to the bathroom, or change clothes?" Determine the last consensual intercourse, last menstrual period, birth control method, medical history, and allergies.
- **B. Signs:** Carefully document all trauma-related lacerations, bruising, bite marks, and scratches. Special attention should be paid to the neck, mouth, breasts, wrists, and thighs. Vagina and anus must be carefully inspected for trauma. Male victims of sodomy may have abrasions on the thorax or the abdomen.
- **C. Workup:** Blood or urine pregnancy test, UA (sperm), Wet mount (trichomonas, gardnerella, sperm), RPR, hepatitis B, HIV, PCR test for *Chlamydia* and gonorrhea. Sperm motility is lost in 12 hours; however, nonmotile sperm can be recovered in 72 hours. Conversely, acid phosphate decreases in 2 to 9 hours. Obtain the victim's underclothes, pubic hair combing, and fingernail clippings as evidence. Acquire rectal or buccal smears to determine whether penetration occurred at that site.

3.2. RX:

- **A.** Assess for and treat injuries.
- **B.** Provide rape counseling and a safe environment for discharge.
- **C.** Provide STD prophylaxis with ceftriaxone, 125 mg IM, and doxycycline, 100 mg po bid for 7 days or azithromycin 1 g po.
- **D.** If positive for gardnerella (bacterial vaginosis) and/or trichomonas treat with metronidazole 2 g po × 1 dose.
- **E.** Provide pregnancy prophylaxis with two tablets of ovral and two additional tablets in 12 hours. Give tetanus if needed. Recommend re-evaluation by the GYN for STD and pregnancy. Consider an empiric antiviral prophylaxis for HIV.
- **F. Disposition:** Arrange outpatient follow-up with their primary MD, gynecologist, and an appropriate counselor. Consider a "safe-house," shelter, or other disposition as needed to ensure a safe environment.

4. Ectopic Pregnancy:

Pregnancy that implants and develops outside the uterine cavity and is the leading cause of first-trimester maternal death. This implantation typically occurs in the lateral two-thirds of the fallopian tube, which ultimately lead to fetal death. The risk factors associated with ectopic pregnancies include tubal abnormalities, previous ectopic, infertility drugs, history of PID, tubal ligation, IUD use, recent abortion, and smoking.

4.1. Clinical Evaluation:

- **A. Symptoms:** Amenorrhea, abdominal pain, followed by vaginal bleeding. Various symptoms based on tubal distention versus rupture.
- **B. Signs:** Diffused or localized abdominal pain, pallor, shoulder (diaphragmatic irritation), adnexal mass, adnexal tenderness, and CMT. Tachycardia, hypotension, tachypnea, and severe pain if a rupture occurs.
- **C. DDX:** PID, UTI, ovarian/cyst, threatened abortion, renal colic, molar pregnancy, appendicitis, and dysfunctional uterine bleeding.
- **D. Workup:** Urine or blood HCG. If positive: quantitative beta-HCG, CBC, LFTs, UA, Type & Rh, pelvic (transvaginal) US. Beta-HCG 1,000 to 1,500 mIU/mL, should see IUP on transvaginal US.

4.2. RX:

A. Support ABCs, IV, O_2, pulse oximeter, and monitor prn.
B. If in shock, two large IVs, infuse NS or LR, give PRBCs if no response, and obtain a state OB/GYN consult.
C. Consider culdocentesis, if US is not available and the patient is unstable. Aspiration of nonclotting blood with hematocrit >15% represents a positive finding.
D. Disposition:
- Stable, unruptured ectopics may be evaluated by OB/GYN for methotrexate therapy (in or outpatient) or laproscopic removal.
- Indeterminate US with a beta-HCG above the discriminatory zone (>1,000 mIU/mL), are usually admitted.
- Indeterminate US with a beta-HCG below the discriminatory zone may be sent home and followed up in 2 days for a recheck of the beta-HCG.
- Patients stable or unstable from a ruptured ectopic require emergent laparotomy.

5. Emergency Delivery:

5.1. Clinical Evaluation:

A. Symptoms: True labor: Regular uterine contractions with increasing intensity and decreasing intervals. Pain in uterine fundus radiates over the uterus into the lower back. "Bloody show" consists of a bloody mucous discharge representing expulsion of the cervical mucous plug and indicates ongoing labor. Spontaneous rupture of membranes also verifies active labor.
- First stage results in cervical dilation and effacement. It continues for 6 to 8 hours in the multiparous patient and for 8 to 12 hours in the primiparous patient.
- The second stage of labor begins with complete cervical dilation and ends with the delivery of the infant.
- The third stage is from delivery of the fetus to delivery of the placenta. This stage lasts for several minutes to 2 hours.

B. Signs: If vaginal bleeding, not just a "bloody show," is present, avoid a pelvic examination but perform a US to assess for placenta previa. Otherwise, perform a sterile speculum examination to confirm ruptured membranes by inspecting vaginal secretions for ferning and for turning Nitrazine paper blue. Check the fetal heart tones with Doppler. Expect FHT 120 to 160 with variation. Monitor continuously, if available, or q 15 minutes in stage 1, q 5 minutes in stage 2, and for 30 seconds after contractions. If prolonged bradycardia or tachycardia occurs after contractions, fetal distress is present. Determine position, presentation (portion of fetus in birth canal), lie (longitudinal vs. transverse) of fetus, and stage of labor. Check for cord prolapse, cervical effacement, cervical dilation (10 cm is complete), and station (relationship of fetal part to ischial spines). A delivery in the second stage presents as crowning, pressure on rectum with urge to defecate, and an uncontrolled bearing down movements of mother.

5.2. RX:

A. For a premature delivery, consider transferring the patient to an institution with obstetrics and neonatal facilities.
B. Call the NICU to assist with impending birth and OB for help with delivery.
C. For fetal distress, position mother on left side. Start IV, O_2, pulse oximeter, and monitor. Arrange for an immediate delivery.
D. For cord prolapse, exert manual pressure through vagina to lift presenting part away from cord. Place patient in knee-chest or deep Trendelenburg position. Use tocolytic agents to stop labor, such as magnesium sulfate, 4 to 6 g IV, **or** terbutaline, 0.25 sq, **or** ritodrine, 0.1 mg/min IV.
E. If ED delivery required:
- Position mother on stretcher in the dorsal lithotomy position with thighs abducted, knees flexed, and feet on stretcher or in stirrups.
- If time permits, cleanse, and drape perineum.

- Place digital traction on the inferior portion of the perineum and consider an episiotomy if needed.
- Control delivery of head with one hand on the occipital area and one hand supporting the mother's perineum. The baby's chin can be lifted from posterior position.
- After delivering the baby's head (suctioning oral cavity with bulb syringe is discouraged if amniotic fluid is clear). Feel for nuchal cord, loosen and slip over head if present.
- Grasp head and exert gentle pressure downward until anterior shoulder appears beneath the pubic symphysis. Lift head upward to aid posterior shoulder delivery. If shoulders are impacted perform episiotomy, anesthetize area with lidocaine and cut from perineum avoiding the anal sphincter.
- After shoulders are delivered, support head with one hand and prepare to catch body and legs with other hand.
- Cut umbilical cord after clamping twice. Send cord blood for infant serology and Rh. Place a sterile cord clamp or tie around cord 1 to 3 cm distal to navel.
- Place the neonate on warm blankets in heated isolette.
- Take 1- and 5-minute APGAR scores.
- Apply pressure above pubic symphysis and minimal traction on cord to deliver placenta. A placental delivery is recognized by a sudden gush of blood umbilical cord protrusion, and uterus contracts and rises.
- Check placenta for completeness and gently massage the uterus.
- Oxytocin, 20 IU in 1 L IV bag, and run at 10 mL/min.
- Methergine 0.2 mg IM.
- Inspect and repair lacerations of cervix, vagina, and episiotomy.

F. Admit OB unit.

G. Special conditions:

- Nuchal cord: Occurs in >25% of deliveries and can cause fetal asphyxia if not identified and treated quickly. With a loose cord, slip over the head in between contractions. For a tight cord deliver quickly and clamp the cord after.
- Cord prolapse: The umbilical cord is seen first, through the cervix or vagina. Put mother in left lateral knee-chest position and apply continuous pressure through vagina on presenting fetal part. Rush to the OR for a stat c-section.

6. Preeclampsia/Eclampsia:

Preeclampsia is the presence of new-onset hypertension (>140/90), proteinuria, and edema in a female >20 weeks of gestation. Eclampsia is preeclampsia with seizures and can occur up to 28 days post delivery.

6.1. Clinical Evaluation:

A. Symptoms: Weight gain, headache, facial and extremity swelling, visual disturbances, mental status changes, abdominal pain, and seizures.

B. Signs: Papilledema, abdominal tenderness, edema, ankle clonus, hyperreflexia, tremulousness, coma. If pulmonary edema is present may see tachypnea, tachycardia, and rales.

C. DDX: Chronic hypertension, gestational hypertension, seizure disorder, SAH, meningitis, or drug ingestion.

D. Workup: CBC, BMP, BNP, LFTs, lipase, PT/PTT/INR, calcium, magnesium, fibrin split products, fibrinogen, uric acid, Type & Rh, UA, CXR, CT head prn.

6.2. RX:

A. Support ABCs, IV, O_2, pulse oximeter, and monitor prn with the understanding the mother's safety is the first priority.

B. For mild to moderate preeclampsia <37 weeks, admit for bed rest, salt restriction, seizure precaution, cardiotocography, and OB/GYN consult for possible delivery.

C. For severe preeclampsia >34 weeks' gestation, admit and consult for delivery.

- Treat HTN with hydralazine 5 mg IV then 5 to 10 mg q 10–20 minutes, or labetalol 10 to 20 mg IV q 10 minutes up to 300 mg.
- Seizure prophylaxis with magnesium sulfate ($MgSO_4$), 4 to 6 g (20% solution) IV over 5 to 10 minutes followed by a 1 to 2 g/h infusion.

D. For eclampsia with seizures:
- Secure an airway, place in left lateral decubitus position, and place on cardiotocographic monitoring.
- Benzodiazepines (lorazepam or diazepam), used to acutely stop the seizure. My use phenytoin or phenobarbital as an alternative.
- Start magnesium sulfate ($MgSO_4$), 4 to 6 g (20% solution) IV over 5 to 10 minutes followed by a 1 to 2 g/h infusion.

7. HELLP Syndrome:

HELLP syndrome (**H**emolysis, **E**levated **L**iver enzymes, **L**ow **P**latelets) is a severe variant of preeclampsia. It is seen in 0.5% of all pregnancies and 5% to 10% of patients with preeclampsia.

7.1. Clinical Evaluation:

A. Symptoms: RUQ pain, N/V, headache, malaise, and edema.
B. Signs: HTN, tachycardia, tachypnea, jaundice, edema, and petechiae.
C. DDX: Hyperemesis gravidarum, eclampsia, preeclampsia, TTP, anemia, hepatitis, thrombocytopenia of pregnancy.
D. Workup: CBC, BMP, BNP, LFTs, PT/PTT/INR, fibrin split products, fibrinogen, Type & Rh, Uric acid, UA, US RUQ and pelvis, monitor fetal heart tones, CXR prn.

7.2. RX:

A. Support ABCs, IV, O_2, pulse oximeter, and monitor prn.
B. Obtain an OB/GYN consult for immediate delivery (70% by c-section).
C. Treat HTN with hydralazine 5 mg IV then 5 to 10 mg q 10 to 20 minutes, or labetalol 10 to 20 mg IV q 10 minutes up to 300 mg.
D. Seizure prophylaxis with magnesium sulfate ($MgSO_4$), 4 to 6 g (20% solution) IV over 5 to 10 minutes followed by a 1 to 2 g/h infusion.
E. Consider dexamethasone 10 mg IV.
F. Consider platelet transfusion if <20,000.
G. Disposition: Admit to OB/GYN.

8. Placenta Previa:

Implantation of the placenta adjacent to or over the os. Presentation is painless, bright red vaginal bleeding after 28 weeks. Bleeding between the placenta and uterine wall can result in significant bleeding with separation resulting in a >50% fetal mortality. Risk factors include multiple surgeries, multiple pregnancies, HTN, smoking, prior previa or abruption, and advance maternal age.

8.1. Clinical Evaluation:

A. Symptoms: Painless, bright red vaginal bleeding.
B. Signs: Soft, nontender uterus, profuse vaginal bleeding, tachycardia, hypotension, and + fetal distress.
C. DDX: Normal labor, uterine rupture, vasa previa, and bloody show, abruption placentae, DIC, cervicitis, vaginitis.
D. Workup: CBC, BMP, LFTs, PT/PTTINR, fibrin split products, fibrinogen, uric acid, Type & Rh, T&C, UA, US.

8.2. RX:

A. Support the ABCs, two IVs, O_2, pulse oximeter, and monitor.
B. Emergent OB/GYN consult.
C. Position patient on left side, start cardiotocography.
D. Consider a tocolytic agent and steroids in consultation with OB/GYN.
E. Rh-isoimmunization prophylaxis as needed.
F. Disposition: Admit to OB/GYN.

9. Abruptio Placenta:

A premature separation of the placenta from the uterine wall. It occurs in 1% to 2% of all pregnancies. Maternal mortality is <1% but fetal mortality is 35% to 50%. Risk factors include HTN, smoking, cocaine use, advance maternal age, multiparity, previous abruption, and abdominal trauma.

9.1. Clinical Evaluation:

- **A. Symptoms:** Painful, dark red, vaginal bleeding, abdominal/pelvic pain, and preterm labor.
- **B. Signs:** Painful tender uterus, rigid abdomen, profuse vaginal bleeding, tachycardia, hypotension, and + fetal distress.
- **C. DDX:** Normal labor, uterine rupture, vasa previa, bloody show, placenta previa, appendicitis, trauma in pregnancy, ovarian torsion.
- **D. Workup:** CBC, BMP, LFTs, PT/PTTINR, fibrin split products, fibrinogen, uric acid, Type & Rh, T&C, UA, US (+ 25% of cases).

9.2. RX:

- **A.** Support the ABCs, two IVs, O_2, pulse oximeter, and monitor.
- **B.** Emergent OB/GYN consult.
- **C.** Position patient on left side, start cardiotocography.
- **D.** Rh-isoimmunization prophylaxis as needed.
- **E. Disposition:** Admit to OB/GYN for possible emergent c-section.

HEENT

1. Ludwig's Angina:

This is a deep space neck infection (mixed aerobic and anaerobic), involving the submandibular, submental, and sublingual spaces resulting in significant swelling to the floor of the mouth. This is due to a dental infection (molars most common), dental procedure, tongue piercing, and fractures.

1.1. Clinical Evaluation:

- **A. Symptoms:** Pain, edema, trismus, drooling dysphonia, and dysphagia.
- **B. Signs:** Brawny edema of submandibular region, displaced tongue, fever, poor dentition, cervical lymphadenopathy.
- **C. DDX:** Epiglottitis, peritonsillar abscess, angioedema.
- **D. Workup:** CBC, BMP, PT/PTT/INR, blood cultures, lateral C-spine x-ray, CT neck.

1.2. RX:

- **A.** Support ABCs, IV, O_2, pulse oximeter, and monitor.
- **B.** Consider awake, nasal, or glide scope intubation.
- **C.** Have a cricothyrotomy kit along with a "difficult airway cart," at the bedside.
- **D.** Emergent ENT consult for I&D.
- **E.** Give penicillin G, 4 million units IV + metronidazole 500 mg IV, **or** clindamycin, 600 to 900 mg IV, **or** cefazolin, 1 to 2 g IV.
- **F. Disposition:** Admit patients to the ICU.

2. Peritonsillar Abscess:

A common infection located in the peritonsillar space due to group A beta-hemolytic streptococcus (*Streptococcus pyogenes*). This is the most common deep head/neck infection (50%).

2.1. Clinical Evaluation:

- **A. Symptoms:** Severe sore throat, dysphagia, odynophagia, fever, trismus, muffled voice, drooling.
- **B. Signs:** Dehydration, fever, tachycardia, fluctuant displaced unilateral tonsil, anterior cervical lymphadenopathy, and uvula deviation.

C. **DDX:** Epiglottitis, retropharyngeal abscess, mononucleosis, pharyngitis.
D. **Workup:** CBC, BMP, monospot, rapid strep, throat culture, lateral C-spine x-ray, CT neck as needed.

2.2. RX:

A. Support ABCs, IV, O_2, pulse oximeter, and monitor.
B. Administer penicillin, or clindamycin, 600 mg IV, or ampicillin/sulbactam.
C. Consult ENT for possible I&D.
D. Have airway equipment at the bedside.
E. If unable to obtain a consult anesthetize, aspirate or incise pus from tonsil.
F. IV rehydration and consider dexamethasone IV/IM.
G. **Disposition:** Admit if toxic, dehydrated, potential airway compromise, or severe trismus.

3. Epiglottitis:

An acute inflammation in the supraglottic region of the oropharynx involving the epiglottis, arytenoids, and aryepiglottic folds. It was caused by *Haemophilus influenzae* type B until the HIB vaccine made it extinct, now streptococcal species are more common. It is more common in males in their 40s and more commonly due to *H. influenzae*, *Haemophilus parainfluenza*, Strep *pneumonia*, and group A streptococci.

3.1. Clinical Evaluation:

A. **Symptoms:** Severe sore throat, dysphagia, odynophagia, muffled voice, stridor, drooling.
B. **Signs:** Dehydration, fever, tachycardia, cough, cervical adenopathy, tachypnea, sitting in tripod position (tongue out and head forward).
C. **DDX:** Retropharyngeal abscess, pharyngitis, laryngotracheobronchitis, laryngitis, peritonsillar abscess.
D. **Workup:** CBC, BMP, monospot, rapid strep, throat culture, blood cultures, lateral C-spine x-ray (thumbprint sign), CT neck as needed.

3.2. RX:

A. Support ABCs, IV, O_2, pulse oximeter, and monitor.
B. Administer ceftriaxone or cefotaxime.
C. Consult ENT and anesthesia for airway help.
D. Have airway equipment at the bedside.
E. If intubation is needed use direct or fiberoptic laryngoscopy.
F. Give dexamethasone 10 mg IV/IM.
G. Consider nebulized epinephrine.
H. **Disposition:** Admit to the ICU.

4. Foreign Bodies Upper Airway:

Usually seen in children <3 y/o. Common FBs include food, coins, and toys. Symptoms depend on the nature and location of the obstruction.

4.1. Clinical Evaluation:

A. **Symptoms:** Stridor, voice changes, dysphagia, coughing episodes, dyspnea, dysphonia.
B. **Signs:** Wheezing, apnea, cyanosis, petechiae, respiratory accessory muscle use, drooling.
C. **Workup:** CXR, AP/lateral, inspiratory/expiratory, C-spine x-ray, CT neck as needed.

4.2. RX:

A. Support the ABCs, IV/IO, O_2, pulse oximeter, and monitor.
B. Immediate airway management must be the first priority.
C. Children with airway obstruction: Back blows, then chest thrusts, Heimlich maneuver for children >12 y/o.

D. Do not attempt to blindly remove an FB in a child.
E. If unable to remove after noninvasive maneuvers, perform laryngoscopy with Magill forceps if patient is cooperative and object is visualized.
F. If unsuccessful, perform a cricothyrotomy or transtracheal jet ventilation (cric contraindicated in children <10 y/o).
G. If FB below the cricoid, may temporize by pushing FB into the bronchus and intubate and ventilate the unobstructed lung.
H. Disposition:
- Obtain an ENT consultation for children with subglottic FBs and for adults with hypopharyngeal FBs that cannot be removed by means of indirect laryngoscopy.
- Consult pulmonary or ENT for bronchoscopy if FB in trachea or bronchus.
- May be discharged with close follow-up after the FB is removed, and the patient is awake and stable.

5. Acute Angle–Closure Glaucoma:

Increased intraocular pressure (IOP) caused by an overproduction of aqueous humor or a decreased in aqueous outflow. With increasing and persistent pressure, optic nerve damage leads to blindness. The patient usually presents with acute, severe, unilateral eye pain.

5.1. Clinical Evaluation:

A. Symptoms: Severe unilateral eye pain, headache, N/V, abdominal pain, seeing "halos" (corneal edema), photophobia.
B. Signs: Decreased visual acuity (VA), red eye, cloudy cornea, IOP >30 mm Hg, mid-dilated pupil, nonreactive pupil, shallow anterior chamber, hard painful globe to palpation.
C. DDX: Conjunctivitis, iritis, open-closure glaucoma, trauma, allergic reactions, keratitis.
D. Workup: Tonometry for IOP, fluorescein staining, slit-lamp examination.

5.2. RX:

A. IV pain medication and place patient in the supine position.
B. Block production of aqueous humor:
- Topical beta-blocker, timolol 0.5%, 1 to 2 drops q 10 to 15 minutes for 3 doses.
- Carbonic anhydrase inhibitor, acetazolamide 500 mg po/IV.
- Alpha-2-agonist, apraclonidine or brimonidine 1 gtt q 30 minutes.

C. Facilitate the outflow of aqueous humor:
- Constrict pupil with pilocarpine 2%, 1 gtt q 15 minutes until pupil constricted.
- Increase uveoscleral outflow with prostaglandin agonist latanoprost intraocular.

D. Reduce vitreous humor volume with mannitol, 1 to 1.5 g/kg IV.
E. Consult ophthalmology immediately.
F. Disposition: Admit. Definitive therapy is surgical iridectomy.

6. Iritis/Uveitis:

Inflammation of the iris or uveal tissue due to trauma, infection, rheumatologic, or autoimmune disorders.

6.1. Clinical Evaluation:

A. Symptoms: Unilateral eye pain, severe photophobia, redness.
B. Signs: Decreased VA, injected conjunctiva, flare + cells on slit-lamp examination, miosis, cornea clear to hazy, pain to accommodation.
C. DDX: Conjunctivitis, angle-closure glaucoma, trauma, allergic reactions, keratitis, optic neuritis, corneal ulcer.
D. Workup: CBC, BMP, ESR, CRP, RPR, ANA, CXR, tonometry, fluorescein staining, slit-lamp examination.

6.2. RX:

A. Treat pain and vomiting.
B. Use a cycloplegic (atropine, cyclogel) to dilate pupil.
C. Treat infection if present.
D. Use a topical corticosteroid in consultation with ophthalmology.
E. Consult ophthalmology.
F. **Disposition:** May require admission for further workup. If stable, may be discharged with prompt ophthalmology follow-up.

7. Endophthalmitis:

Inflammatory condition of the intraocular structures. It may be endogenous (infection from hematogenous spread) or exogenous (ocular surgery, penetrating trauma). Decreased or loss of vision is a common complication.

7.1. Clinical Evaluation:

A. **Symptoms:** Visual loss, eye pain, headache, photophobia, red eye, ocular discharge.
B. **Signs:** Eyelid swelling, injected conjunctiva, hypopyon, chemosis, proptosis, cotton-wool spots, purulent discharge, fever, cell and flare on slit-lamp examination.
C. **DDX:** Corneal abrasion, corneal laceration corneal ulceration, globe rupture, herpes zoster ophthalmicus, iritis/uveitis, lupus, postoperative inflammation.
D. **Workup:** CBC, BMP, ESR, CRP, blood culture, tonometry, slit-lamp examination, CXR, cardiac echo (endocarditis), ocular ultrasound, CT/MRI orbits.

7.2. RX:

A. Treat pain.
B. Give antibiotics. Vancomycin + aminoglycoside or cephalosporin.
C. Consult ophthalmology.
D. Use topical cycloplegic drops.
E. Consider topical corticosteroids in consultation with ophthalmology.
F. **Disposition:** Admit patient for possible intravitreal antibiotics.

8. Central Retinal Artery Occlusion (CRAO):

Abrupt cessation of blood flow to the central retinal artery. Common causes include embolized atheromatous plaque, hyperviscosity syndrome (multiple myeloma), trauma (fat emboli), sickle cell disease, DM, and temporal arteritis. Permanent damage can occur if vision loss persists longer than 2 hours. Life expectancy of patients with CRAO is 5.5 years compared to 15 years for an age-matched population without CRAO.

8.1. Clinical Evaluation:

A. **Symptoms:** Sudden painless monocular visual loss. May have a history of jaw claudication, headaches, weight loss, scalp tenderness, anorexia.
B. **Signs:** Decrease or absent VA, afferent pupillary defect, cherry red spot (nonedematous fovea), pale fundus (edema), boxcar segmentation of retinal arteries and veins, temporal tenderness.
C. **DDX:** Retinal detachment, central retinal vein occlusion, vitreous hemorrhage, amaurosis fugax, diabetic retinopathy.
D. **Workup:** CBC, BMP, ESR, CRP, PT/PTT/INR, blood cultures, tonometry, slit-lamp examination, CXR, cardiac echo (endocarditis), carotid ultrasound, fluorescein angiogram, MRI/MRA head and neck, CT head.

8.2. RX:

A. Goals are to lower IOP, increase retinal perfusion, and oxygen delivery to ischemic tissues.
B. Consult ophthalmology STAT.

C. Give acetazolamide 500 mg IV and timolol topical, to decrease IOP.
D. Digital massage of globe may help dislodge the embolus.
E. Rebreath CO_2 in an attempt to vasodilate retinal arterioles by breathing in a paper bag 10 to 15 minutes each hour.
F. **Disposition:** Admit patient for further workup.

HEMATOLOGY/ONCOLOGY

Transfusion Products

- **Cryoprecipitate:** Cold-insoluble portion of FFP that precipitates when FFP is thawed. It contains fibrinogen, factor VIII, factor XIII, and Von Willebrand factor. Each unit contains approximately 150 mg of fibrinogen and 100 units of factor VIII in a final volume of 20 mL. (1 unit bag). Transfuse to achieve a fibrinogen level of 100 mg/dL, which will take 2 U/10 kg of cryoprecipitate.
- **Fresh frozen plasma:** 1 unit of FFP is the amount of plasma taken from 1 unit of whole blood in the process of making PRBCs. FFP contains all the clotting factors and 4 units are required to adequately change the coagulation status.
- **Platelets:** Used to correct the prolonged bleeding time associated with factor V deficiency as well as thrombocytopenia. Platelets should also be considered when bleeding time is prolonged (>9 minutes). Each unit of platelets should increase platelet count to 5,000 to 10,000/μL.
- **Prothrombin-complex concentrate:** This is a pooled plasma product that contains factors II, VII, IX, and X plus protein S and C. This is the treatment of choice for warfarin anticoagulation in the setting of life-threatening hemorrhage.

1. Anemia:

Anemia can be induced by a large variety of diseases and is defined as a decrease in RBC mass. Anemia is a symptom that requires investigation to determine the underlying etiology. There are three primary causes of anemia (1) blood loss, (2) increased RBC destruction, (3) decreased RBC production.

1.1. Chemical Evaluation:

A. **Symptoms:** Malaise, DOE, fatigue, angina, claudication, syncope/near syncope.
B. **Signs:** Pallor, tachycardia, orthostasis, wide-pulse pressure, murmur, icterus, petechiae, ecchymosis, and hepatosplenomegaly.
C. **DDX:** Aplastic anemia, sickle cell disease, hemolytic anemia, iron deficiency anemia, pernicious anemia, thalassemia, GI bleed, trauma, cancer.
D. **Workup:** CBC with differential, reticulocyte count, peripheral smear, iron, TIBC, and/or ferritin, LFTs, PT/PTT/INR, BMP, BNP, and cardiac enzymes as needed.

1.2. RX:

A. Support ABCs, IV, O_2, pulse oximeter, and monitor.
B. Resuscitate patients presenting with hypovolemic shock.
C. Chronic anemia and anemia secondary to chronic disease or iron deficiency is usually tolerated well and outpatient management may be appropriate.
D. **Disposition:** Admit for active bleeding, severe hypovolemia, shock, ischemia from low blood volume, or when a transfusion is required.

2. Disseminated Intravascular Coagulation (DIC):

DIC is a disorder characterized by activation of blood coagulation, causing generation and deposition of fibrin, leading to thrombi in various organs, contributing to multiple organ dysfunction syndrome. DIC is not a specific disease but a complication of another disorder. Mortality rates very depending on the precipitating event, but can be as high as 70%.

2.1. Clinical Evaluation:

A. **Symptoms:** Fever, fatigue, weakness, dyspnea, cough, abdominal pain, fever, possible chest pain.
B. **Signs:** Bleeding from puncture sites, hematuria, ecchymosis, petechia are displayed. Thrombotic manifestations include renal failure, bowel infarction, pulmonary insufficiency, cyanosis, hypoxemia, and change in mental status.
C. **DDX:** Sepsis, malignancy, OB complications, trauma, heat stroke, hemolytic-uremic syndrome, TTP, ITP.
D. **Workup:** CBC with peripheral smear, BMP, LFTs, PT/PTT/INR, fibrin split products, fibrinogen, hemoccult stools, ECG, CXR, and further test as needed depending on disorder.

2.2. RX:

A. Treat the underlying disorder. Manage severe hemorrhage with fluids, blood, and platelets. Evacuate uterus in a septic abortion. Treat hypovolemia, sepsis, acidosis, and hypoxia.
B. For a patient at high risk of bleeding or actively bleeding with biochemical evidence of DIC, replace fibrinogen, platelets, and clotting factors with cryoprecipitate (fibrinogen and factor VIII), FFP (clotting factors), and platelets (maintain platelets >50,000/μL) as appropriate. Provide whole blood, if necessary. Consider aminocaproic acid for refractory DIC, 5 to 10 g slow IV push, followed by 2 to 4 g/h for 24 hours or until bleeding stops. Use concurrent heparin treatment.
C. Consider management of thrombotic complications with heparin **except** for common ED presentations of DIC after surgery or trauma, with abruption, or when other bleeding risks are present.
D. Treat infection with appropriate antibiotic.
E. Consider obtaining a hematology consultation.
F. **Disposition:** Admit to the ICU.

3. Sickle Cell Crisis (SCD):

SCD is an autosomal recessive defect in the beta-globulin chains of hemoglobin. Chains change causing abnormal hemoglobin. These patients are at a higher risk for deoxygenation, polymerization of Hgb, and sickling of RBCs. These sickle cells cause vaso-occlusive ischemic tissue injury.

- Acute chest syndrome: A life-threatening complication caused by pulmonary vascular infarction and/or infection. Most common infectious agents are *Chlamydia pneumoniae*, *Mycoplasma pneumoniae*, RSV, *S. aureus*, and *Streptococcus pneumoniae*. It has a 5% to 12% mortality rate and is hard to differentiate from pneumonia.
- Aplastic crisis: Sudden failure of the bone marrow to produce enough RBCs to compensate for the ones destroyed. Parvovirus B-19 is a common cause and this is a self-limiting disorder.
- Sepsis: This is the leading cause of death in sickle cell patients. These patients are susceptible to many different organisms and infection can come from various organ systems.

3.1. Clinical Evaluation:

A. **Symptoms:** Severe pain in the back, abdomen, chest, or extremities, chest pain, dyspnea, ± associated fever, and jaundice.
B. **Signs:** Pallor, icterus, meningeal signs, focal neuro deficits, pulmonary findings of CHF and/or pneumonia, abdominal pain to palpation.
C. **DDX:** Sepsis, septic arthritis, lupus, pneumonia, anemia, osteomyelitis, PE, leukemia.
D. **Workup:** CBC, BMP, reticulocyte count, Type & cross, blood cultures, UA, ABG, ECG, CXR, bone x-ray (prn), CT/MRI head prn.

3.2. RX:

A. Support ABCs, IV, O_2, pulse oximeter, and monitor.
B. For patients with vaso-occlusive crisis, place on O_2 if hypoxic, hydrate with 0.9 NS IV fluid, and administer analgesics (NSAIDs, narcotics).
C. For severely anemic patients, treat with IV fluids and transfuse PRBCs.
D. Treat infections with appropriate antibiotics.
E. **Disposition:** Admit the patient for transfusion, antibiotics, hydration, and pain control.

4. Hypercalcemia:

The most common cause is malignancy followed by hyperparathyroidism, dysproteinemias, vitamin D intoxication, milk-alkali syndrome, and sarcoidosis. This can lead to pancreatitis, nephrolithiasis, and heart block.

4.1. Clinical Evaluation:

- **A. Symptoms:** Weakness, N/V, anorexia, mental status changes, back pain, constipation, malaise, abdominal pain, psychosis, seizure, coma.
- **B. Signs:** Muscle weakness, dehydration, hypertension, abdominal pain to palpation, confusion.
- **C. DDX:** Hyperkalemia, hypernatremia, dehydration, sepsis, narcotic overdose, adrenal insufficiency
- **D. Workup:** CBC, BMP, LFTs, PT/PTT/INR, lipase, calcium, ionized calcium, magnesium, phosphate, TSH, T_4, ECG, CXR, CT head (prn).

4.2. RX:

- **A.** Support ABCs, IV, O_2, pulse oximeter, and monitor.
- **B.** For coma, naloxone 2 mg IV, check glucose.
- **C.** NS 1 to 2 L over 2 to 3 hours.
- **D.** Consider Lasix 20 mg IV.
- **E.** Hydrocortisone 100 mg IV.
- **F.** Dialysis if in renal failure.
- **G. Disposition:** Admit symptomatic patients with a corrected calcium >13 mg/dL to a monitored be. Severe symptoms with high calcium requires an ICU admit.

INFECTIOUS DISEASES

1. Encephalitis:

Encephalitis is an infection/inflammation of the brain parenchyma caused by a viral or bacterial source. Although bacterial, fungal, and autoimmune disorders can occur, most cases are due to a virus with arboviruses being the most common class.

1.1. Clinical Evaluation:

- **A. Symptoms:** Headache, fever, neck stiffness, photophobia, lethargy, confusion, behavioral changes.
- **B. Signs:** AMS, focal neurologic findings, papilledema, meningeal signs, flaccid paralysis, tachycardia, tachypnea.
- **C. DDX:** CNS tumor, CNS syphilis, Ehrlichiosis, CVA, intracranial hemorrhage, head trauma, acute confusional state (drugs, toxins, psychosis), hepatic encephalopathy, hypoglycemia, brain abscess.
- **D. Workup:** CBC, BMP, LFTs, PT/PTT/INR, UA, LP (glucose, protein, Gram stain, culture, viral PCR, cryptococcal antigen, india ink, acid-fast bacillus), CRP, ESR, consider Lyme/RMSF testing, CXR, CT head as needed.

1.2. RX:

- **A.** Support ABCs, IV, O_2, pulse oximeter, and monitor.
- **B.** Give empiric antibiotics (ceftriaxone, cefotaxime), early because an overlap exists between bacterial and viral presentations.
- **C.** General treatment measures for hydrocephalus and increased ICP: Elevating head of the bed, treat fever and pain, prevent seizures (phenytoin), prevent hypotension.
- **D.** Severe increase in ICP: Intubation with hyperventilation (pCO_2 30 mm Hg), mannitol 1 g/kg IV or Lasix 20 mg IV.
- **E.** Dexamethasone 10 mg IV, for edema surrounding a space-occupying lesion.
- **F.** Empiric treatment for suspected organisms:
  - Herpes simplex virus (HSV) and varicella zoster (VZV), acyclovir 10 mg/kg IV.
  - CMV, ganciclovir 5 mg/kg IV q 12 hours.
- **G.** For treatments of arthropod-borne viruses, refer to "Rocky Mountain spotted fever" and "Lyme's disease" sections.
- **H. Disposition:** Admit to the ICU.

2. Meningitis:

Meningitis is an infection or inflammation of the meninges caused by a virus, bacteria, fungi, or autoimmune phenomena. Meningitis is caused by a variety of pathogens that have the potential of infecting different age groups.

2.1. Clinical Evaluation:

A. **Symptoms:** HA, fever, nuchal rigidity, photophobia, N/V, AMS, confusion, irritability, coma.
B. **Signs:** Fever, Kernig's and Brudzinski's signs, nuchal rigidity, papilledema, petechial, hyperreflexia, AMS. A change in mental status may occur, including confusion, lethargy, coma, seizure, cranial nerve, or other focal neurologic findings.
C. **DDX:** CNS tumor, CNS syphilis, seizure, sepsis, intracranial hemorrhage, febrile illness, delirium tremens, encephalitis, brain abscess.
D. **Workup:** CBC, BMP, LFTs, PT/PTT/INR, UA, LP (glucose, protein, Gram stain, culture, viral PCR, cryptococcal antigen, india ink, acid-fast bacillus, VDRL), CRP, ESR, consider Lyme/RMSF testing, CT head as needed.
   - Guidelines for a CT before LP includes; immunocompromised state, history of CNS disease (mass, stroke, focal infection), seizure within 1 week, papilledema, AMS, focal neuro deficit.

2.2. RX:

A. Support ABCs, IV, O_2, pulse oximeter, and monitor.
B. NS bolus for shock or hypotension.
C. Early empiric antibiotics are mandatory. *S. pneumoniae* (most common), *N. meningitides*, and *Listeria monocytogenes* are the most common organisms.
   - Vancomycin 1 g IV + ceftriaxone 1 g IV (or cefotaxime).
   - Give ampicillin if concerned about *Listeria*.
   - Consider empiric treatment with acyclovir IV for suspected herpes virus.
   - Cryptococcus is treated with amphotericin + flucytosine.
D. Give prophylactic medication (rifampin or ciprofloxacin), to health professionals and family in close contact with a patient with *N. meningitidis*.
E. Give dexamethasone 0.15 mg/kg IV.
F. **Disposition:** Admit to the ICU.

3. Endocarditis, Infectious:

Endocarditis is an infection of the endocardial lining of the heart and valves. High-risk groups include IV drug abusers (IVDA), prosthetic heart valves, mitral valve prolapse, previous endocarditis, pacemakers, and those with recent invasive procedures. Mortality rate is 10% to 50% depending on the organism involved. Death usually comes from emboli going to the coronaries, brain, and kidneys and if left untreated this disorder is universally fatal. For native valve endocarditis, *Streptococcus viridans* and *bovis* make up >70% of infections, followed by enterococcus and Staphylococcus species. In prosthetic valve and IVDA endocarditis, *S. aureus* (MRSA and MSSA) accounts for >50% reported cases, followed by Strep species, *Pseudomonas, Serratia marcescens*, and *Candida albicans*.

3.1. Clinical Evaluation:

A. **Symptoms:** Low-grade fever, nonspecific complaints, myalgias, arthralgias, heart disease, anorexia, weight loss.
B. **Signs:** Osler's nodes (painful red nodules on fingers), Janeway lesions (nontender plaques on the palms and soles), subungual splinter hemorrhages, petechia, Roth's spots (white spots surrounded by hemorrhage in the retina), murmur, CHF signs.
C. **DDX:** Septicemia, rheumatic fever, pericarditis, pneumonia, TB, meningitis, intra-abdominal infection, glomerulonephritis, cerebrovascular accident, SLE, cancer, congestive heart failure, multiple pulmonary embolisms, DIC.
D. **Workup:** CBC, BMP, PT/PTT/INR, D-dimer, UA, blood cultures × 3, ESR, CRP, ECG, CXR, echocardiogram.

3.2. RX:

A. Support ABCs, IV, O_2, pulse oximeter, and monitor.
B. For native valve endocarditis give penicillin G 4 million units or ceftriaxone 1 g IV + gentamicin and/or vancomycin 30 mg/kg/d IV bid for Staph species.
C. For prosthetic valve and IVDA patients, give penicillin G 4 million units or ceftriaxone 1 g IV + gentamicin and/or vancomycin 1 g IV bid.
D. Disposition: Admit stable patients to a monitored bed. If the patient is toxic, admit to the ICU.

4. Erysipelas:

Skin infection involving the dermis and lymphatics usually caused by Group *A beta-hemolytic Streptococcus*. A break in the skin (trauma, insect bite, leg ulcer) allows the infection to occur. Most cases are easily treated but in neonates, elderly, and those immunocompromised septic emboli, gangrene, sepsis, abscess formation, pneumonia, and death can occur.

4.1. Clinical Evaluation:

A. Symptoms: Small wound, local infection to widespread involvement, abrupt onset of fever/chills, N/V, myalgias, headache, arthralgias.
B. Signs: Rash is red, shiny, hot, raised, tense, painful, indurated, and well demarcated. Fever, lymphadenopathy, tachycardic, tachypnea.
C. DDX: Cellulitis, sinusitis, erysipeloid (hands), contact dermatitis, angioneurotic edema, lupus, and necrotizing fasciitis.
D. Workup: CBC with differential, BMP, lactate, CRP, ESR, x-ray as needed, blood cultures as needed.

4.2. RX:

A. Support ABCs, IV, O_2, pulse oximeter, and monitor as needed.
B. Hydrate with NS, treat pain and vomiting.
C. Treat with Penicillin G or Nafcillin or second/third-generation cephalosporin. Consider vancomycin if concerned about MRSA.
D. Disposition: Admit patients with widespread infection, clinical toxicity, and social issues preventing effective outpatient therapy. If nontoxic, discharge with a po antibiotic regimen, and close follow-up.

5. Necrotizing Fasciitis (NF):

NF is a rapidly progressive infection of the fascia with secondary necrosis of the subcutaneous tissue. Fournier's gangrene is a form of NF that is localized to the scrotum and perineal region. Usually this infection is polymicrobial and rapidly progressive. When due to a single organism consider group A beta-hemolytic *Strep* (flesh-eating bacteria), *Clostridial* myonecrosis and *Vibrio vulnificus* (saltwater infection) as the leading cause. Mortality is 70% to 80% in high-risk patients (DM, immunocompromised, trauma).

- Clostridial myonecrosis (gas gangrene): A subset of necrotizing myositis due to a Clostridium species and associated with a high morbidity and mortality. Deep trauma and surgery are the most common causes. The infection is aggressive and shock like symptoms may be present within 24 hours of exposure.

5.1. Clinical Evaluation:

A. Symptoms: Sudden severe pain (out of proportion to examination), fever, chills, warm erythematous skin, weakness, malaise.
B. Signs: Fever, erythema to black skin, vesicles/bullae, severe pain to palpation of infected tissue, edema, crepitus, tachycardia, tachypnea, hypotension
C. DDX: Myonecrosis, cellulitis, erysipelas, phlegmasia cerulea dolens, hernias, toxic shock syndrome, testicular torsion.
D. Workup: CBC, BMP, lactate, PT/PTT/INR, ABG/VBG, blood cultures, wound culture (prn), CT/x-ray (r/o subcutaneous air).

5.2. RX:

A. Support ABCs, IV, O_2, pulse oximeter, and monitor.
B. Emergent surgical consult.
C. Give ampicillin/sulbactam (Unasyn), 1.5 to 3 g IV + gentamicin 3 to 6 mg/kg/d q 8 hours IV or ceftriaxone or vancomycin (MRSA coverage).
D. Consider tetanus prophylaxis if indicated.
E. **Disposition:** Transfer the patient to OR for debridement and then admit to the ICU.

6. Pneumonia:

Community-acquired pneumonia (CAP), and influenza remain a leading cause of death in the United States. Inhalation of infectious aerosols is the most common mode of infection. Pneumonia is classified into types:

- CAP is a pneumonia not acquired in a hospital or long-term care facility. The most common organisms include *S. pneumoniae*, *M. pneumoniae*, and *Haemophilus influenzae* RSV, and *influenza*. Mortality rate is around 10%.
- Hospital-acquired pneumonia (HAP) is a nosocomial infection that occurs >48 hours after admission, and was not incubating at the time of admission. Multidrug-resistant organisms, *Pseudomonas*, and *S. aureus* are common. Mortality rates are 20%.
- Healthcare-associated pneumonia (HCAP) is a nosocomial infection seen in nursing home patients, those hospitalized in a hospital for >2 days or within the last 90 days, and received wound care or chemotherapy within the past 30 days. Organisms are the same as those seen with HAP. The mortality rate is around 20%.
- Ventilator-associated pneumonia (VAP) is a pneumonia that occurs within 48 hours or longer after intubation and has 30% mortality.

6.1. Clinical Evaluation:

A. **Symptoms:** URI symptoms, cough, sputum production, wheezing, dyspnea, fever, malaise, pleuritic chest pain/abdominal pain, anorexia N/V, obtundation.
B. **Signs:** Fever, tachypnea, tachycardia, retractions, splinting, wheezing, rhonchi, consolidation, friction rub, dullness to percussion, ± egophony, ± hypotension.
C. **DDX:** CHF, tumor, pulmonary contusion, pleural effusion (cirrhosis, CHF, uremia), aspiration pneumonia, pneumothorax, influenza, ACS.
D. **Workup:** CBC with differential, BMP, LFTs, ABG blood cultures, sputum for Gram stain and C&S, PCR viral studies, CXR, CT chest prn.

6.2. RX:

A. Support ABCs, IV, O_2, pulse oximeter, and monitor.
B. Follow the American Thoracic Society's guidelines.
C. Hydrate with NS and treat fever with an NSAID or acetaminophen.
D. CAP stable outpatient therapy azithromycin, doxycycline, or fluoroquinolone for patient with comorbidities.
E. Inpatient non-ICU patient give a fluoroquinolone po/IV or azithromycin IV or ceftriaxone IV.
F. Inpatient ICU patient give a third-generation cephalosporin plus a fluoroquinolone.
G. HAP, HCAP, or VAP patient, give a carbapenem or third-generation cephalosporin or zosyn + gentamicin or a fluoroquinolone + vancomycin.
H. **Disposition:** Admit patients based on clinical, social, and/or a risk stratifying score (Pneumonia severity index [PSI] or CURB-65). Admit to the ICU if signs of sepsis are present. Mild CAP may be discharged if no comorbidities and adequate follow-up is available.

7. Systemic Inflammatory Response (SIRS), Sepsis, Septic Shock:

SIRS describes the clinical manifestations that result from the systemic response to infection. Criteria for SIRS are met by having two of the four criteria.

- Fever of more than 38°C (100.4°F) or less than 36°C (96.8°F)
- Heart rate >90 beats per minute
- RR >20 breaths per minute or $PaCO_2$ <32 mm Hg.
- WBC >12,000 or <4,000 or bands >10%.

Sepsis is the presence of an infection in association with SIRS.

Sepsis = 2 SIRS criteria + 1 documented infection + at least 1 sign of organ dysfunction.

- AMS
- Hypoxemia (PaO_2 <72 mm Hg, with pulmonary disease not being the direct cause).
- Elevated lactate level (≥4 mmol/L)
- Oliguria (urine output <30 mL or 0.5 mL/kg for at least 1 hour)

Severe Sepsis
Sepsis complicated by end-organ dysfunction that responds to fluids.

- BP <90 mm Hg or >40 mm Hg drop from baseline.
- Elevated Cr.
- DIC

Septic Shock = Severe sepsis + hypotension that does not respond to fluid)

7.1. Clinical Evaluation:

A. Symptoms: Fever, malaise, headache, and arthralgias/myalgias, weakness, tachypnea, cough, dysuria, headache, N/V/D.

B. Signs: Fever, hypotension, wide-pulse pressure, tachycardia, tachypnea, hypothermia (4%).

C. DDX: RMSF, typhus, typhoid fever, endocarditis, vasculitis, PE, AMI, DKA, toxic shock, pancreatitis.

D. Workup: CBC, BMP, LFTs, PT/PTT/INR, CRP, ESR, lactate, UA with culture, blood cultures, LP if needed, CXR, CT head/abdomen/pelvis as needed.

7.2. RX:

A. Support ABCs, two IVs, O_2, pulse oximeter, and monitor.

B. Head to toe examination in order to find the source of infection.

C. Assume any catheter anywhere in the body could be the source (Foley, central line, PICC line), and treat accordingly.

D. Start early goal-directed therapy;

- Intubate if needed to maintain oxygenation, and decrease work of breathing (tidal volume 6 cc/kg).
- Maximize BP with NS or LR fluid boluses (usually requires >4 L). If unsuccessful, use an inotropic agent (dopamine, norepinephrine). Keep the MAP >65 mm Hg.
- Consider a central line to measure CVP (8–12 mm Hg), $ScvO_2$ (>70%). *Controversial.*
- Consider a Foley catheter, keep urine output >0.5 mL/kg/h.
- Transfuse PRBCs for an Hct <30% and persistent $ScvO_2$ <70%.
- Early antibiotic therapy is the most important single measure at reducing mortality. Should be given within the first 4 to 6 hours of presentation.

E. When the source of infection is not immediately obvious, use a broad-spectrum antibiotic that covers gram-positive and gram-negative bacteria.

- Aminoglycoside + beta-lactam + vancomycin (MRSA coverage)

F. IV corticosteroids are controversial. May be of benefit to the patient who does not response to adequate fluid resuscitation and vasopressor administration.

G. Disposition: Admit all patients to the ICU.

8. Septic Arthritis:

Septic arthritis is a monoarticular arthritis most commonly caused by *S. aureus*. *N. gonorrheae* is the most common cause in adolescents and young adults. This commonly result from hematologic spread of bacteria, but may result from contiguous spread or direct inoculation. Larger joints are affected most often; Knee > hip > shoulder > ankle > wrist.

8.1. Clinical Evaluation:

A. Symptoms: Fever, chills, limp, refusal to walk, arthralgias/myalgias.
B. Signs: Pain with active/passive joint movement, possible effusion, fever, red and warm, maculopapular rash,
C. DDX: Rheumatoid arthritis, gout, osteoarthritis, osteomyelitis, SLE, slipped capital femoral epiphysis, transient synovitis, trauma, Osgood Schlatter.
D. Workup: CBC, BMP, ESR, CRP, uric acid, blood cultures, STD tests, VDRL, joint aspiration (WBC count, crystals, culture, Gram stain, glucose), plain x-ray, bone scan as needed, MRI.

8.2. RX:

A. IV, treat sepsis as appropriate if present.
B. Consult orthopedic immediately.
C. For gram-negative bacilli use a third-generation cephalosporin. For gram-positive cocci use vancomycin. Treat GC with ceftriaxone + Zithromax or doxycycline.
D. Customize treatment for the compromised adults, such as an IV drug abuser, HIV patient, and the debilitated.
E. Treat pain.
F. Disposition: Admit with orthopedic consult. If unsure, admit and treat pending C&S.

METABOLIC/ELECTROLYTE DISORDERS

Acid–Base Disturbances

1. Metabolic Acidosis:

In metabolic acidosis the pH is <7.35 and the pCO_2 is low.

1.1. Clinical Evaluation:

A. Elevated AG: A MUDPILE CAT (refer section in this chapter).
B. Normal AG: Hypochloremic–RTA, diarrhea, pancreatic fistula, ileostomy, ureteroenterostomy, TPN, NH_4Cl, and drugs, such as acetazolamide, Sulfamylon, cholestyramine, spironolactone.

1.2. RX:

A. Support ABCs, IV, O_2, pulse oximeter, and monitor.
B. Start NS or LR, for volume expansion.
C. Implement a specific therapy for a given metabolic derangement or toxic ingestion.
D. Consider bicarbonate therapy when the pH is <7.1 or HCO_3^- <4.

2. Metabolic Alkalosis:

In metabolic alkalosis, the pH is >7.40 and the HCO_3^- is high.

2.1. Clinical Evaluation:

A. NaCl responsive: Contraction alkalosis, vomiting, NG suction, villous adenoma, penicillin (large dose), diuretics, rapid correction of chronic hypercapnia (most common).
B. NaCl unresponsive: Mineralocorticoid excess in primary hyperaldosteronism, hyperreninism, licorice ingestion, Cushing's syndrome, Barter's syndrome, and adrenal hyperplasia.

2.2. RX:

A. For NaCl nonresistant cases:
- Support ABCs, IV, O_2, pulse oximeter, and monitor.
- Correct hypovolemia with NS.
- Correct hypokalemia with 20 to 40 mEq/L KCl, IV/po.

B. For NaCl resistant cases:
- Support ABCs, IV, O_2, pulse oximeter, and monitor.
- Start 20 to 40 mEq/L KCl IV/po.
- Consider giving spironolactone and/or acetazolamide to enhance HCO_3 excretion.
- Consult for dialysis as indicated for renal failure.

3. Respiratory Acidosis:

In respiratory acidosis the pH is <7.35 and the pCO_2 his high. In chronic lung disease the HCO_3^- will increase to compensation the persistently low pH.

- Acute: Expect increase $HCO_3^- = (CO_2)/10$.
- Chronic: Expect increase $HCO_3^- = (CO_2) \times 4.0$.

3.1. Clinical Evaluation:

Acute airway obstruction, lung disease, pleural effusions, pnuemothorax, thoracic cage abnormalities, hypoventilation, hypokalemia, hypophosphatemia, hypomagnesemia, and muscular dystrophy.

3.2. RX:

A. Support ABCs, IV, O_2, pulse oximeter, and monitor.
B. Improve alveolar ventilation and oxygenation by using bronchodilators, postural drainage, noninvasive, and invasive respiratory support, and antibiotics when necessary.
C. Metabolic acidosis may be coincident resulting from anaerobic metabolism.
D. Cautiously adjust oxygen supplements and assisted ventilatory rates in chronic acidosis to avoid CO_2 retention narcosis and posthypercapneic metabolic alkalosis, respectively.

4. Respiratory Alkalosis:

In respiratory alkalosis the pH is >7.35 and the pCO_2 (acute) is low. Over time, the HCO_3 decreases to compensate for the high pH.

- Acute: Expect HCO_3^- decrease $= pCO_2 \times 0.2$ (a drop of HCO_3^- of 2 for every decrease CO_2 of 10).
- Chronic: Expect HCO_3^- decrease $= pCO_2 \times 0.5$ (a drop of HCO_3^- of 5 for every decrease CO_2 of 10).

4.1. Clinical Evaluation:

Hyperventilation, anxiety, pain, cerebrovascular accident, head trauma, early sepsis, fevers, pulmonary embolism, congestive heart failure, pneumonia, interstitial lung disease, hepatic insufficiency, pregnancy, ASA toxicity, thyrotoxicosis, hypoxemia, and ventilation-induced.

4.2. RX:

Treat underlying problem.

5. Anion Gap Metabolic Acidosis:

Normal anion gap = Na − (HCO_3^- + Cl) (8–12 mEq/L).

A MUDPILE CAT.

A = alcohol

M = methanol

U = uremia

D = DKA

P = paraldehyde

I = iron and isoniazid

L = lactic acidosis

E = ethylene glycol, ethanol

C = carbon monoxide

A = aspirin

T = toluene

History and physical examination of the patient greatly assist in narrowing this list down. Also, a large anion gap, >35 mEq/L, is usually caused by ethylene glycol, methanol, or lactic acidosis. There are only three endogenous causes of an anion gap acidosis: Lactate, ketones, and uremia. All other causes are exogenous.

The "osmolar gap" can serve as an aid in diagnosing the onset of an anion gap acidosis. Osmolar gap is the difference between the measured osmolality and the calculated osmolarity.

Measured osmolality – calculated osmolarity = osmolar gap.

(Normal = 275–285 mOsm/L and normal gap <10 mOsm/L)

$$\textit{Calculated Osmol}\,(mOsm/L) = 2(Na) + \frac{glucose}{18} + \frac{BUN}{2.8}$$

5.1. Clinical Evaluation:

A. AMS with a high anion gap use the osmolar gap as a screening test for unmeasured osmoles, like methanol or ethylene glycol.
B. Isopropyl will cause a high osmolar gap but no anion gap.

6. Hyperkalemia:

Causes of hyperkalemia include acidosis, tissue necrosis, hemolysis, blood transfusion, GI bleed, renal failure, pseudohyperkalemia (leukocytosis), thrombocytosis, spironolactone, triamterene, amiloride, excess po potassium, RTA, high-dose penicillin, beta-blockers, captopril, laboratory error, and decreased mineralocorticoid activity, such as Addison's hypoaldosteronism. The ECG shows peaked T-waves, ST depression, diminished R-wave, prolonged PR interval, small p wave, sine waves, cardiac ventricular fibrillation, asystole, and cardiac arrest.

6.1. Clinical Evaluation:

A. Symptoms: Weakness, paresthesias, fatigue, cramps, paralysis.
B. Signs: Decreased DTRs, tetany, focal neuro deficits, dysrhythmias.
C. DDX: Hypocalcemia, pseudohyperkalemia, dehydration, Addison's disease.
D. Workup: CBC, BMP, ABG/VBG, calcium, magnesium, ECG.

6.2. RX:

A. Support ABCs, IV, O_2, pulse oximeter, and monitor.
B. Treat as follows:

- Calcium chloride, 10 mL of 10% solution, or 10 mL of 10% calcium gluconate, IV. If digitalis toxicity is suspected, administer over 30 minutes or omit entirely.
- $NaHCO_3$ 1 amp IV, only if acidotic.
- Regular insulin, 10 to 20 units IV.
- 1 amp 50% glucose (25 g), IV.
- Kayexalate (controversial), 15 to 30 g po/pr.
- Furosemide, 20 to 40 mg IV.

- Albuterol, 10 to 20 mg by nebulizer.
- Consider emergent dialysis for cardiac/pulm complications and renal failure.

C. Disposition: Admission to ICU for ECG changes, otherwise admit to monitored bed.

7. Hypernatremia:

- Excess free H_2O loss from renal (diabetes insipidus and osmotic diuresis); GI, skin, and respiratory origins.
- Inadequate free H_2O intake arising from coma, reset osmotic regulator, and poor po intake.
- Excess Na^+ gain from iatrogenic agents ($NaHCO_3$, hypertonic saline, and exogenous steroids), hyperaldosteronism, Cushing's, and congenital adrenal hyperplasia.
- Laboratory error.

7.1. Clinical Evaluation:

A. Symptoms: Headache, thirst, confusion, seizures, muscle irritability, weakness.
B. Signs: Orthostatic hypotension, ataxia, tachycardia, poor skin turgor, dry mucous membranes, seizures, coma.
C. Workup: CBC, BMP, LFTs, PT/PTT/INR, calcium, phosphate, magnesium, serum protein, UA, urine osmolality.

7.2. RX:

A. Support ABCs, IV, O_2, pulse oximeter, and monitor.
B. Rehydrate with NS starting with a 1-L bolus.
C. If severe CNS symptoms (seizure, coma), correct rapidly.
D. If correction is too rapid, CNS edema and seizures may result.
E. Body water deficit (L) = $(0.6 \times [\text{weight kg}] \times ([\text{serum Na}] - 140))/140$
F. Replete 30% over the first 24 hours.
G. Disposition: Most patients require admission.

8. Hypokalemia:

Hypokalemia is the most common electrolyte abnormality. The causes include alkalosis, insulin use, beta-2-agonist therapy, periodic paralysis, diuretics, low magnesium, Batter's, RTA, vomiting, diarrhea, pica, bile, and laboratory error. ECG finding includes T-wave flattening or inversion, U-wave prominence, ST-segment depression, and PVC's.

8.1. Clinical Evaluation:

A. Symptoms: Weakness, paresthesia, abdominal distention, polyuria, and paralysis.
B. Signs: Hyporeflexia, rhabdomyolysis, orthostatic hypotension, ileus, paralysis.
C. D/DX: Hypocalcemia, infection, ALS, Guillain–Barré syndrome, MS, botulism, myasthenia gravis.
D. Workup: CBC, BMP, calcium, magnesium, UA, ECG.

8.2. RX:

A. Support ABCs, IV, O_2, pulse oximeter, and monitor.
B. If serum potassium is >2.5 mEq/L and ECG changes are absent, treat with KCl, 10 to 20 mEq/h IV or 40 mEq po.
C. If potassium is <2.5 mEq/L and ECG abnormalities are present, treat with KCl, 30 to 40 IV mEq/h (prefer central line). May combine with 30 to 40 mEq po. 10 mEq will raise the K^+ by 0.1 mEq/L with a goal of >3.5 mEq/L.
D. Correct magnesium deficiency with 2 g IV over 20 to 30 minutes.
E. Disposition: Admit to the ICU for malignant cardiac dysrhythmias, digitalis toxicity, profound weakness, impending respiratory insufficiency, K^+ <2.0 mEq/L.

9. **Hyponatremia:**

- Hypovolemic hyponatremia is due to diuretic excess, mineralocorticoid deficiency, nephritis, RTA, ATN, vomiting, diarrhea, burns, pancreatitis, and traumatized muscle.
- Euvolemic hyponatremia is due to Addison's disease, hypothyroidism, pain, drugs (NSAIDs, TCA), SIADH secretion.
- Hypervolemic hyponatremia is due to CHF, cirrhosis, nephrotic syndrome, renal failure.
- Over aggressive correction may cause central pontine myelinolysis (CPM) (CN palsies, quadriplegia, or coma).

9.1. Clinical Evaluation:

A. **Symptoms:** Lethargy, apathy, disorientation, muscle cramps, anorexia, N/V, headache.
B. **Signs:** AMS, depressed DTRs, hypothermia, pseudobulbar palsy, seizures, and Cheyne–Stokes respiration.
C. **D/DX:** Cirrhosis, CHF, hypothyroidism, renal failure, SIADH, adrenal crisis, sepsis.
D. **Workup:** CBC, BMP, LFTs, PT/PTT/INR, calcium, magnesium, BNP, UA, ECG, CXR.

9.2. RX:

A. Support the ABCs, IV, O_2, pulse oximeter, and monitor.
B. If it develops slowly correct slowly. Goal is to raise $Na^+ > 125$.
C. If severe CNS symptoms (seizures, COMA), hypertonic saline 3%, 300 to 500 mL IV over 6 hours. Give Lasix 20 mg to lessen volume load.
D. Mild symptoms; restrict free water and give NS IV.
E. Over aggressive correction may cause osmotic demyelination syndrome formerly known as central pontine myelinolysis (CPM) (CN palsies, quadriplegia, or coma).
F. **Disposition:** Admit if $Na^+ < 130$, and to the ICU if Na^+ is < 120 or seizures or AMS exists.

NEUROLOGY

1. **Altered Mental Status and Coma:**

The history of present illness is often not available. This is the time to utilize friends, family, paramedics, nursing home staff and records, and family doctor. Obtaining a past medical history, social history, and use of medication, herbs, supplements, and drugs may help with the etiology.

1.1. Clinical Evaluation:

A. **Symptoms:** Progressive confusion, disorientation, stupor, obtundation, coma, ± fevers.
B. **Signs:**
  - Alcohol or fruity breath: Alcohol intoxication, DKA.
  - Young, healthy patient: overdose, intoxication.
  - Jaundice: Hepatic failure.
  - Petechial hemorrhage: ITP, DIC, leukemia, meningitis, and hepatic/renal failure.
  - Fecal/urine incontinence: Cerebrovascular accident, seizures, head injury.
  - Barrel chest/emphysematous, pursed lip breathing: Respiratory failure, hypercapnia.
  - Diaphoretic, cold, or hypothermic: Hypoglycemia, hypothermia, adrenal crisis, sepsis.
  - Tachypnea: Respiratory failure, acidosis.
  - Meningismus, Kernig's/Brudzinski's signs: Meningitis, sepsis, and subarachnoid hemorrhage.
  - Rhinorrhea, otorrhea, Battle's sign, raccoon's eyes: Basilar skull fracture.
  - Needle tracks: IV drug abuser/overdose.
  - Tongue laceration: Seizure.

C. **DDX:** AEIOU TIPS
  - A: Alcohol abuse.
  - E: Endocrine, encephalopathy, epilepsy, electrolyte.
  - I: Insulin (overdose, DKA, hypoglycemia).
  - O: Oxygen (lack of), opiates, overdose.

- U: Uremia.
- T: Trauma, temperature, tumors.
- I: Infection.
- P: Poisoning, psychiatric, pills.
- S: Shock, stroke, space-occupying lesions, SAH.

D. Workup: CBC, BMP, BNP, LFTs, CPK, PT/PTT/INR, ABG/VBG, calcium, phosphorus, blood cultures, UA, urine culture urine myoglobin, lactate, ETOH, urine drug screen, toxic alcohols, acetaminophen, salicylate, CT head as needed, CXR, ECG.

1.2. RX:

A. Support ABCs, IV, O_2, pulse oximeter, and monitor.
B. Bedside glucose test or D_{50}, 1 to 2 amp IV for adults. For children younger than 8 y/o give D_{25}, 0.5 to 1.0 g/kg IV.
C. Narcan, 0.4 to 2 mg IV.
D. Give specific antidotes based on clinical toxidrome.
E. Consider broad-spectrum antibiotics for suspected sepsis/meningitis.
F. Obtain the appropriate consult based on the condition.
G. Disposition: Admit patients with suspected prolonged detoxification, infection, trauma, intractable, or those seizing for the first time.

2. Cerebrovascular Accident (CVA):

Ischemic stroke accounts for 80% of strokes, and is due to a thrombotic or embolic occlusion of a cerebral artery. It is important to clearly determine the onset time to properly identify thrombolytic candidates.

2.1. Clinical Evaluation:

A. Symptoms: Weakness, paralysis, vertigo, aphasia, facial droop, AMS.
B. Signs:

- Middle cerebral artery: Contralateral hemiplegia where the upper extremity weakness > lower extremity, hemianesthesia, and homonymous hemianopsia. Contralateral conjugate gaze is affected. Aphasia with dominant hemispheric involvement is displayed.
- Anterior cerebral artery: Contralateral extremity weakness, lower > upper, gait apraxia, abulia, and incontinence.
- Posterior cerebral artery: Contralateral homonymous hemianopsia, hemiparesis, hemisensory, ipsilateral CN III, and memory loss.
- Vertebrobasilar artery: Ipsilateral CN, cerebellar ataxia, contralateral hemiplegia, and hemisensory loss, N/V, nystagmus, vertigo, and tinnitus/hearing loss.
- Basilar artery: Quadriplegia, upward gaze/"locked-in" syndrome.
- Cerebellar: Ataxia, especially with vermis infarct, vertigo, tinnitus, N/V, and nystagmus.
- Lacunar: Lipohyalinotic, cystic infarcts off penetrating cerebral arterioles within internal capsule. Specific syndromes include midpons–dysarthria/clumsy hand, pons/internal capsule—ataxia, leg paresis or pure motor hemiplegia, and thalamus—pure sensory syndrome.
- Transient global amnesia: Amygdaloid/hippocampus infarcts, commonly in patients older than 60 years, that last minutes to hours with complete resolution. Patient's somatic/speech, cognition, and long-term memory are intact during and after an episode, but the patient has no knowledge of event. Hemorrhagic events include subarachnoid and intracerebral. (Refer also the "Intracranial Hemorrhage" section.)

C. DDX: Concussion, epidural/subdural hematoma, cerebral contusion, neoplasm, infection, abscess, metabolic abnormalities (e.g., hyponatremia), toxidromes (narcotics, phenothiazines, cyclic antidepressants, cholinesterase inhibitors/pesticides), seizures, complex migraine, hypoglycemia.
D. Workup: CBC, BMP, LFTs, PT/PTT/INR, ESR, ABG/VBG, calcium, magnesium, ammonia, blood cultures, UA, urine culture, ± LP, CT head, ECG, CXR.

2.2. RX:

A. Support ABCs, IV, O_2, pulse oximeter, and monitor.
B. Control BP (SBP <185 mm Hg and DBP <110 mm Hg). Use labetalol 10 mg IV q 10 minutes or esmolol 500 μg/kg or nitroprusside 1 μg/kg/min.
C. Correct hypoglycemia if it exists.
D. Manage increased ICP if present.
E. Do the NIH stroke scale and review tPA inclusion/exclusion criteria.

Inclusion criteria for rt-PA Administration:

- Ischemic stroke.
- Presentation within 3 hours of symptom onset (ECASS III extended it to 4.5 hours).
- CT negative for hemorrhage.

Exclusion criteria:

- Substantial edema, mass effect or midline shift on CT scan.
- Intracranial surgery in past 3 months.
- Intracranial neoplasm.
- AV malformation or aneurysm.
- Uncontrolled hypertension >190 mm Hg systolic and >100 mm Hg diastolic.
- Subarachnoid hemorrhage or hx of ICH.
- Major surgery in the past 2 weeks.
- Platelet count <100,000.
- GI bleed in the past 3 weeks.
- Known bleeding diathesis and prolonged PT/PTT/INR.
- Heparin use within the last 48 hours.

3- to 4.5-hour exclusion criteria

- 80 y/o
- History of stroke with diabetes.
- All patients taking anticoagulation regardless of the INR.
- NIH stroke scale >25.

Obtain a neurology consult for possible use of thrombolytics.

Consult interventional radiology for possible intra-arterial tPA.

If you decide on thrombolytic therapy, the drug of choice is t-PA 0.9 mg/kg (maximum dose of 90 mg), 10% as a bolus dose, and the remainder given over 60 minutes.

Disposition: Admit to ICU if tPA given. All stable strokes admit to a monitored bed.

3. Temporal Arteritis:

Giant cell arteritis (temporal arteritis) is the most common systemic inflammatory vasculitis in older adults. The etiology is unknown and it most commonly affects superficial temporal arteries. The examination may a reveal a tender, pulseless temporal artery. Symptoms worsen with arterial compression. If a temporal artery is involved, there is a very high risk that a retinal artery is also involved which may lead to blindness. Do not misdiagnose this as a migraine! ESR is usually >50.

3.1. Clinical Evaluation:

A. **Symptoms:** Unilateral headache, facial pain, ± jaw/tongue pain, unilateral eye pain, ± vision changes, fatigue, malaise, fever, neck.
B. **Signs:** Tender pulseless temporal artery, ptosis, nystagmus, pupillary abnormality, CN abnormalities.
C. **DDX:** Glaucoma, iritis, uveitis, migraine headache, retinal artery occlusion, retinal vain occlusion, TIA.
D. **Workup:** CBC, BMP, ESR, CRP, color duplex US, consult for biopsy, CT head as needed.

3.2. RX:

A. Start steroids ASAP. Prednisone 50 mg po or solumedrol 125 mg IV.
B. Ophthalmology/rheumatology consult.
C. Control pain.
D. **Disposition:** Admit patients with severe symptoms. Outpatient management for minor symptoms.

4. Subarachnoid Hemorrhage (SAH):

SAH can be due to trauma, a ruptured aneurysm (80%), AVM, and dissection. The mortality rate is 10% to 15% before reaching medical care and 25% within the next 2 weeks. There is no combination of history and physical examination findings that rule out a SAH. Complications include hydrocephalus, rebleeding, vasospasm, seizures, and cardiac dysfunction.

4.1. Clinical Evaluation:

A. **Symptoms:** Headache (sudden onset, worst in life), sentinel headache, dizziness, orbital pain, neck pain, N/V, photophobia.
B. **Signs:** Seizures, focal neuro deficit, tachycardia, papilledema, retinal hemorrhage, fever, meningeal signs.

Grading scale for SAH:
- Grade I: Change in mental status, focal deficit, mild HA, and meningismus.
- Grade II: Mild change in mental status, some focal deficit, severe HA, and meningismus.
- Grade III: Major change in mental status or major focal deficit.
- Grade IV: Semicomatose or comatose.

C. **DDX:** Metabolic abnormality, meningitis, encephalitis, brain tumor or abscess, migraine, TIA, hypertensive intracranial hemorrhage, seizure.
D. **Workup:** CBC, BMP, PT/ PTT/INR, D-dimer, fibrinogen, FDP, T&S, ABG/VBG, cardiac enzymes, CXR, CT head, LP (if CT negative), consider CT angiography.

4.2. RX:

A. Support ABCs, IV, O_2, pulse oximeter, and monitor.
B. For evidence of elevated ICP or impending herniation, perform RSI.
C. Neurosurgical consult.
D. If not intubating, NPO, elevate head of bed
E. BP management: Titrate to SBP <150 mm Hg or DBP <90 mm Hg or within 5% of baseline. Esmolol 500 μg/kg bolus then 50 μg/kg/min drip **or** hydralazine, 10 to 20 mg IV **or** Labetalol, 20 mg IV q 10 minutes up to 300 mg.
F. Ventilate to a pCO_2 of 30 to 35 mm Hg, and consider mannitol, 1 g/kg.
G. Consider seizure prophylaxis with phenytoin 15 to 20 mg/kg IV.
H. Nimodipine 60 mg po to prevent vasospasm.
I. **Disposition:** Admit to the ICU.

5. Guillain–Barré Syndrome:

An acute idiopathic inflammatory demyelinating polyradiculoneuropathy characterized by a progressive motor weakness. This weakness starts distally in the legs and ascends to involve the trunk, upper extremities, and respiratory muscles. It usually occurs 1 to 2 weeks after a viral illness, especially gastroenteritis, and may require months to recover.

5.1. Clinical Evaluation:

A. **Symptoms:** Progressive motor weakness, numbness, dysphagia, tachypnea, dyspnea.
B. **Signs:** Decreased or absent DTRs, muscle weakness, CN abnormalities, motor weakness, tachycardia, orthostatic hypotension.
C. **DDX:** Tick paralysis, poliomyelitis, hypokalemia periodic paralysis, acute transverse myelitis, radiculopathies, polymyositis, botulism, tetanus, diphtheria, myasthenia gravis.

D. **Workup:** CBC, BMP, calcium, magnesium, CPK, LFTs, ABG, LP (high protein), ECG, CT/MRI head/spine as needed.

5.2. RX:

A. Support ABCs, IV, O_2, pulse oximeter, and monitor.
B. Consider IV IgG in consultation with neurology.
C. **Disposition:** Admit all suspected cases. Admit to the ICU if respiratory issues exist.

6. **Myasthenia Gravis:**

An autoimmune disease that attacks acetylcholine receptor at the neuromuscular junction. Destruction and poor neurotransmission at the motor end plate results in weakness and eventual respiratory failure. There are two types of myasthenic crises as described below.

- **Myasthenic:** Usually occurs in an undiagnosed patient with severe weakness resulting from a functional lack of acetylcholine. Administer edrophonium (Tensilon), 2 mg IV, followed by 8 mg IV slow, will improve symptoms.
- **Cholinergic:** Occurs in patients undergoing treatment for myasthenia with excess acetylcholine esterase (anticholinesterase). Severe muscle weakness occurs. Edrophonium increases symptoms! Examine for muscarinic symptom-SLUDGE. Administer atropine, 1 mg IV and prn, for bradycardia, low BP, wheezing/rales, or SLUDGE.

6.1. Clinical Evaluation:

A. **Symptoms:** Muscle weakness (worsened by prolonged activity), ocular ptosis (most common symptom), diplopia, blurred vision, tachypnea, dysphagia.
B. **Signs:** Ptosis, CN findings, motor weakness, diminished DTRs, tachypnea, tachycardia.
C. **DDX:** Eaton–Lambert syndrome, MS, thyroid disease, botulism, Guillain–Barré syndrome, tick paralysis, familial periodic paralysis, polymyositis, MS, ALS.
D. **Workup:** CBC, BMP, LFTs, ESR, CRP, ABG, thyroid studies, LP as needed, CXR, MRI/CT head (MS), CT chest (thymoma), electromyography (test of choice for diagnosis).

6.2. RX:

A. Support ABCs, IV, O_2, pulse oximeter, and monitor.
B. Consider BiPAP or intubation for even mild respiratory failure.
C. Give pyridostigmine 60 mg po.
D. Prednisone 50 to 100 mg po.
E. Treat fever as it exacerbated MG.
F. Consider IVIg and plasmapheresis in consult with neurology.
G. **Disposition:** Admit to the ICU.

7. **Cauda Equina Syndrome:**

This is a serious complication of lumbar disc disease resulting in compression of several lumbosacral nerve roots. It is characterized by neuromuscular and urogenital symptoms and may be irreversible if not operated on quickly. Other causes include a mass lesion, fracture with hematoma, and infection.

7.1. Clinical Evaluation:

A. **Symptoms:** Low back pain, sciatica, bowel and bladder complaints, muscle weakness, fever, saddle anesthesia, weight loss, night sweats.
B. **Signs:** Muscle weakness, decreased/absent sphincter tone, decreased DTRs, distended bladder, decreased sensation.
C. **DDX:** ALS, Guillain-Barré syndrome, multiple sclerosis, infection, acute transverse myelitis, radiculopathies, polymyositis, botulism, tetanus, myasthenia gravis.
D. **Workup:** CBC, BMP, calcium, magnesium, LFTs, blood cultures, PT/PTT/INR, LP, UA, ABG/VBG, MRI spine, CT spine, T&L spine x-rays.

7.2. RX:

- **A.** Support ABCs, IV, O_2, pulse oximeter, and monitor.
- **B.** If due to infection use antibiotics that cover for *S. aureus*.
- **C.** Neurosurgical consult.
- **D.** Consider steroids for severe paralysis in consultation with neurosurgery.
- **E.** Consult radiation oncology for radiation therapy if a cancerous lesion.
- **F.** **Disposition:** Admit all suspected cases. Admit to the ICU if respiratory issues exist.

8. Seizures:

Seizures result from excessive and disordered neuronal firing. They may be a primary disorder or secondary to an underlying medical condition (toxins, trauma, tumor, infection, fever, eclampsia). A detailed history is the most important factor in figuring out the etiology. Start antibiotics early if a fever exists, and stop the seizure first then make the diagnosis. Seizure categories are as follows:

- Partial (focal) seizures: Begin in a localized area of the brain is brief, and are without alteration of consciousness.
  - Complex partial: Involve the temporal lobe and present with AMS, confusion, hallucinations, automatisms and a postictal
  - Secondary generalized: Partial seizure that spreads throughout the brain causing a generalized seizure.
- Generalized seizure: Begin in both hemispheres and do not have an inciting focus. There is an associated AMS with a postictal period. Absence seizures are in this group.

8.1. Clinical Evaluation:

- **A.** **Symptoms:** Fever, AMS, Todd's paralysis (focal weakness/paralysis after seizure lasting up to several days), urine/stool incontinence, headache, myalgias, syncope.
- **B.** **Signs:** Head/facial abrasions, contusions, lacerations, tongue lacerations or bruising, AMS/coma, focal neuro deficits.
- **C.** **DDX:** Drug intoxication/withdrawal, hypoglycemia, hyper/hyponatremia, hypocalcemia, infection, TIA/CVA, syncope, cataplexy, narcolepsy, myoclonia, TBI, pseudoseizures.
- **D.** **Workup:** Glucose, CBC, BMP, LFTs, ammonia, PT/PTT/INR, beta-HCG (female), calcium, magnesium, ETOH, urine drug screen, UA, CPK, lactate, acetaminophen, salicylate, anticonvulsant levels, LP as needed, ECG, CXR, CT/MRI head as needed.

8.2. RX:

- **A.** Support ABCs, IV, O_2, pulse oximeter, elevate head of bed, roll on side, and monitor.
- **B.** Glucose check or give D_{50} IV.
- **C.** Give naloxone 2 to 4 mg IV.
- **D.** Acute seizure lasting >5 minutes, give a benzodiazepine (lorazepam, diazepam, midazolam).
- **E.** Start back on chronic medication if blood levels are subtherapeutic. Consider dosing alteration in consultation with neurology.
- **F.** Give pyridoxine (vitamin B6) for isoniazid overdose.
- **G.** Give thiamine 1 mg IV/IM/po, multivitamin, and magnesium 1 to 2 mg IV over 20 minutes, to those in withdrawal or at risk for a deficiency.
- **H.** Refer to the OB/GYN section for treatment of eclampsia.
- **I.** **Disposition:**
  - Admit status epilepticus patients to the ICU.
  - Discharge individuals with first-time seizures, negative workup, and no additional activity during 6 hours of observation. Obtain neurology follow-up in 24 to 48 hours for EEG and MRI. Provide instructions such as no driving, swimming, or other high-risk behavior.
  - Discharge patients with known seizure disorders not related to drug intoxication or withdrawal pending therapeutic anticonvulsant levels.
  - Observe patients with a question of drug intoxication/withdrawal as etiology for seizures for a minimum of 6 hours. There are no data currently available that supports a shorter length of stay.

9. Status Epilepticus:

Seizure lasting >5 minutes or recurrent seizures without resolution of postictal state. Typically seen in children <2 y/o and adults >60 y/o. Etiology 25% idiopathic, 25% febrile, 25% chronic (known seizure disorder), and 25% acute etiology (trauma, infection, tumor, toxin, metabolic).

9.1. Clinical Evaluation:

A. Symptoms: Fever, AMS, Todd's paralysis (focal weakness/paralysis after seizure lasting up to several days), urine/stool incontinence, headache, myalgias, syncope.
B. Signs: Head/facial abrasions, contusions, lacerations, tongue lacerations or bruising, AMS/coma, focal neuro deficits.
C. DDX: Drug intoxication/withdrawal, hypoglycemia, hyper/hyponatremia, hypocalcemia, infection, TIA/CVA, syncope, cataplexy, narcolepsy, TBI, pseudoseizures.
D. Workup: Glucose, CBC, BMP, LFTs, ammonia, PT/PTT/INR, beta-HCG (female), calcium, magnesium, ETOH, urine drug screen, ABG, UA, CPK, lactate, acetaminophen, salicylate, anticonvulsant levels, LP as needed, ECG, CXR, CT/MRI head as needed.

9.2. RX:

A. Support ABCs (low threshold for intubation), IV, O_2, pulse oximeter, elevate head of bed, roll on side, and monitor.
B. Glucose check or give D_{50} 1 amp IV.
C. Give naloxone 2 to 4 mg IV.
D. STOP THE SEIZURE.
E. Benzodiazepines are the first-line acute therapy lorazepam 1 to 2 mg IV or diazepam 5 to 10 mg IV/IM/pr or midazolam 0.05 to 0.2 mg/kg IV/IM.
F. Second-line acute therapy is phenytoin 15 to 20 mg/kg IV or fosphenytoin 15 to 20 mg IV/IM.
G. If seizure continues after above therapy, give phenobarbital 10 to 20 mg/kg IV or valproic acid 15 to 30 mg/kg IV or propofol 2 mg/kg loading dose then 0.1 to 0.2 mg/kg/min IV infusion.
H. If seizure persists, consider continuous infusion of pentobarbital or diazepam or midazolam, or inhaled isoflurane.
I. Give thiamine 1 mg IV/IM/po, multivitamin, and magnesium 1 to 2 mg IV over 20 minutes, to those in withdrawal or at risk for a deficiency.
J. Disposition: Admit to the ICU.

Pediatric Pearls

1. Parkland formula:	Weight (kg) × percent burn × 4 mL = 24-hour total (give half over the first 8 h followed by the other half over the next 16 h). Don't forget to add the hourly maintenance.
2. ETT size:	(16 + age)/4
3. Pediatric weight:	(Age × 3) + 6 = Wt in Kg
4. Pediatric BP:	<1year of age < 90 systolic BP >1year of age 80 + (2 × age) = Systolic BP Diastolic BP = two-thirds of the systolic BP
5. Pediatric fluid bolus:	20 mL/kg
6. Blood (PRBCs):	10 mL/kg in children

7. Fluid maintenance:	4 mL/kg/h	first 10 kg of weight			
	2 mL/kg/h	second 10 kg of weight			
	1 mL/kg/h	for each kg over 20			
8. Foley catheter and nasogastric tube sizes:	age	0–5 y	8 y	10 y	12 y
	size	5 F	8 F	10 F	12 F
9. Chest tube sizes:	age	0–6 y	6–10 y 1	0–12 y	
	size	10–20 F	0–30 F	30–38 F	
10. APGAR	(1) Appearance (0–2 points)				
	Pink (2)	Acrocyanotic (1)	Cyanotic (0)		
	(2) Pulse (0–2 points)				
	>100/min (2)	50–<100 (1)		<50 (0)	
	(3) Grimace				
	Present (2)	Weak (1)		None (0)	
	(4) Activity/tone (0–2 points)				
	Good (2)	Mild hypotonic (1)	None (0)		
	(5) Respiratory effort (0–2)				
	Good cry (2)	Weak effort (1)	None (0)		

PEDIATRICS

1. **Neonatal Resuscitation:**

Newborn resuscitation focuses almost entirely on management of airway and breathing because the majority of cardiorespiratory compromise is because of hypoxia. Bradycardia leading to asystole from hypoxemia causes the majority of cardiac dysrhythmias. V-tach/V-fib are rare but if present are usually due to a cardiac anomaly.

- Birth to 30 seconds
  - Immediately after delivery only suction the airway if an obvious obstruction is present or the infant is not responding with meconium-stained amniotic fluid.
  - Assess for breathing, heart rate, and crying.
  - Assess for color and muscle tone.
  - Dry newborn, provide tactile stimulation, and place in warmer.
  - If the heart rate is <100 and poor tone, intubate and suction.
  - If heart rate <60 despite adequate assisted ventilation for 30 seconds start CPR at a rate of 3:1
    - Check pulse at brachial or femoral artery.
    - Compress at lower half of sternum between nipples, two-thumb technique. Depth of one-third anteroposterior chest diameter with at least 100 compressions per minute.
- 30 to 60 seconds
  - APGAR: Appearance, pulse, grimace, activity, respiratory effort.
  - If heart rate >100 proceed to routine care.
  - If heart rate <100 clear airway, provide positive pressure ventilation at 40 to 60 breaths per minute with bag-valve-mask.
  - Give supplemental O_2.
- 5 minutes
  - APGAR at 5 minutes.
  - If poor respiratory effort or bradycardia, intubate and give positive pressure ventilation. Use a 2.5 to 3.5 uncuffed ETT.

1.1. Common Drug Doses:

- Epinephrine, 0.01 to 0.03 mg/kg 1:10,000 IV/IO.
- Atropine, 0.02 mg/kg (min 0.1 mg).
- Naloxone, 0.1 mg/kg IV/IO/ET/IM/sq.
- $NaHCO_3^-$, 0.5 mEq/mL IV/IO.
- D_{10} 2 g/kg IV/IO (glucose <40 mg/dL).
- Fluid bolus 10 mL/kg NS or LR over 10 minutes.

2. Pediatric Resuscitation:

Review and know the PALS algorithms. Start all assessments by practicing universal precautions and have a Broselow tape available.

2.1. Airway:

A. ETT size = (16 + age)/4 or size of little finger. Use a straight blade for <6 y/o. Cuffed tubes are appropriate at all ages. Tube depth is 3× the tube size (cm).
B. Premedication: Atropine 0.01 mg/kg IV (min dose 0.1 mg).
C. RSI medications: Paralytic—Succinylcholine 1 to 2 mg/kg or vecuronium or rocuronium. Sedating agent of choice (etomidate, midazolam, ketamine).
D. Confirm placement: Listen, CXR, end tidal CO_2 monitor.
E. Cricothyroidotomy is contraindicated in children <10 y/o, perform needle cricothyroidotomy.

2.2. RX:

A. Common Drug Doses:

- Adenosine 0.1 mg/kg IV/IO rapid push. Second dose 0.2 mg/kg IV/IO rapid push.
- Epinephrine 0.01 mg/kg 1:10,000 IV/IO.
- Epinephrine 0.1 mg/kg 1:1000 ET.
- Epinephrine 0.01 mg/kg 1:1000 IM for anaphylaxis q 15 minutes.
- Atropine 0.02 mg/kg (min 0.1 mg, max 0.5 mg child, 1.0 mg adolescent).
- Lidocaine 1 mg/kg, repeat up to 3 mg/kg.
- Amiodarone 5 mg/kg IV.
- Naloxone 0.01 mg/kg.
- D_{50} 0.5 to 1 g/kg IV/IO.
- D_{25} 2 to 4 mL/kg IV/IO.
- $NaHCO_3^-$, 1 mEq/kg of 8.4% solution IV or IO.
- $NaHCO_3^-$, 0.5 mEq/mL solution for neonates.
- Epinephrine, 0.1 to 1.0 μg/kg/min.
- Isoproterenol, 0.1 to 1.0 μg/kg/min.
- Lidocaine, 20 to 50 μg/kg/min.
- NAVEL drugs can go down the ET tube, such as lidocaine, atropine, naloxone, epinephrine, and valium or versed.

2.3. Algorithms

A. Asystole:

- Start CPR (hard and fast 100/min).
- IV/IO access.
- Consider an advanced airway.
- Give epinephrine, 0.01 mg/kg of 1:10,000 IV/IO, repeat 3 to 5 minutes.
- Treat reversible causes.
- Confirm asystole in two leads and/or US of the heart before terminating code.

B. Bradycardia:
- Identify and treat underlying cause.
- Support ABCs, IV/IO access, O_2, pulse oximeter, monitor.
- ECG if available, do not delay therapy.
- For cardiopulmonary compromise (heart rate <60, poor perfusion despite oxygenation and ventilation), start CPR.
- Administer atropine, 0.02 mg/kg (minimum 0.1 mg). Repeat one time.
- Start epinephrine, 0.01 mg/kg of 1:10,000 IV/IO q 3 to 5 minutes, or 0.1 mg/kg 1:1000 ET, if IV/IO not available.
- Consider pacing.

C. PEA:
- Start CPR (hard and fast 100/min).
- IV/IO access.
- Consider an advanced airway.
- Give epinephrine, 0.01 mg/kg of 1:10,000 IV/IO or epinephrine, 0.1 mg/kg of 1:1,000 ETT q 3 to 5 minutes.
- Identify and treat cause (6 Hs, 5Ts) hypoxia, hypovolemia, hydrogen ion (acidosis, hypo/hyperkalemia, hypoglycemia, hypothermia, toxins, tension pneumothorax, tamponade, thrombosis (PE, MI), trauma.

D. SVT:
- Support ABCs, IV/IO access, O_2, pulse oximeter, monitor, search, and treat cause.
- ECG if available, do not delay therapy.
- Consider vagal maneuvers.
- If unstable, sedate and synchronize cardiovert at 0.5 to 1 J/kg. If not effective cardiovert at 2 J/kg.
- Give adenosine 0.1 mg/kg rapid IV/IO. If not effective, give 0.2 mg/kg IV/IO.

E. V-fibrillation/pulseless V-tachycardia:
- Start CPR (hard and fast 100/min).
- Shock, 2 J/kg.
- CPR for 2 minutes, IV/IO access.
- Rhythm check and shock at 4 J/kg.
- CPR for 2 minutes. Consider an advanced airway.
- Give epinephrine, 0.01 mg/kg of 1:10,000 IV/IO.
- Rhythm check and shock at 4 J/kg.
- CPR for 2 minutes, give amiodarone 5 mg/kg IV/IO (may repeat two more times).
- Treat reversible causes.

F. V-tachycardia, stable:
- Support ABCs, IV/IO access, O_2, pulse oximeter, monitor, search, and treat cause.
- ECG if available, do not delay therapy.
- Consider adenosine 0.1 mg/kg rapid IV/IO. If not effective, give 0.2 mg/kg IV/IO.
- Give amiodarone or procainamide.

3. Acute Life-Threatening Event (ALTE):

ALTE is also known as infant apnea and is characterized by some combination of apnea, color change, change in muscle tone, and a choking episode. There is no correlation with SIDS, and the challenge is to make the diagnosis based on history. Possible causes include GERD, central apnea, cardiac arrhythmia, seizure disorder, child abuse, sepsis, or obstructive sleep apnea.

3.1. Clinical Evaluation:

A. Symptoms: Infant found unconscious, unresponsive, ± cyanosis, and apneic. Patient aroused spontaneously or via tactile stimulation. ± history of recent URI, and gastroenteritis, vomit on clothing or bed.

B. Signs: Unconscious, unresponsive, apneic, ± cyanotic, wheezing, murmur, bulging fontanelle, rash, extremity deformity. Examination is usually normal.

C. DDX: Seizure, hypoglycemia, sepsis, meningitis, cardiomyopathy, apnea, arrhythmia, botulism.
D. Workup: CBC, BMP, CRP, ABG/VBG, UA, urine culture, blood cultures, LP as needed, CXR, skeletal survey, CT head as needed, carboxyhgb, ECG.

3.2. RX:

A. Support ABCs, IV/IO, O_2, pulse oximeter, and monitor.
B. For toxic-appearing child start antibiotics.
C. Disposition: Admit for monitoring and further workup. Transfer if the facility has no pediatric ICU.

4. Bronchiolitis:

Bronchiolitis is an infection of the lower airways most commonly due to respiratory syncytial virus (RSV). It usually occurs during the winter in infants 3 to 12 m/o. The presentation can vary from a minor URI to severe respiratory distress. Age (<8 weeks), and comorbidities (prematurity, congenital heart/lung disease), are important historical features.

4.1. Clinical Evaluation:

A. Symptoms: Poor appetite, dyspnea, rhinorrhea, cough, fever, apnea.
B. Signs: Tachypnea, tachycardia, fever, wheezing, intercostal retractions, hypoxia, grunting, post-tussive emesis.
C. DDX: Asthma, pneumonia, cystic fibrosis, croup, FB aspiration.
D. Workup: CBC, BMP, nasal swab for RSV, ABG as needed, CXR (peribronchiolar cuffing, hyperinflation).

4.2. RX:

A. Support ABCs, IV/IO, O_2, pulse oximeter and monitor as needed.
B. Steroid and bronchodilators have no evidence of usefulness.
C. Antibiotics are not indicated unless signs of an infection exist (WBC >15,000, infiltrate on CXR, positive UA).
D. Disposition: Admit for hypoxia, toxic appearance, moderate/severe respiratory distress, apnea, unreliable caretaker, premature, age <6 weeks, poor feeding, and social reasons.

5. Fever 0 to 28 days:

Fever is the most common pediatric chief complaint and is defined as a rectal temperature >100.4°F (38.0°C). Evaluation and disposition are determined by age, medical conditions (cancer, immunosuppression), and immunization status. The most common serious bacterial organisms arise from maternal vaginal flora. An immature immune system along with being unvaccinated places these newborn at significant risk. In the first 2 weeks the common organisms are group B *strep*, *E. coli*, *L. monocytogenes*, HSV, and *C. pneumoniae*. Between 2 weeks and 28 days, group B *Strep* and *E. coli* predominate.

5.1. Clinical Evaluation:

A. Symptoms: Fever, vomiting, diarrhea, poor feeding, seizure, dehydration, lethargy, irritability, apnea, respiratory distress, grunting respirations.
B. Signs: Bulging fontanelle, poor skin turgor, rash (petechial, vesicles), umbilical redness (omphalitis), jaundice, cyanosis, tachycardia, tachypnea.
C. DDX: Herpes encephalitis, UTI, pneumonia, meningitis, RSV, gastroenteritis with dehydration, congenital heart disease, hypoglycemia, child abuse, metabolic derangement.
D. Workup: CBC, BMP, LFTs, blood culture, LP, UA, urine culture, herpes culture, CXR, stool for WBC and culture.

5.2. RX:

A. Support ABCs, IV/IO, O_2, pulse oximeter, and monitor.
B. If dehydrated, give NS 20 mL/kg IV/IO, over 20 minutes.
C. Give empiric antibiotics: Ampicillin 50 mg/kg IV + gentamicin 2.5 mg/kg IV or cefotaxime 50 mg/kg q 12 hours.
D. Give acyclovir if HSV is suspected.
E. Disposition: Admit all patients for continued antibiotic therapy and further workup.

6. Fever 29 to 90 days:

Evaluation and disposition of this group is more controversial. The immune system is still not fully competent, so a high index of suspicion for severe infection should be the rule. *H. influenzae* B, *N. meningitides*, *S. pneumoniae*, and enterovirus are the most common organisms. It requires at least two doses of HIB vaccine before you can be considered at low risk for invasive disease.

6.1. Clinical Evaluation:

A. Symptoms: Fever, vomiting, diarrhea, poor feeding, seizure, dehydration, lethargy, irritability, apnea, respiratory distress, grunting respirations.
B. Signs: Bulging fontanelle, poor skin turgor, rash (petechial), hypotension, cyanosis, tachycardia, tachypnea, hypotonia.
C. DDX: Encephalitis, UTI, pneumonia, meningitis, RSV, gastroenteritis with dehydration, congenital heart disease, hypoglycemia, child abuse, metabolic derangement.
D. Workup: CBC, BMP, LFTs, blood culture, PT/PTT/INR, LP, UA, urine culture, CXR, stool for WBC and culture, risk stratify with Philadelphia criteria or Rochester criteria.
- Philadelphia criteria: **Age** 29 to 60 days, **temp** >100.7°F (38.2°C), **well appearing**, **normal PE**, **WBC**, 15,000, **band/neutrophil ratio** <0.2, **UA** normal, **CSF** normal, **CXR** normal, **Stool** normal.
- Rochester criteria: **Age** <60 days, **temp** >100.4°F (38°C), **well appearing**, **normal PE**, **WBC** >5,000 and <15,000, **absolute band count** <1500, **UA** <10 WBC/HPF, **Stool** normal.

6.2. RX:

A. Support ABCs, IV/IO, O_2, pulse oximeter, and monitor as needed.
B. If dehydrated, give NS 20 mL/kg IV/IO, over 20 minutes.
C. If at least one screening test is positive give antibiotics:
- UTI/pyelonephritis: Ampicillin 50 mg/kg IV + gentamicin 2.5 mg/kg IV.
- Pneumonia: Ceftriaxone 50 to 100 mg/kg IV/IM.
- Meningitis: Ampicillin 50 mg/kg IV + ceftriaxone 50 to100 mg/kg IV/IM, + vancomycin 15 mg/kg IV, and/or gentamicin 2.5 mg/kg IV.

D. Disposition: If the septic workup and screening criteria are negative; consider a single dose of ceftriaxone 50 mg/kg IV/IM (if LP performed), and discharge with follow-up within 24 hours. Toxic-appearing or meningitic infants require admit with empiric antibiotics described above.

7. Fever 3 to 36 months:

Fever in this group is more commonly due to a virus than a bacterium. The common bacterial pathogens are *S. pneumoniae*, *E. coli*, and *N. meningitides*. The immune system is more competent and evaluation is tailored to clinical presentation, temperature, and vaccine status. The history and physical examination are more reliable in making an accurate diagnosis in the ED. A UTI is the most common bacterial infection in this age group.

7.1. Clinical Evaluation:

A. Symptoms: Fever, vomiting, diarrhea, poor feeding, seizure, dehydration, lethargy, irritability, apnea, respiratory distress, grunting respirations.
B. Signs: Poor skin turgor, rash (petechial), hypotension, cyanosis, tachycardia, tachypnea, hypotonia, bulging fontanelle, abdominal pain to palpation, abnormal breath sounds, meningeal signs.
C. DDX: Viral URI, otitis media, roseola, bronchitis, croup, UTI, pneumonia, meningitis, RSV, gastroenteritis with dehydration, pyelonephritis, intussusception, epiglottitis, metabolic derangement.
D. Workup: CBC, BMP, LFTs, blood culture, PT/PTT/INR, LP, UA, urine culture, CXR, stool for WBC and culture.

7.2. RX:

A. Support ABCs, IV/IO, O_2, pulse oximeter, and monitor as needed.
B. If dehydrated, give NS 20 mL/kg IV/IO, over 20 minutes.

C. If patient appears toxic do a full septic workup and give empiric antibiotics:
   - Toxic patient: Cefotaxime 50 mg/kg IV + vancomycin 15 mg/kg IV or ceftriaxone + vancomycin.
   - UTI/pyelonephritis: Ceftriaxone 50 mg/kg IV/IM.
   - Pneumonia: Ceftriaxone 50 to 100 mg/kg IV/IM.
   - Meningitis: Ceftriaxone (or cefotaxime) 50 to 100 mg/kg IV/IM + vancomycin 15 mg/kg IV. Consider dexamethasone 0.15 mg/kg IV/IM.

D. **Disposition:** If the septic workup is negative and the patient does not appear toxic, consider a single dose of ceftriaxone 50 mg/kg IV/IM, and discharge with follow-up within 24 hours. Admit toxic-appearing or meningitic patients and give empiric antibiotics described above.

8. Laryngotracheobronchitis (Croup):

This is a common illness of the upper airway in children age 3 months to 5 y/o, caused by parainfluenza, adenovirus, RSV, and rhinovirus. Croup presents as a barking cough, in middle of the night, which gets much better on the trip to the ED.

8.1. Clinical Evaluation:

A. **Symptoms:** Sudden onset of fever, barking cough, rhinorrhea, inspiratory stridor, hoarseness, respiratory distress, agitation.

B. **Signs:** Wheezing, stridor, intercostal retractions, fever, tachycardia, tachypnea, cyanosis.

C. **DDX:** Epiglottitis, inhalation injury, peritonsillar abscess, bacterial tracheitis, mononucleosis, diphtheria, epiglottitis, airway FB.

D. **Workup:** CBC, ABG (respiratory fatigue), nasal swab for RSV, influenza, AP neck x-ray (steeple sign), CXR (FB), lateral C-spine (concern for epiglottitis).

8.2. RX:

A. Support ABCs, pulse oximeter, O_2, and monitor as needed.

B. Treat symptomatic patients with blow-by humidified O_2.

C. Start racemic epinephrine 0.5 mL of 2.25% solution, in 4 mL NS, via nebulizer.

D. Give all patients with croup dexamethasone 0.15 mg/kg IV/IM/po.

E. RSI for a patient with severe disease that does not respond to therapy. Consider using an ETT 0.5 size smaller than normal.

F. **Disposition:** Observe all patients that require racemic epinephrine for 2 to 6 hours. Admit patients who do not respond to therapy or appear dehydrated. Most patients can be discharged with close follow-up.

9. Orbital/Periorbital Cellulitis:

Orbital cellulitis is an infection of the soft tissues of the orbit posterior to the orbital septum, and is most common in children. The most likely cause is direct extension of an infection from the ethmoids sinuses (90% of cases). The most common organisms include *Streptococcus* species, *S. aureus*, and *H. influenzae*. Periorbital (preseptal) cellulitis is an infection of the soft tissue of the eyelids and periocular area anterior to the orbital septum. This is most commonly due to *S. aureus* (MRSA, MSSA), *S. epidermidis, Streptococcus* species, and anaerobes. Approximately 10% of patients will sustain permanent visual loss with orbital cellulitis.

9.1. Clinical Evaluation:

A. **Symptoms:** Unilateral eye lid swelling and pain, diplopia, rhinorrhea, visual loss.

B. **Signs:** Fever, periorbital erythema, edema, warmth, and tenderness, closure of palpebral fissure, mucopurulent discharge, orbital chemosis, proptosis, ophthalmoplegia, pupillary sluggishness or paralysis, decreased VA, pain with EOM movement.

C. **DDX:** Orbital versus periorbital cellulitis, allergy, trauma, orbital abscess, cavernous sinus thrombosis, neoplasm, thyroid ophthalmopathy, bug bite.

D. **Workup:** CBC, BMP, blood cultures, CT orbits, measure IOP.

9.2. RX:

A. IV NS bolus if needed.
B. For periorbital cellulitis consider a second- or third-generation cephalosporin.
C. For orbital cellulitis may use nafcillin + metronidazole or ticarcillin-clavulanate or nafcillin + ceftazidine. Consider adding vancomycin is suspect MRSA.
D. Obtain an immediate ophthalmologic consultation.
E. **Disposition:** Admit children and all but the mildest adult cases.

10. Retropharyngeal Abscess:

This is a mixed flora infection posterior to the pharynx, more commonly seen in children 3 to 5 y/o. The high mortality rate is due to the complications like airway obstruction, mediastinitis, aspiration pneumonia, epidural abscess, jugular venous thrombosis, and sepsis. The disease is most commonly due to trauma (falling onto popsicle/lollipop stick), or an upper respiratory infection.

10.1. Clinical Evaluation:

A. **Symptoms:** Sore throat, dysphagia, trismus, stridor, neck pain, nuchal rigidity, fever, toxic appearing, and drooling.
B. **Signs:** Hyponasal voice, noisy breathing, toxic appearance, dehydration, stiff and painful neck, redness, or swelling to the pharyngeal wall.
C. **DDX:** Pharyngitis, FB, epiglottitis, croup, tonsillar abscess, submandibular abscess, parapharyngeal abscess, Ludwig's angina, diphtheria.
D. **Workup:** CBC, BMP, ESR, CRP, throat culture, blood cultures, lateral C-spine x-ray (prevertebral soft tissue swelling), CT neck as needed.

10.2. RX:

A. Support ABCs, IV, O_2, pulse oximeter, and monitor.
B. Airway, including cricothyrotomy set at the bedside.
C. ENT consult for surgical I&D.
D. Give a cephalosporin or ampicillin/sulbactam or nafcillin + clindamycin.
E. Consider dexamethasone 10 mg IV.
F. **Disposition:** Admit, either to ICU or directly to the OR.

11. Meningitis:

Meningitis is an infection or inflammation of the meninges caused by a virus, bacteria, fungi, or autoimmune phenomena. Meningitis is caused by a variety of pathogens that have the potential of infecting different age groups.

11.1. Clinical Evaluation:

A. **Symptoms:** Headache, fever, nuchal rigidity, photophobia, N/V, AMS, irritability, coma, lethargy, hypothermia, poor feeding, hypotonia, shrill cry.
B. **Signs:** Fever, Kernig's + Brudzinski's signs, papilledema, petechial, hyperreflexia, AMS, seizure, cranial nerve or other focal neurologic deficits, bulging fontanelle, paradoxic irritability, jaundice, hypotonia.
C. **DDX:** Viral syndromes, encephalitis, brain abscess, lead encephalopathy, sepsis, seizures, brain tumor.
D. **Workup:** CBC, BMP, LFTs, CRP, PT/PTT/INR, blood cultures, UA, urine culture, CXR, CT/MRI brain as needed, LP (cell count, culture, Gram stain, protein, glucose, viral PCR).

11.2. RX:

A. Support ABCs, IV, O_2, pulse oximeter, monitor, and start antibiotics immediately.
B. Give NS 20 mL/kg bolus over 20 minutes, may repeat prn hypotension or dehydration.
C. Neonate (0–1 m/o): Group B *Strep.* (70%), *L. monocytogenes* (20%), *E. coli* (10%). Give ampicillin 50 mg/kg IV + cefotaxime 50 mg/kg IV or gentamicin 2.5 mg/kg IV. Consider empiric coverage with acyclovir 20 mg/kg IV, for HSV.

D. Infant/child (1 month–12 y/o): *S. pneumoniae*, *N. meningitidis*, *H. influenzae* (unvaccinated). Give ceftriaxone 50 mg/kg IV + vancomycin 15 mg/kg IV. Consider dexamethasone 0.15 mg/kg IV, before the first dose of antibiotic.
E. Adolescent: *N. meningitidis* and *S. pneumoniae*. Give ceftriaxone 50 mg/kg IV + vancomycin 15 mg/kg IV. Consider dexamethasone 0.15 mg/kg IV, before the first dose of antibiotic.
F. Treat seizures with a benzodiazepine and phenytoin.
G. **Disposition:** Admit to the ICU, if necessary.

12. Kawasaki Disease (Mucocutaneous Lymph Node Syndrome):

Medium vessel vasculitis of unknown etiology leading to coronary artery aneurysms, pericarditis, and dysrhythmias if not treated. For diagnosis the child must have a 5-day history of fever, plus 4 of the following: mucous membrane changes, cracked red lips, strawberry tongue, pharyngeal erythema, conjunctival injection, morbilliform or maculopapular rash, peripheral edema, erythema hands/feet, desquamation of hand/feet, unilateral cervical lymphadenopathy.

12.1. Clinical Evaluation:

A. **Symptoms:** Fever, conjunctival injection, rash, edema, cough, irritability, abdominal pain, headache, arthralgias.
B. **Signs:** Fever, polymorphous rash, cervical lymphadenopathy, friction rub, possible meningeal signs, mucous membrane abnormalities, strawberry tongue, jaundice, hepatomegaly.
C. **DDX:** Toxic shock syndrome, RMSF, TEN, measles, SSSS, scarlet fever.
D. **Workup:** CBC, BMP, LFTs, PT/PTT/INR, ESR, CRP, cardiac enzymes, blood cultures, UA, ECG, cardiac echo as needed, CXR.

12.2. RX:

A. Support ABCs, IV, O_2, pulse oximeter, and monitor.
B. Give IVIG 2 g/kg over 12 hours.
C. Give aspirin 80 to100 mg/kg/d po, q 6 hours.
D. Treat fever and pain.
E. Consult cardiology for echo.
F. **Disposition:** Admit all patients to monitored bed. Admit to PICU for abnormal ECG, large coronary artery aneurysms, or AMI.

13. Pyloric Stenosis:

Pyloric stenosis is the most common cause of gastric outlet obstruction in infants and the etiology is unknown. The classic presentation is a 3 to 6 w/o infant with nonbilious, postprandial vomiting. Vomiting increases in frequency and force (projectile), leading to profound dehydration. Hypokalemic, hypochloremic, metabolic alkalosis are the classic electrolyte findings.

13.1. Clinical Evaluation:

A. **Symptoms:** Fussy, weight loss, dry mucous membranes, lethargic, vomiting.
B. **Signs:** Palpable "olive" in RUQ, weight loss, poor skin turgor.
C. **DDX:** Gastroenteritis, volvulus, esophagitis, GERD, duodenal atresia, UTI, hiatal hernia.
D. **Workup:** CBC, BMP, LFTs, PT/PTT/INR, UA, abdominal ultrasound (4 mm pyloric thickness), barium swallow (string or beak sign).

13.2. RX:

A. Support ABCs, IV, O_2, pulse oximeter, and monitor.
B. Give NS, 20 mL/kg bolus over 20 minutes then reassess hydration status, repeat if needed.
C. NPO.
D. Consider K^+ replacement if needed.
E. Consult surgery
F. **Disposition:** Admit for surgical correction. Admit to PICU if unstable after fluid rehydration.

14. Intussusception:

Intussusception occurs when a proximal portion of bowel telescopes into a distal portion. The classic triad is intermittent, severe, colicky abdominal pain, vomiting, and currant jelly stools. The pain is sudden and severe and resolves spontaneously. The typical age is 6 to 18 months, and it is the most common cause of a bowel obstruction between 3 to 12 m/o.

14.1. Clinical Evaluation:

- **A. Symptoms:** Vomiting, intermittent abdominal pain, hematochezia, lethargy, low-grade fever.
- **B. Signs:** Pallor, abdominal pain to palpation, hemoccult + stool.
- **C. DDX:** Gastroenteritis, Mekel's diverticulum, appendicitis, volvulus, incarcerated hernia, testicular/ovarian torsion.
- **D. Workup:** CBC, BMP, LFTs, PT/PTT/INR, UA, abdominal ultrasound, KUB (crescent sign), barium, or air enema.

14.2. RX:

- **A.** Support ABCs, IV, O_2, pulse oximeter, and monitor.
- **B.** Give NS, 20 mL/kg IV bolus over 20 minutes then reassess hydration status, repeat if needed.
- **C.** NPO and NG tube.
- **D.** Surgical consult.
- **E.** Barium/air enema.
- **F. Disposition:** Admit to surgical service even if reduced on barium/air enema.

15. Volvulus:

A malrotation of the midgut causing it to twist on itself, leading to a bowel obstruction and vascular compromise. The majority of cases occur within the first month of life and bilious vomiting is the hallmark finding. Bilious vomiting in an infant is always considered serious and requires a surgical consult, even if the patient appears nontoxic.

15.1. Clinical Evaluation:

- **A. Symptoms:** Fussy, bilious vomiting, sudden onset abdominal pain, feeding intolerance, constipation/diarrhea.
- **B. Signs:** Abdominal distention, bloody stools, abdominal mass, shock, jaundice.
- **C. DDX:** Gastroenteritis, intussusception, hernia, pyloric stenosis, peritonitis, NEC, duodenal atresia, Hirschsprung's disease.
- **D. Workup:** CBC, BMP, LFTs, PT/PTT/INR, UA, hemoccult stool, KUB (bowel overriding liver, double bubble-sign), abdominal ultrasound, Upper GI (test of choice).

15.2. RX:

- **A.** Support ABCs, IV, O_2, pulse oximeter, and monitor.
- **B.** Give NS, 20 mL/kg bolus over 20 minutes then reassess hydration status, repeat if needed.
- **C.** GI decompression with NG tube.
- **D.** Consider starting triple antibiotics (ampicillin, clindamycin, gentamicin).
- **E.** Consult surgery STAT.
- **F. Disposition:** Admit for surgical correction. Admit to PICU if unstable after fluid rehydration.

16. Slipped Capital Femoral Epiphysis (SCFE):

SCFE is a posterior and inferior displacement of the proximal femoral epiphysis on the metaphysis. The typical patient is an obese, adolescent who can walk (stable SCFE), or is unable to walk (unstable SCFE). The greater the degree of slippage, the greater the pain and risk of complications (avascular necrosis, nonunion).

16.1. Clinical Evaluation:

A. **Symptoms:** Pain in hips for <3 weeks, pain with passive motion, unable to bear weight, obese.
B. **Signs:** External rotational deformity, limited ROM, shortening of leg, antalgic gait (unilateral disease), Trendelenburg gait (bilateral disease)
C. **DDX:** Muscle strain, transient synovitis, osteomyelitis, septic joint, hip/femur fracture.
D. **Workup:** CBC, BMP, ESR, CRP, AP/lateral/frog leg views of hip, CT/MRI if high clinical suspicion with negative x-ray.

16.2. RX:

A. Treat pain.
B. No weight bearing; crutches, wheelchair, bed rest.
C. Ortho consult.
D. **Disposition:** Discharge with next day follow-up unless it is the acute form.

PULMONARY

Airway Management and Intubation

There is no single guideline for managing the airway. Differences in clinical presentation and condition, patient anatomy, and physician and institution practices mandate that airway management be individually customized. The following are rational indications: hypercapnia, agonal shallow respirations, apnea, hypoxia, AMS, GCS <8, absent gag reflex, impending airway obstruction (angioedema), impending respiratory failure, and the uncooperative trauma patient with life-threatening injuries.

1. Orotracheal Intubation:

A. Asses for a difficult airway.
   - **LEMON** rule
     - ☐ Look externally: Small mandible, large tongue, short neck.
     - ☐ Evaluate 3–3–2 rule. Three fingers between teeth, 3 finger breadths between hyoid and mentum, 2 finger breadths between hyoid and thyroid cartilage.
     - ☐ Mallampati score: Class 1, see oropharynx; class 4, see nothing.
     - ☐ Obstruction: Difficulty swallowing, stridor, muffled (hot potato) voice.
     - ☐ Neck mobility: Stiff neck affects visualization of the glottis opening.

B. ETT size (interior diameter):
   - Women: 7.0 to 9.0 mm.
   - Men: 7.5 to 10.0 mm.
   - Peds: (Age + 16)/4 mm.

C. Prepare equipment, including suction, O_2, bag-valve-mask, ET tubes, bougie, video laryngoscopy equipment, cricothyrotomy or needle-jet equipment, CO_2 indicator, laryngoscope, and pulse oximeter.

D. If sedation and/or paralysis is required, prepare all meds, including those required for a rapid sequence induction, if so planned. These may include:
   - Fentanyl (Sublimaze), 1 to 5 μg/kg.
   - Midazolam (Versed), 0.2 mg/kg IV.
   - Ketamine 1 to 2 mg/kg IV.
   - Atropine, 0.02 mg/kg pretreatment in patients <10 y/o.
   - Etomidate 0.3 mg/kg IV over 30 seconds;
     - ☐ Vecuronium, 0.015 mg/kg defasciculating dose, and 0.1 mg/kg paralytic dose.
   - Succinylcholine, 1.5 mg/kg. There is a risk for vomiting and aspiration; therefore, apply cricoid cartilage pressure as soon as the patient is unable to protect airway (Sellick maneuver). Considerable expertise is required for use of paralyzing agents and rapid sequence intubation.

E. Position patient's head in a "sniffing" position with head flexed at lower neck and extended at the occiput.
F. Preoxygenate by allowing patient to breathe 100% oxygen. Avoid unnecessary gastric filling by minimizing assisted bag-valve-mask ventilation.
G. Hold laryngoscope handle with the left hand. Insert along the right side of mouth to the base of tongue and push tongue to the left. Advance to the vallecula (superior to epiglottis, if using curved blade) and lift anteriorly. If a straight blade is used, place it beneath the epiglottis and lift anteriorly.
H. Intubate until cuff disappears behind vocal cords. If unsuccessful after 30 seconds, stop and resume bag-valve-mask ventilation before reattempting.
I. Inflate cuff with syringe and attach the tube to an Ambu bag or ventilator.
J. Confirm ETT location by checking for equal bilateral breath sounds, no sounds over epigastric region, end tidal CO_2 detector, direct laryngoscopy, and CXR. Secure tube in place.

2. **Noninvasive ventilation:**

- Constant positive airway pressure (CPAP): This provides constant airway pressure throughout the respiratory cycle thereby decreasing preload and afterload, improving lung compliance, and decreasing the work of breathing. Used in COPD and CHF with an initial setting of 5 cm H_2O.
- Bilevel positive airway pressure (BiPAP): Augments inspiratory and expiratory pressures throughout the respiratory cycle and has benefits similar to CPAP. Used in COPD, CHF, asthma, and pneumonia. Usual setting is IPAP of 10 cm H_2O, and EPAP of 5 cm H_2O.

3. **Asthma:**

A syndrome of reversible airway obstruction, bronchial hyperresponsiveness, and airway inflammation. High-risk patients include those with previous ICU admits, multiple ED visits, previous intubations, illicit drug use, presently on steroids, low socioeconomic status, and those with COPD.

3.1. Clinical Evaluation:

A. **Symptoms:** Wheezing, dyspnea, AMS, diaphoresis, chest pain, cough.
B. **Signs:** Anxious, tachypnea, tachycardia, accessory muscle use, cyanosis, hypertension, pulsus paradoxus, increase I/E ratio.
C. **DDX:** Pneumonia, bronchitis, croup, bronchiolitis, COPD, congestive heart failure, pulmonary embolism, allergic reaction, upper airway obstruction.
D. **Workup:** CBC, BMP, ABG, BNP, D-dimer, peak flow, CXR as needed.

3.2. RX:

A. Support ABCs, IV, O_2, pulse oximeter, and monitor as needed.
B. All that wheezes is not asthma, be aware that there may be another diagnosis.
C. Treatment may include:
   - Albuterol (Ventolin), 2.5 mg, in 3 mL of saline q 20 minutes or 10 to 20 mg continuous over 60 minutes.
   - Epinephrine, 0.3 to 0.5 mL of 1:1,000 sq or nebulized q 20 minutes × 3 doses.
   - Ipratropium bromide (atrovent), 0.5 mg q 20 minutes times 3 doses.
   - Give methylprednisolone (Solu-Medrol), 60 to 120 mg IV or prednisone 1 mg/kg po.
   - Consider BiPAP.
   - Magnesium sulfate 2 g IV over 20 minutes (questionable benefit).
   - Heliox (80% Helium + 20% O_2) may help with few side effects.
   - If intubation is required use ketamine and succinylcholine. Allow permissive hypercapnia to minimize barotrauma and breath stacking. Use high FiO_2, low tidal volume (6–8 mL/kg), low vent rate, low or no PEEP, and give in-line bronchodilator.

D. Disposition: If the patient responds well to therapy, discharge with close follow-up, corticosteroids, and a beta agonist MDI. Admit patients who do not improve, have comorbid conditions (pneumonia), or are in severe distress.

4. Chronic Obstructive Pulmonary Disease (COPD):

COPD is a progressive disorder that results from a combination of chronic bronchitis and emphysema. Chronic bronchitis is defined as a chronic productive cough for 3 consecutive months in 2 consecutive years. Emphysema is defined as abnormal enlargement and destruction of the airspaces distal to the terminal bronchioles.

4.1. Clinical Evaluation:

A. Symptoms: Cough, purulent sputum, DOE, wheezing

B. Signs: ± obese, ± central cyanosis, pursed lip breathing, rales, rhonchi, wheezing. S4, S3, systolic murmur, tachycardia, tachypnea.

C. DDX: Pneumonia, asthma, congestive heart failure, cardiogenic shock, ARDS, pulmonary embolism, FB, aspiration pneumonitis, cancer.

D. Workup: CBC, BMP, BNP, cardiac enzymes, ECG, ABG, CXR.

4.2. RX:

A. Support ABCs, IV, O_2, pulse oximeter, and monitor as needed.

B. Give beta-agonist, albuterol by MDI or nebulizer.

C. Give anticholinergic, ipratropium by MDI or nebulizer.

D. Give corticosteroids, prednisone 40 to 60 mg po **or** methylprednisolone 60 to 125 mg IV.

E. Give antibiotics for acute exacerbations who have a change in sputum amount, consistency, or color.
- Outpatient treatment: Doxycycline, TMP/SMX, azithromycin, levofloxacin, cefdinir.
- Inpatient treatment: Levofloxacin, ceftriaxone, cefepime, ceftazidine, zosyn.

F. Consider BiPAP for moderate to severe respiratory distress. Intubate if condition worsens.

G. Disposition: Admit patients who do not improve, feel uncomfortable with being discharged, or have severe symptoms. Discharge if patient feels back to "normal." Arrange close follow-up and start on steroids, antibiotics, and appropriate MDIs.

5. Hemoptysis:

Hemoptysis is defined as the coughing up of blood from the lower respiratory tract. Massive hemoptysis is defined as >100 mL/h acutely or >600 mL/24 hours. 25% are due to non-TB infections (bronchitis), 25% are due to cancer, 25% are due to a misc cause (TB, cardiovascular disease), and 25% have no identifiable cause.

5.1. Clinical Evaluation:

A. Signs: Cough, URI symptoms, weight loss, night sweats, DOE, chest pain, fever.

B. Symptoms: Wheeze, rhonchi, tachypnea, tachycardia, cachexia, petechial, bruises.

C. DDX: Lung cancer, PE, CHF, bronchitis, pneumonia, mitral stenosis, AV fistula, vasculitis, Goodpasture's syndrome, trauma, cystic fibrosis, SLE, epistaxis, DIC.

D. Workup: CBC, BMP, BNP, LFTs, PT/PTT/INR, PPD test, T&S (possible T&C 4–6 units PRBCs for massive bleeding), cardiac enzymes, D-dimer, ESR, ABG, sputum (Gram stain, C&S, AFB, fungal, cytology), CXR, ECG, consider VQ scan, and/or CT angiogram chest.

5.2. RX:

A. Support ABCs, IV, O_2, pulse oximeter, and monitor as needed.

B. Keep patient in lateral decubitus (bleeding side down) and Trendelenburg positions.

C. Correct coagulopathy if it exists.

D. Intubate the unaffected lung if possible in massive bleeds.

E. Consult CT surgery, pulmonary, and interventional radiology for possible angiography and embolization.

F. **Disposition:** Admit patient with massive bleeding to the ICU. Healthy patients with blood-streaked sputum can be discharged with close follow-up.

TOXICOLOGY

1. **General:**

Toxicity results from the ingestion of a toxic substance or from an overdose of prescription or nonprescription drugs. To determine what was taken consider calling friends, family, pharmacy personal physician, medical records, and send paramedics or police back to the scene. Ask if there are any other people living with the patient, and if they take medications (beta-blockers, calcium channel blockers, digoxin).

1.1. GI decontamination:

A. **Induced Emesis:** This utilizes syrup of ipecac to induce vomiting thereby emptying the stomach and decreasing absorption. This has largely been abandoned.

B. **Gastric Lavage:** Removal of stomach contents via an NG/OG tube.
- Indication: <1 hour of ingestion, substances not bound by charcoal, substances with no effective antidote and if benefits outweigh risks.
- Contraindications: Spontaneous emesis, substances not meeting above indications, AMS, ingestion of hydrocarbons or caustic acids, FB ingestion, high risk for gastric or esophageal injury.
- Procedure: Protect airway, position on left lateral decubitus and Trendelenburg positions. Insert a 36- to 40-Fr orogastric tube and lavage with 200 mL aliquots after conformation of proper placement.

C. **Activated Charcoal:** AC is ingested in order to absorb poisons within the GI tract. The cathartic sorbitol is mixed with AC, and this helps speed transit time of toxins through the GI tract. Dose is 1 g/kg with only one 50 g dose having sorbitol. No sorbitol in children.
- Indications: Patient presents within 1 to 2 hours after ingestion. Ingestion of a dangerous amount of poison that is absorbed by charcoal.
- Contraindications: Ingested substances poorly absorbed (iron, lithium, heavy metals, toxic alcohols, pesticides). AMS, present >2 hours after ingestion, ingestion of a caustic agent.

D. **Whole-Bowel Irrigation:** Flushes the GI tract to decrease the transit time of luminal contents. Polyethylene glycol (PEG) is given at a rate of 1 to 2 L/h po/NG/OG. Endpoints for therapy are clear rectal effluent or total irrigation volume of 10 L.
- Indications: Sustained release or enteric coated pills, ingested illicit drug packets, drugs not absorbed by charcoal (arsenic, iron, lithium).
- Contraindications: AMS, bowel obstruction or perforation, GI bleed, ileus, intractable vomiting.

E. **Enhanced Elimination:**
- Urinary alkalinization: An $NaHCO_3$ infusion can increase renal elimination of some substances by increasing the urine pH (aspirin, phenobarbital, formic acid).
- Multi-dose charcoal: Drugs that have enterohepatic or enteroenteric circulation, sustained release agents, and those that form concretions can possibly be removed (phenobarbital, phenytoin, carbamazepine, theophylline, aspirin).
- Hemodialysis: This directly removes toxins from the patient's plasma, using a standard dialysis machine. Toxins that are removable by hemodialysis must be water soluble, have a low molecular weight, low protein binding, and a small volume of distribution (isopropyl, salicylates, methanol, barbituates, lithium, ethylene glycol).

1.2. Risk stratification: Most overdoses can be observed and if no symptoms occur within 6 hours, the patient will be alright. Some substances may present in a delayed fashion and require prolonged monitoring (acetaminophen, sustained-release drugs, toxic alcohols, mushrooms, iron, paraquat).

2. Acetaminophen:

Acetaminophen is metabolized in the liver. A small dosage of the drug is metabolized via the cytochrome P-450 oxidase system to a final toxic metabolite. This metabolite is detoxified by glutathione and excreted in urine. In the case of an overdose (>140 mg/kg or 7.5–10 g) of acetaminophen, glutathione is depleted and the toxic metabolite accumulates causing hepatic necrosis.

- Phase I (to 24 hours): Anorexia, nausea, and vomiting.
- Phase II (24–72 hours): Abdominal pain.
- Phase III (3–5 days): Jaundice, hypoglycemia, coagulopathy, and encephalopathy.
- Phase IV (1 week): Resolution if Phase III is not lethal.

2.1. Clinical Evaluation:

A. Symptoms: N/V, abdominal pain, diaphoresis, malaise, jaundice, AMS.
B. Signs: AMS, jaundice, hepatomegaly, RUQ tenderness, pallor, bruising.
C. DDX: Alcoholic hepatitis, viral hepatitis, cholecystitis, amanita mushroom poisoning.
D. Workup: CBC, BMP, PT,/PTT/INR, LFTs, ammonia, lactate, phosphate, calcium, ABG, UA, urine pregnancy test, urine drug screen, serum osmolality, acetaminophen level (4 hours post ingestion, plot on Rumack nomogram), salicylate level, ETOH, ECG, CXR.

2.2. RX:

A. Support ABCs, IV, O_2, pulse oximeter, and monitor.
B. If AMS check or give glucose and naloxone.
C. If ingestion within 1 to 2 hours, give activated charcoal with sorbitol 1 g/kg po (max 50 g).
D. If patient ingested a toxic dose, give N-acetylcysteine (NAC), 140 mg/kg po, then give 70 mg/kg po q 4 hrs × 17 doses. If unable to tolerate po, give NAC 150 mg/kg in 200 mL of D_5W over 1 hour. This followed by 50 mg/kg in 500 mL D_5W over 4 hours, then 100 mg/kg in 1L D5W over 16 hours.
E. Treat nausea and vomiting.
F. Consider a psych consult.
G. Disposition: Admit all patients requiring NAC, have liver function abnormalities, or took a toxic dose regardless of laboratory results.

3. Methanol:

Methanol (wood alcohol) is found in antifreeze, paint solvents, canned fuels (Sterno), gasoline additives, and home heating fuels. It is metabolized in the liver to formic acid. Formic acid is the toxic substance that causes an anion gap metabolic acidosis, putamen damage, and retinal toxicity.

3.1. Clinical Evaluation:

A. Symptoms: Photophobia, blindness, abdominal pain, N/V, AMS, seizures, coma.
B. Signs: Tachypnea, tachycardia/bradycardia, hypotension, fixed and dilated pupils, ataxia, papilledema, hyperventilation.
C. DDX: Seizures, head injury, hyperammonemia, viral encephalitis, meningitis, ethylene glycol intoxication, ethanol intoxication, CO poisoning.
D. Workup: CBC, BMP, lactate, LFTs, PT/PTT/INR, calcium, phosphate, acetaminophen/salicylate level, ammonia, serum osmolality, urine drug screen, toxic alcohol screen, ETOH, lipase (pancreatitis), ABG, UA, ECG, CXR, calculate osmolar and anion gap.

3.2. RX:

A. Support ABCs, IV, O_2, pulse oximeter, and monitor.
B. Give naloxone, thiamine, and check or give glucose.
C. Fomepizole (antizol) loading dose 15 mg/kg IV followed by 10 mg/kg IV q 12 hours. This has become the agent of choice.

D. Alternative antidote: Ethanol 75 mL/kg of a 10% ethanol in D_5W over 30 minutes, then IV infusion to reach a goal of 150 mg/dL.
E. Gastric lavage for ingestion <2 hours and activated charcoal if a coingestion occurred.
F. Consider hemodialysis for visual complaints, high osmolar gap, persistent acidosis, methanol level >25 to 50 mg/dL.
G. Give $NaHCO_3$ for pH <7.20 to 7.25, and folate 50 mg IV.
H. **Disposition:** Admit all patients poisoned with methanol to the ICU. Obtain a renal, ophthalmology, and psychiatric consult.

4. Ethylene Glycol:

Ethylene glycol (EG) is found in antifreeze, de-icing solutions, latex paints, hydraulic fluids, solvents, and cleaning products. EG is metabolized to glycolic acid and oxalic acid, which lead to an anion gap metabolic acidosis and renal failure. The fluorescence added to antifreeze is excreted in the urine and can be detected by Wood's lamp.

4.1. Clinical Evaluation:

A. **Symptoms:** Intoxicated, ataxia, AMS, N/V, hematuria, dyspnea, flank pain, coma.
B. **Signs:** Tachypnea, tachycardia, hypotension, nystagmus, abdominal tenderness, ataxia, respiratory depression.
C. **DDX:** Seizures, head injury, hyperammonemia, viral encephalitis, meningitis, methanol intoxication, ethanol intoxication, CO poisoning.
D. **Workup:** CBC, BMP, lactate, LFTs, PT/PTT/INR, calcium, phosphate, acetaminophen, salicylate, serum osmolality, ammonia, urine toxicology screen, toxic alcohol screen, ETOH, ABG, UA (oxalate crystals), ECG, CXR, calculate osmolar and anion gap.

4.2. RX:

A. Support ABCs, IV, O_2, pulse oximeter, and monitor.
B. Give naloxone 2 mg IV, thiamine 100 mg IV, and check or give glucose.
C. Fomepizole (antizol) loading dose, 15 mg/kg IV followed by 10 mg/kg IV q 12 hours. This has become the agent of choice.
D. Alternative antidote: Ethanol 75 mL/kg of a 10% ethanol in D_5W over 30 minutes, then IV infusion to reach a goal of 150 mg/dL.
E. Consider hemodialysis for persistent acidosis, ethylene glycol level >50 mg/dL, renal failure.
F. Give pyridoxine 100 mg IV.
G. Give $NaHCO_3$ for pH <7.20 to 7.25.
H. **Disposition:** Admit all patients poisoned with EG to the ICU. Obtain a renal and psychiatric consult if needed.

5. Isopropyl Alcohol:

Isopropyl alcohol is found in rubbing alcohol, perfumes, and hand sanitizers. It is metabolized to acetone, which is twice as potent as ethanol but does not cause an acidosis. There will be an osmolar gap but no anion gap metabolic acidosis.

5.1. Clinical Evaluation:

A. **Symptoms:** Ataxia, AMS, coma, abdominal pain, N/V, GI bleed.
B. **Signs:** Intoxication, nystagmus, miosis, hypotension, fruity breath, abdominal tenderness, tachycardia, respiratory depression.
C. **DDX:** Seizures, head injury, hyperammonemia, viral encephalitis, meningitis, methanol intoxication, ethylene glycol intoxication, ethanol intoxication, CO poisoning.
D. **Workup:** CBC, BMP, lactate, LFTs, PT/PTT/INR, calcium, phosphate, acetaminophen/salicylate level, CPK, ammonia, serum osmolality, urine drug screen, toxic alcohol screen, ETOH, ABG, UA (oxalate crystals), acetone, hemoccult stool, ECG, CXR, calculate osmolar and anion gap.

5.2. RX:

- **A.** Support ABCs, IV, O_2, pulse oximeter, and monitor.
- **B.** Give naloxone 2 mg IV, thiamine 100 mg IV, and check or give glucose.
- **C.** Gastric lavage is <2 hours from ingestion. Give activated charcoal 1 g/kg po/ng.
- **D.** Consider hemodialysis for shock or an isopropyl level >400 mg/dL.
- **E.** Give norepinephrine or dopamine for persistent hypotension.
- **F.** **Disposition:** If asymptomatic after 3 hours discharge. Admit symptomatic patients.

6. Anticholinergics:

A wide variety of prescription and nonprescription drugs have anticholinergic properties. These drugs include antidepressants, diphenhydramine, scopoloamine, dicyclomine, ipratropium, oxybutynin, atropine, hydroxyzine, benztropine, antiparkinson meds, ophthalmoplegics, and over-the-counter cough and cold meds. Parasympathetic blockade creates a clinical picture of:

Hot as hades.
Blind as a bat.
Dry as a bone.
Red as a beet.
Mad as a hatter.

6.1. Clinical Evaluation:

- **A.** **Symptoms:** Red flushed skin, AMS, seizures, visual complaints, fever, urinary retention, increased thirst, dry mouth.
- **B.** **Signs:** Fever, tachycardia, hypertension, respiratory depression, mydriasis, poor VA, decreased bowel sounds, disorientation/confusion, warm/dry skin.
- **C.** **DDX:** CNS infection, dehydration, psychiatric disorder, sepsis, malignant hyperthermia, cocaine or amphetamine intoxication, serotonin syndrome.
- **D.** **Workup:** CBC, BMP, CPK, ETOH, UA, urine drug screen, TCA screen, ABG, CXR, ECG.

6.2. RX:

- **A.** Support ABCs, IV, O_2, pulse oximeter, and monitor.
- **B.** Perform conservative and supportive care.
- **C.** For uncontrollable agitation, seizures, coma, life-threatening arrhythmias, treat with physostigmine 1 mg over 2 minutes q 30 minutes as needed. This drug is dangerous, use is controversial so have atropine at bedside for potential cholinergic crisis.
- **D.** Give a benzodiazepine for seizures.
- **E.** Treat hyperthermia with a cooling blanket.
- **F.** **Disposition:** Observe patient in the ED until condition resolves. Admit for severe symptoms or complications. Obtain a psychiatric consultation as appropriate.

7. Neuroleptic Malignant Syndrome (NMS):

NMS follows the initiation or increased dosing of an antipsychotic (neuroleptic) drug, and is characterized by hyperthermia, rigidity, and autonomic dysregulation. Patients with this condition carry a 20% mortality and death occurs from renal failure, DIC, dysrhythmias, and respiratory failure.

7.1. Clinical Evaluation:

- **A.** **Symptoms:** AMS, fever, muscular rigidity, diaphoresis, tremor, dyspnea, agitation, incontinence, pallor.
- **B.** **Signs:** Hyperthermia, tachycardia, tachypnea, orthostatic hypotension, dystonias, lead pipe rigidity, tremor, shuffling gait, akathisia.

C. **DDX:** Malignant hyperthermia, heatstroke, extrapyramidal reaction, hyperthyroidism, meningitis, encephalitis, schizophrenia, serotonin syndrome.
D. **Workup:** CBC, BMP, calcium, phosphate, PT/PTT/INR, LFTs, UA, CPK, ECG, CXR.

7.2. RX:

A. Support ABCs, IV, O_2, fingerstick glucose, pulse oximeter, and monitor.
B. Stop the offending medication.
C. Treat hypotension with NS followed by norepinephrine if unsuccessful.
D. For dystonia, diphenhydramine (Benadryl), 50 mg IM/IV, or benztropine (Cogentin), 2 mg IM. Bromocriptine and dantrolene may be used but of questionable benefit.
E. Active cooling for hyperthermia.
F. Considering alkalinizing urine if rhabdomyolysis is present.
G. Use benzodiazepines to treat the rigidity and assist in sedation and relaxation.
H. **Disposition:** Admit to the ICU.

8. Beta-Blockers:

A **beta-blocker** overdose causes hypoglycemia, bradycardia, decreased myocardial contractility, and hypotension. The ingestion of one pill can cause death in a child.

8.1. Clinical Evaluation:

A. **Symptoms:** Chest pain, lethargy, N/V, AMS, seizure.
B. **Signs:** Bradycardia, hypotension, bradyarrhythmias, rales (pulmonary edema), coma.
C. **DDX:** Digoxin toxicity, cholinergic toxicity, tricyclic antidepressant OD, hyperkalemia, cardiogenic shock, sepsis, calcium channel blocker OD.
D. **Workup:** CBC, BMP, calcium, phosphate, magnesium, acetaminophen/salicylate level, serum osmolality, urine drug screen, ETOH, ABG, UA, ECG, CXR.

8.2. RX:

A. Support ABCs, IV, O_2, pulse oximeter, fingerstick glucose, and monitor.
B. Gastric lavage if early presentation.
C. Give activated charcoal 1 g/kg po (50 g max).
D. Consider whole-bowel irrigation with PEG 1 to 2 L/h per ng (500 mL/h in peds), especially for sustained release drugs.
E. Treatment for severe bradycardia and hypotension:
   - NS fluid bolus followed by a vasopressor if unsuccessful.
   - Atropine 0.5 to 1 mg IV
   - Glucagon 5 to 10 mg IV.
   - Calcium chloride 10 mL (10% solution) IV or calcium gluconate 10 mL (10% solution) IV.
   - High dose insulin infusion (0.1 to 1 U/kg/h), along with glucose replacement.
   - Consider pacing and intra-aortic balloon pump.
F. **Disposition:** Discharge patients with mild toxicity after 4 to 6 hours with or without a psychiatric consultation as necessary. For more severe cases, admit to the ICU and obtain a psychiatric consult if needed.

9. Calcium Channel Blockers (CCB):

CCB obstruct calcium influx leading to vasodilatation, decreased SA node activity, decreased cardiac contractility, and slowing of AV nodal conduction. These medications are widely used for hypertension, angina, arrhythmias, SVT, migraine headaches, CHF, and cardiomyopathy.

9.1. Clinical Evaluation:

A. **Symptoms:** Lethargy, N/V, dyspnea, fewer CNS effects than with beta-blockers.
B. **Signs:** Bradycardia, hypotension, bradyarrhythmias, respiratory depression, apnea.

C. **DDX:** Digoxin toxicity, cholinergic toxicity, tricyclic antidepressant OD, hyperkalemia, cardiogenic shock, sepsis, beta-blocker OD.
D. **Workup:** CBC, BMP, calcium, phosphate, magnesium, acetaminophen/salicylate level, serum osmolality, urine toxicology screen, ETOH, ABG, UA, ECG, CXR.

9.2. RX:

A. Support ABCs, IV, O_2, pulse oximeter, fingerstick glucose, and monitor.
B. Gastric lavage if early presentation.
C. Give activated charcoal 1 g/kg po (50 g max).
D. Consider whole-bowel irrigation with PEG 1 to 2 L/h per ng (500 mL/h in peds), especially for sustained release drugs.
E. Treatment for severe bradycardia and hypotension:
- NS fluid bolus followed by a vasopressor if unsuccessful.
- Atropine 0.5 to 1 mg IV
- Glucagon 5 to 10 mg IV.
- Calcium chloride 10 mL (10% solution) IV or calcium gluconate 10 mL (10% solution) IV.
- High-dose insulin infusion (0.1 to 1 U/kg/h), along with glucose replacement.
- Consider pacing and intra-aortic balloon pump.

F. **Disposition:** Discharge patients with mild toxicity after 4 to 6 hours with or without a psychiatric consultation as necessary. For more severe cases, admit to the ICU and obtain a psychiatric consult if needed.

10. Cyanide (CN):

Cyanide poisoning can occur from inhalation of wool and plastics during a house fire, ingestion of artificial nail remover, nitroprusside use, and pit/seed ingestion (apricot). It binds to cytochrome oxidase inhibiting cellular respiration leading to cellular hypoxia and lactic acidosis.

10.1. Clinical Evaluation:

A. **Symptoms:** Headache, seizures, dyspnea, confusion, abdominal pain, blurred vision, N/V.

B. **Signs:** Hypotension, tachycardia (followed by bradycardia), cherry-red skin, cyanosis, coma, mydriasis, pulmonary edema.

C. **DDX:** Methemoglobinemia, organophosphate toxicity, toxic alcohol ingestion, encephalitis, meningitis, smoke inhalation.

D. **Workup:** CBC, BMP, BNP, cardiac enzymes, lactate, ETOH, PT/PTT/INR, ABG/VBG, UA, carboxyhemoglobin, methemoglobin, serum osmolality, toxic alcohol screen, acetaminophen/salicylate level, CXR, ECG.

10.2. RX:

A. Support ABCs, IV, O_2, pulse oximeter, and monitor.
B. Administer naloxone, thiamine, and check or give glucose.
C. Give hydroxocobalamine 5 g IV. This binds can and converts it to vitamin B12.
D. Cyanide antidote kit (this is being phased out).
- Amyl nitrite pearls. Break and inhale 0.3 mL until IV is started.
- Sodium nitrite 300 mg IV over 5 minutes.
- Sodium thiosulfate 12.5 g IV over 10 minutes.

E. Gastric lavage if <1 hour from ingestion.
F. Give activated charcoal 1 g/kg po (max 50 g).
G. Consider hemodialysis and hyperbaric oxygen in refractory cases.
H. Dopamine or norepinephrine infusion for persistent hypotension.
I. **Disposition:** Admit all symptomatic patients to the ICU.

11. Carbon Monoxide:

Carbon monoxide is a colorless, odorless gas with a 240× higher affinity for hemoglobin than O_2. It is the most common cause of poisoning morbidity and mortality in the United States. Toxic exposure occurs from smoke inhalation during a fire or from improperly vented exhausts from stoves, furnaces, and automobiles. CO binding to hemoglobin causes cellular hypoxia, lactic acidosis, lipid peroxidation, and neurolgic damage. The half-life is 4 to 5 hours if breathing room air and 1 to 1.5 hours on 100% O_2.

11.1. Clinical Evaluation:

A. **Symptoms:** Headache, dizziness, and nausea are the most common symptoms.
- 5% to 15%: Moderate headache, dyspnea, nausea, and dizziness.
- 15% to 25%: Severe headache, vomiting, fatigue, poor judgment, palpitations, tinnitus, visual complaints, memory disturbance.
- >25%: Confusion, syncope, tachypnea, tachycardia, syncope, seizures, and coma, convulsions, respiratory failure, arrhythmias, death.

B. **Signs:** Tachycardia, tachypnea, hypertension/hypotension, hyperthermia, cherry red skin (rare), papilledema, nystagmus, psychosis, cyanosis, rales/rhonchi, AMS, coma.

C. **DDX:** Meningitis, lactic acidosis, migraine headache, opiate toxicity, toxic alcohol ingestion, encephalitis, DKA.

D. **Workup:** CBC, BMP, arterial/venous COHb, lactate, cardiac enzymes, ETOH UA, urine drug screen, CPK, ABG, CXR, ECG, CT/MRI brain as needed.

11.2. RX:

A. Support ABCs, IV, O_2 100% nonrebreather mask, pulse oximeter, fingerstick glucose, and monitor.

B. During O_2 therapy, recheck COHb level q 2 hours.

C. **Disposition:**
- Admit all patients with COHb levels of 25% to 30%, with cardiac, pulmonary or neurologic disease, and with anemia.
- Transport patients who are unconscious, seizing, have COHb levels >25%, had prolonged CO exposure, have evidence of end-organ damage, are pregnant (level >15%) or have cardiac complications (ischemia), to a hyperbaric chamber.
- Psychiatric consult as needed.
- Discharge nonpregnant patients who are asymptomatic with a COHb level <10%.

12. Cocaine:

Cocaine is a natural alkaloid that causes release of catecholamines, and inhibits its reuptake. It may be injected, inhaled, insufflated, or ingested. Nearly every organ system is affected by cocaine and aside from alcohol, it is the most common cause of drug-related ED visits.

12.1. Clinical Evaluation:

A. **Symptoms:** Palpitations, chest pain, nervousness, abdominal pain, psychosis, headache, tics, hallucinations.

B. **Signs:** Agitation, AMS, hyperthermia, tachycardia, tachypnea, hypertension, mydriasis, bruxism, tremor, coma.

C. **DDX:** Angina, delirium tremens, hypertensive encephalopathy, NMS, heat exhaustion/heatstroke, sepsis, epilepsy, hemorrhagic stroke, amphetamine intoxication, bath salt intoxication, ecstasy intoxication, thyrotoxicosis, alcohol withdrawal, anticholinergic toxicity.

D. **Workup:** CBC, BMP, calcium, phosphate, magnesium, CPK, urine drug screen, ETOH, ABG, UA, ECG, CXR, CT head as needed.

12.2. RX:

A. Support ABCs, IV, O_2, pulse oximeter, and monitor.

B. Give diazepam, 2.5 to 5 mg IV or Ativan 1 to 2 mg IV prn agitation. Avoid beta-blockers' use.

C. Nitroglycerine or nitroprusside for hypertension not controlled by benzodiazepines.
D. Consider phentolamine in conjunction with consultation with poison control.
E. Body packers ingest large numbers of well-sealed packages of cocaine to transport them undetected. Treatment includes whole-bowel irrigation and supportive care.
F. Body stuffing is the ingesting of a small numbers of poorly sealed packages. Treatment includes whole-bowel irrigation and supportive care.
G. **Disposition:** Observe the patient in the ED for 3 to 6 hours and discharge mild cases. Admit individuals with sustained chest pain, altered vital signs, and ECG changes.

13. Tricyclic Antidepressants:

The primary mechanism of toxicity is the blockade of norepinephrine reuptake resulting in an anticholinergic effect, and an α-adrenergic blockade effect. Tricyclic antidepressants primarily affect the cardiovascular and central nervous systems. The main toxic effects of an overdose are cardiac arrhythmias/heart blocks (QRS widening >100 msec), seizures, hypotension, and a decreased level of consciousness.

13.1. Clinical Evaluation:

A. **Symptoms:** Palpitations, dry mouth, blurred vision, urinary retention, agitation, convulsions, coma, slurred speech, seizures, drowsiness.
B. **Signs:** Tachycardia, tachypnea, hypertension/hypotension, decreased bowel sounds, mydriasis, respiratory distress, hyperthermia, mydriasis, dry mouth, flushed face, decreased abdominal sounds, hyperreflexia, myoclonus and disorientation.
C. **DDX:** Hypocalcemia, second-+ third-degree heart block, heat exhaustion, heat stroke, hyperkalemia, hyponatremia, metabolic acidosis, antihistamine toxicity, digitalis toxicity, withdrawal syndromes, WPW syndrome, MDMA toxicity, salicylate toxicity.
D. **Workup:** CBC, BMP, PT/PTT/INR, urine drug screen, toxic alcohol screen, urine drug screen, ETOH, TCA toxicology, ABG, ECG (arrhythmias, blocks, widened QRS), serum acetaminophen and salicylate level, and toxicology screen.

13.2. RX:

A. Support ABCs, IV, O_2, pulse oximeter, and monitor.
B. Consider early intubation to avoid respiratory acidosis. Give diazepam, 2.5 to 5 mg IV or Ativan 1 to 2 mg IV prn agitation.
C. Perform gastric lavage and charcoal if early.
D. Give IV NS boluses for hypotension.
E. Consider $NAHCO_3$ infusion 1 to 2 mEq/kg until improvement then start drip.
- Rightward deviation of the terminal 40 msec of the QRS
- QRS >100 msec.
- Ventricular dysrhythmias.
- Hypotension unresponsive to fluid.

F. Benzodiazepines for seizures.
G. Norepinephrine for hypotension unresponsive to fluid.
H. **Disposition:** Observe the patient in the ED for 6 hours and discharge mild cases. Admit individuals with sustained symptoms >6 hours.

14. Digoxin:

Digoxin is a cardiac glycoside that is used to increase myocardial contractility and decrease SA/AV conduction in atrial fibrillation. The therapeutic-toxic window is narrow (0.5–2.0 ng/mL), and is eliminated via renal excretion. To get an accurate digoxin level it must be drawn 6 hours following an acute ingestion. Hyperkalemia in acute digoxin toxicity is a predictor of poor outcome.

14.1. Clinical Evaluation:

A. Symptoms: Fatigue, anorexia, disorientation, confusion, photophobia, seizures, tinnitus, delirium, GI upset, green/yellow visual halos, tremors, N/V.

B. Signs: AMS, brady/tachy arrhythmias, tremors, abdominal tenderness, hemoccult + stool, hypotension, decreased VA, PVCs.

C. DDX: Sepsis, gastroenteritis, meningitis, sinus node dysfunction, heart failure, syncope, hyperkalemia, hypokalemia, hyper/hypocalcemia, hyponatremia, glaucoma, TCA OD, beta-blocker OD, calcium channel blocker OD.

D. Workup: CBC, BMP (hyperkalemia- acute, hypokalemia- chronic), serum digoxin level, LFTs, calcium, phosphate, magnesium, PT/PTT/INR, cardiac enzymes, digoxin level, acetaminophen/salicylate level, ECG (PVCs most common arrhythmia).

14.2. RX:

A. Support ABCs, IV, O_2, pulse oximeter, and monitor.

B. For AMS give naloxone, consider thiamine, and check or give glucose.

C. Give activated charcoal with airway protection if taken within 1 to 2 hours.

D. For severe bradycardia give atropine and consider pacing.

E. Antidote: Digoxin Fab (Digibind) indications:
- Ventricular dysrhythmias
- K^+ >5.0.
- Life-threatening CV instability.
- Serum digoxin level >10 ng/mL at 6 hours post ingestion.
- Ingestion of >10 mg in a digoxin naive adult.
- Ingestion of >4 mg in a child.

F. Digoxin Fab (Digibind) dosing:
- Quick estimation of number of vials needed = Serum digoxin concentration × Wt (kg)/100.
- Empiric therapy for acute poisoning is 10 to 20 vials.
- 1 vial binds to 0.5 mg of digoxin.

G. Disposition: Admit to monitored bed if patient is stable or to ICU, if unstable.

15. Organophosphate (OP)/Carbamate:

Organophosphate and carbamate insecticides are inhibitors of acetylcholinesterase which result in varying degrees of acetylcholine (ACH) accumulation and over stimulation at muscarinic and nicotinic synapses. Poisoning typically occurs as a result of accidental agricultural exposure to one of the common agents (chlorothion, parathion, diazinon, malathion). OP can be absorbed cutaneously, inhaled or ingested. Most of those exposed become symptomatic within 12 hours after exposure, but this varies depending on the nature and type of compound.

Mnemonics are SLUDGE and DUMBELS:

S = Salivation	**D** = Diarrhea
L = Lacrimation	**U** = Urination
U = Urination	**M** = Miosis
D = Diarrhea	**B** = Bronchospasm
G = GI cramps	**E** = Emesis
E = Emesis	**L** = Lacrimation
	S = Salivation

15.1. Clinical Evaluation:

A. Symptoms: Headache, dizziness, blurred vision, weakness, tremors, diarrhea, abdominal cramping, wheezing, incontinence, anxiety.

B. **Signs:** Confusion, coma, AMS, bradycardia, tachycardia, tachypnea, garlic odor to breath, diaphoresis, miosis, salivation, abdominal tenderness, increased bowel sounds, muscle weakness, ataxia, seizure, dysarthria.
C. **DDX:** Opiate OD, phencyclidine OD, nerve agents (VX, soman, tabum), mushroom poisoning, myasthenia gravis, Eaton-Lambert syndrome, Guillain-Barré syndrome, botulism, nicotine poisoning.
D. **Workup:** CBC, BMP, BNP, cardiac enzymes, lactate, PT/PTT/INR, ABG, UA, urine drug screen, RBC cholinesterase levels, plasma pseudocholinesterase levels, serum osmolality, toxic alcohol screen, acetaminophen/salicylate level, CXR, ECG.

15.2. RX:

A. Support ABCs, IV, O_2, pulse oximeter, and monitor.
B. Remove contaminated clothing and clean skin and hair.
C. Antidotes:
   - Atropine 2 to 6 mg IV q 2 to 5 minutes (0.05 mg/kg in peds). This competitively block acetylcholine and use until bronchial secretions clear.
   - Pralidoxime (Protopam, 2-PAM), 2 g IV loading dose (25–50 mg/kg max 1 g in peds), followed by a 250 to 500 mg/h infusion (5–10 mg/kg/h in peds). This reactivates inhibited cholinesterase.
D. Consider activated charcoal without cathartic and gastric lavage if taken within 2 hours.
E. NS bolus for hypotension followed by norepinephrine or dopamine for refractory cases.
F. Treat bronchospasm with ipratropium bromide.
G. Avoid succinylcholine or other cholinergic medications.
H. **Disposition:** Admit asymptomatic patients with significant exposure, and symptomatic patients. Discharge asymptomatic patients after decontamination, and 8 to 12 hours of observation.

16. Iron:

Iron toxicity is caused by the ingestion of iron supplements and is one of the most common causes of poisoning deaths in children <6 y/o. Common formulations and percent weight of elemental iron are as follows: ferrous gluconate (12%), ferrous lactate (19%), ferrous sulfate (20%), ferrous chloride (28%), and ferrous fumarate (33%). Toxicity is by either direct corrosive damage to the GI tract (>20 m/kg), or shock from multiorgan failure (>50 mg/kg). There are five clinical stages of iron poisoning:

- Stage 1 (0–6 hours): N/V/D, GI bleeding, abdominal pain, shock. If no vomiting within 6 hours then no toxicity.
- Stage 2 (6–24 hours): GI symptoms subside and improvement seen over 12 hours.
- Stage 3 (6–48 hours): Multisystem organ failure ensues, return of GI symptoms, elevated anion gap metabolic acidosis, hypovolemic shock, oliguria, anuria, coagulopathy, seizures, coma, hepatic failure, hematemesis, melena.
- Stage 4 (1–4 days): Fulminant liver failure may develop. May have clinical recovery.
- Stage 5 (2–8 weeks): Delayed onset of vomiting due to obstructions from strictures in the stomach or small bowel.

16.1. Clinical Evaluation:

A. **Symptoms/Signs:** Refer to the different stages previously stated.
B. **DDX:** DKA, gastroenteritis, arsenic toxicity, acetaminophen toxicity, toxic alcohol ingestion, salicylate toxicity, theophylline toxicity.
C. **Workup:** CBC, BMP, T&C 2 to 4 units PRBCs, LFTs, calcium, phosphate, magnesium, PT/PTT/INR, cardiac enzymes, acetaminophen/salicylate level, UA, urine drug screen, toxic alcohol screen, serum osmolality, serum iron level (4–6-hr post ingestion), calculate osmolar and anion gap, CXR, KUB (pill fragments), ECG.

16.2. RX:

A. Support ABCs, IV, O_2, pulse oximeter, and monitor.
B. Avoid charcoal, ipecac, and gastric lavage. May consider whole-bowel irrigation if pills are present on KUB.
C. NS bolus followed by vasopressors if hypotensive.

D. Antidote is deferoxamine 10 to15 mg/k/h IV. Indications for use include signs of toxicity, metabolic acidosis, serum iron level >500 μg/dL, or pills present on KUB.
E. **Disposition:** Admit patient to the ICU, if symptomatic and chelation therapy is required.

17. Lithium:

Lithium is a mood stabilizer used to treat bipolar disorder. It has a narrow therapeutic window that predisposes patients to toxicity with minor changes in medications or health status. Risk factors for toxicity include hyponatremia, dehydration, renal insufficiency, elderly, and pediatric patients. Toxicity occurs with levels >2.0 to 3.0 mEq/L with fatalities occurring at levels >4.0 mEq/L.

17.1. Clinical Evaluation:

A. **Symptoms:** History should include drug name, concentration, dosage, time of last ingestion, medical and psychiatric history, and other meds. Nausea, vomiting, diarrhea, tremors, agitation, confusion, and drowsiness are common early symptoms.
B. **Signs:** AMS, polyuria, weakness, lethargy, blurred vision, incontinence, stupor, aphasia, dysarthria, tinnitus, tremor, N/V/D, abdominal pain, seizure, coma.
C. **DDX:** Neuroleptic malignant syndrome, dementia, toxic alcohol ingestion, mercury toxicity, gastroenteritis, cerebrovascular insufficiency, seizure disorder, TCA toxicity, schizophrenia.
D. **Workup:** CBC, BMP, LFTs, lithium level, calcium, phosphate, magnesium, PT/PTT/INR, cardiac enzymes, CPK, acetaminophen/salicylate level, UA, urine drug screen, toxic alcohol screen, serum osmolality, calculate osmolar and anion gap (decreased), CXR, KUB (pill fragments), ECG (increased QT interval, T wave inversion, heart blocks).

17.2. RX:

A. Support ABCs, IV, O_2, pulse oximeter, and monitor.
B. Gastric lavage <1 hour post ingestion or whole-bowel irrigation may enhance gut elimination. Charcoal is not recommended since it does not bind lithium.
C. Initiate saline diuresis with NS. Sodium exchange enhances lithium excretion. Do not use diuretics to augment urinary excretion.
D. Consider sodium polystyrene sulfonate (kayexalate), 30 to 60 g po.
E. Perform hemodialysis in patients with severe poisoning (>4.0 mEq/L), seizures, coma, arrhythmias, or renal failure.
F. **Disposition:** Admit to the ICU. Obtain a psychiatric consult as needed.

18. Narcotics (opioids):

Opioids are found in a wide variety of prescription medications and are commonly abused, and have become one of the most common causes of accidental death in the United States. The opioid toxidrome may result from prescription medication (fentanyl, methadone, oxycodone), over-the-counter medications (diphenoxylate, dextromethorphan), or illicit drugs (heroin). Narcotics stimulate opiate receptors in the CNS, which lead to pain control but also cause toxic effects when taken in excess.

18.1. Clinical Evaluation:

A. **Symptoms:** Confusion, lethargy, coma, respiratory depression.
B. **Signs:** Pinpoint pupils, hypothermia, pulmonary edema, hypotension.
C. **DDX:** DKA, alcohol intoxication, hypercalcemia, hypernatremia/hyponatremia, hypoglycemia, meningitis, CVA, sedative intoxication, cyanide poisoning, toxic alcohol ingestion, HHNK.
D. **Workup:** CBC, BMP, LFTs, calcium, phosphate, magnesium, PT/PTT/INR, cardiac enzymes, CPK, ABG/VBG, acetaminophen/salicylate level, UA, urine drug screen, toxic alcohol screen, serum osmolality, calculate osmolar and anion gap (decreased), CXR (noncardiogenic pulmonary edema), KUB (pill fragments), ECG.

18.2. RX:

A. Support ABCs, IV, O_2, pulse oximeter, and monitor.
B. Give naloxone (Narcan), 2 mg IV/IM/SC, slowly (larger doses may be required for diphenoxylate, extended release opiates, methadone, pentazocine, and fentanyl). Pediatric dose is 0.01 mg/kg IV/IM/SC.
C. Charcoal has no proven benefit and the patient may aspirate if mental status deteriorates.
D. Special considerations:
- Methadone, tramadol (Ultram), and fentanyl do not show up on a standard urine drug screen.
- Give naloxone slowly to prevent agitation.
- Look for opiate patches.
- Check acetaminophen/salicylate levels due to combination medications.
- Tramadol, tapentadol (Nucynta), and meperidine may not induce miosis and causes seizures and serotonin syndrome.

E. Disposition: Admit all patients with pulmonary edema, coma, respiratory depression, persistent naloxone requirement, and unstable vital signs. Observe at least 6 hours after last naloxone dose because the half-life is shorter than the commonly available oral opiates.

19. Petroleum Distillates:

Petroleum distillates (hydrocarbons) include gasoline, kerosene, lighter fluid, mineral oil, turpentine, diesel fuel, motor oil, toluene, xylene, benzene, and carbon tetrachloride. Their toxicity is based on viscosity, volatility, surface tension, and chemical side chains. The low viscosity solutions with low surface tension cause the most frequent and serious adverse effects (chemical pneumonitis from aspiration). Unintentional exposure makes up 95% of cases with 5% due to intentional "huffing" of inhalants.

19.1. Clinical Evaluation:

A. Symptoms: N/V, euphoria, hallucinations, headache, dizziness, confusion, coma, dyspnea, lethargy, lacrimation, chest pain, abdominal pain.
B. Signs: AMS, ataxia, tachycardia, tachypnea, dusky appearance, oral lesions, dysphagia, drooling, nasal flaring, stridor, coughing, wheezes, rales.
C. DDX: ETOH intoxication, toxic alcohol ingestion, cocaine abuse, head injury, thyrotoxicosis, confusional states, epilepsy.
D. Workup: CBC, BMP, LFTs, ABG, calcium, phosphate, magnesium, pregnancy test, PT/PTT/INR, cardiac enzymes, COHb, CPK, acetaminophen/salicylate level, UA, urine drug screen, toxic alcohol screen, serum osmolality, calculate osmolar and anion gap, CXR (immediate and delayed 4 –6 hours), ECG.

19.2. RX:

A. Start ABCs, IV, O_2, pulse oximeter, and monitor.
B. Call poison control or pharmacy for unknown chemicals.
C. Remove contaminated clothing.
D. Give naloxone if indicated.
E. Activated charcoal is not helpful and gastric emptying is contraindicated (aspiration).
F. Treat bronchospasm with beta-agonists.
G. Special considerations:
- Halogenated hydrocarbons can cause "sudden sniffing death" due to myocardial sensitization to catecholamines. Give no epinephrine or norepinephrine.
- For severe poisoning, intubate and place on PEEP.
- Treat dysrhythmias with beta-blockers.
- Consider using N-acetylcysteine for carbon tetrachloride ingestion.

H. Disposition: Discharge home, if the patient is asymptomatic for 6 hours and the second CXR is normal. Admit symptomatic patients to the ICU as needed.

20. Salicylates:

Salicylate is found in many over-the-counter and prescription products. Salicylic acid is a weak acid that at normal pH is ionized, preventing it from crossing the blood brain barrier or renal tubules. As the blood becomes more acidic, a nonionized form develops, allowing it to cross the blood brain barrier and decreasing renal excretion. A toxic level stimulates the respiratory center (hyperventilation), and chemoreceptor trigger zone (vomiting), uncouples oxidative phosphorylation (lactate production, acidosis, hyperthermia), increases fatty acid metabolism (ketone production), and causes cerebral and pulmonary edema.

20.1. Clinical Evaluation:

- **A. Symptoms:** N/V, abdominal pain, anorexia, vertigo, tinnitus, fever, diaphoresis, lethargy, confusion, disorientation, hallucinations, seizures.
- **B. Signs:** AMS, coma, fever, tachycardia, hyperpnea, hypotension, flushing or pallor, rales, hematochezia, dehydration, respiratory depression, deafness.
- **C. DDX:** Theophylline toxicity, iron poisoning, caffeine toxicity, PE, schizophrenia, toxic alcohol ingestion, meningitis, encephalitis, hydrocarbon toxicity, DKA, AKA, anxiety, cerebrovascular disease, sepsis, alcohol withdrawal.
- **D. Workup:** CBC, BMP, lactate, LFTs, PT/PTT/INR, T&S, calcium, phosphate, acetaminophen/salicylate level, CPK, serum osmolality, urine drug screen, toxic alcohol screen, ETOH, ABG, UA, serum ketone, hemoccult stool, ECG, CXR, KUB (pill fragments), calculate osmolar and anion gap.

20.2. RX:

- **A.** Support ABCs, IV, O_2, pulse oximeter, finger stick glucose, and monitor.
- **B.** Give NS IV to maintain renal perfusion (no forced diuresis).
- **C.** Give multiple-dose activated charcoal or whole-bowel irrigation after a massive ingestion or ingestion of sustained-release products.
- **D.** Start alkaline diuresis with $NaHCO_3$ 1 to 2 mEq/kg IV bolus, followed by an infusion at 2 to 4 mL/kg/h with 40 mEq of KCl to ensure hypokalemia does not occur.
- **E.** Consider hemodialysis for an acute salicylate level >100 mg, chronic salicylate level >60 mg/dL, coma, seizure, cerebral/pulmonary edema, or renal failure.
- **F.** Check urine pH, serum K^+, and serum salicylate levels every 2 hours.
- **G.** Special considerations:
  - Done nomogram should not be used because toxicity does not correlate with serum concentration.
  - If intubation occurs, hyperventilate to maintain respiratory alkalosis.
  - Levels >30 mg/dL are toxic with levels >100 mg/dL life threatening. Serial measurements are required.
  - Be aware of possible chronic toxicity in the elderly.
- **H. Disposition:** Admit all symptomatic patients to the ICU as needed. Consider a psychiatric consult as needed.

21. Serotonin Syndrome:

Serotonin syndrome is most commonly due to the use of multiple serotonergic agents or overdose of these medications. Most common medications implicated are MAO inhibitors, amphetamine analogs (ecstasy), and SSRIs.

21.1. Clinical Evaluation:

- **A. Symptoms:** AMS, confusion, hallucinations, hyperthermia, muscular rigidity, diaphoresis, tremors, agitation, diarrhea.
- **B. Signs:** Tachycardia, tachypnea, hypertension, fever, myoclonus, autonomic instability, hyperreflexia.
- **C. DDX:** Neuroleptic malignant syndrome, malignant hyperthermia, anticholinergic OD, encephalitis, meningitis, thyroid storm, alcohol withdrawal.
- **D. Workup:** CBC, BMP, PT/PTT/INR, LFTs, ABG, serum osmolality, lactate, U/A, urine drug screen, acetaminophen level, salicylate level, TCA blood screen, CPK, ETOH, urine myoglobin, CXR, ECG.

21.2. RX:

- **A.** Support ABCs, IV, O_2, pulse oximeter, and monitor.
- **B.** Give naloxone 2 mg IV, consider thiamine 100 mg IV, and give or check glucose.
- **C.** Consider cyproheptadine 4 to 8 mg po (serotonin antagonist).
- **D.** If normal mental status and low aspiration risk, give activated charcoal po.
- **E.** Treat hypertension with nitroprusside, esmolol, or NTG IV.
- **F.** For muscle rigidity (fever inducing) and seizures use a benzodiazepine (lorazepam, diazepam, midazolam).
- **G.** **Disposition:** Admit all serotonin syndrome patients.

TOXICOLOGY MNEMONICS

Dialysis Criteria (AEIOU)

Note: Mnemonic AEIOU also used in "Causes of Coma"

A	**A**cidosis
E	**E**lectrolyte abnormalities (↑K^+)
I	**I**ngestion of toxins (**I**sopropanol, **B**arbiturates, **A**mphetamines, **I**NH, **L**ithium, **T**heophylline, **E**thylene glycol, **A**SA, **m**ethanol)
O	**O**verload-fluid
U	**U**remic Pericarditis

INDICATIONS FOR DIALYSIS OF TOXINS (I BAIL TEAM)

Dialysis Can BAIL Your Medical TEAM out of a Life-Threatening Situation

I	**I**sopropanol (isopropyl alcohol, rubbing alcohol; note: normal AG ↑ osmolar gap) [12, 4th ed. pg 769]
B	**B**arbiturates → long acting (charcoal hemoperfusion); **B**eta blockers (water soluble = atenolol)
A	**A**mphetamines
I	**I**NH
L	**L**ithium (level >4 mEq/L or 2–4 if poor clinical condition)
T	**T**heophylline (charcoal hemoperfusion)
E	**E**thylene glycol (levels >20 mg/dL; nephrotoxicity; metabolic acidosis is present; Triad = history, clinical presentation and laboratory results consistent with Ethylene glycol poisoning)
A	**A**SA (if seizures, CNS alteration, acidosis, serum levels ≥100 mg/dL)
M	**M**ethanol (visual or CNS dysfunction; methanol levels >20 mg/dL; ingestion >30 ml; pH <7.15) **M**ushrooms = Amanita (charcoal hemoperfusion)

Charcoal Ineffective (MP LICE)

M	**M**etals-heavy (Treatment = whole-bowel irrigation = PEG (polyethylene glycol)
P	**P**etroleum distillates (Hydrocarbons)
L	**L**ithium
I	**I**ron
C	**C**austics
E	**E**thylene glycol (Also → ethanol, methanol and isopropyl alcohol)

Radiopaque Substances (BET A CHIP)

B Barium
E Enteric coated ASA
T TCA's
A Antihistamines
C Chloral hydrate
H Heavy metals (Iron, lead, etc. *Note:* MVI with Iron-not seen on x-ray)
I Iodine
P Phenothiazine → *Examples:* chlorpromazine (Thorazine), prochlorperazine (Compazine), mesoridazine (Serentil), thioridazine (Mellaril) and promethazine (Phenergan)

Substances Causing an Osmolar Gap (I MADE GAS)

Note: You would too, if you ate GYROS everyday!

I Isopropyl alcohol
M Methanol / Mannitol
A Alcohol (ETOH)
D DKA (due to acetone)
E Ethylene Glycol
G Glycerol
A Acetone
S Sorbitol

Poisoning Associated with Fever (SALT ASAP)

S	**S**alicylates		
A	**A**mphetamines		
L	**L**SD (rare) [12, p. 781]	**L**ithium	
T	**T**CA's	**T**heophylline	**T**hyroxine
A	**A**nticholinergics (antihistamines, phenothiazine, TCAs)		
S	**S**ympathomimetics (cocaine, amphetamines)	**S**eizures	
A	**A**ntihistamines		
P	**P**henothiazine	**P**CP (may be hypo-or hyperthermic)	
MAO Inhibitor overdose			

Poisoning Associated with Hypothermia (COOLS)

C Carbon monoxide
O Opiates
O Oral hypoglycemics, insulin
L Liquor
S Sedative hypnotics (barbiturates, benzodiazepines, chloral hydrate, etc.)

Diaphoretic Skin (SOAP)

S	Sympathomimetics
O	Organophosphates
A	ASA (salicylates)
P	PCP

Substance Causing Nystagmus (PCP PETS MEALS)

If you want to see your pets go crazy and demonstrate nystagmus, add PCP to your pets' meals

PCP	PCP (Phencyclidine)
P	Phenytoin
E	ETOH
T	(1) Tegretol (2) Thiamine depletion
S	Solvents
M	Methanol
E	Ethylene glycol
A	Alcohols (isopropyl alcohol)
L	Lithium [10, 4th ed. p.. 1392]
S	Sedative hypnotics

Miosis (COPS)

C	**C**lonidine	**C**holinergics
O	**O**piates	**O**rganophosphates
P	**P**henothiazine	**P**ilocarpine
S	**S**edative hypnotics	**S**troke (pontine bleed)

Horner syndrome = miosis.

Mydriasis (4—AAAA)

A	Antihistamines
A	Antidepressants (TCAs)
A	ANTI-cholinergics
A	Amphetamines and other Sympathomimetics (cocaine)

Noncardiogenic Pulmonary Edema (MOP CDs)

M	**M**ethamphetamine [12, p. 780] smoking met	**M**ountain sickness (HAPE = high-altitude pulmonary edema)
O	**O**piates (heroin, methadone)	**O**verwhelming Sepsis
P	**P**henobarbital	**P**ancreatitis
C	**C**arbon Monoxide [12, p. 916]	**CVA** (neurogenic pulmonary edema)
D	**D**rugs	**D**rowning [12, p. 891]
s	**S**ympathomimetics (smoking cocaine or methamphetamines) **S**alicylates (more common in *chronic* poisoning and *adults* more common than peds) [12, p. 784]	

Causes of Seizures (U HIT OTIS CAMPBELL)

TOXICOLOGY
Otis Campbell = The "town drunk" on "The Andy Griffith Show"

O	Organophosphates	Opiates
T	TCAs	Theophylline
I	INH	Iron
S	Sympathomimetics	Salicylates
C	Cocaine	CO (CN, Camphor)
A	Amphetamines	Anticholinergics
M	Meperidine (Demerol)	Mushrooms (Gyromita)
P	PCP	Physostigmine Propoxyphene (Darvon)
B	Beta-blockers	Benadryl
E	ETOH withdrawal	Etomidate
L	Lithium	LSD [12, p. 781]
L	Lead	Lidocaine Lindane

- Toxic odors:
  - Fruity—isopropanol, DKA
  - Pear like—chloral hydrate
  - Garlic—arsenic, organophosphates, DMSO, selenium
  - Rotten eggs—hydrogen sulfide, sulfur dioxide
  - Fresh hay—phosgene
  - Wintergreen mint—methylsalicylate
  - Moth balls—camphor, naphthalene

TRAUMA

Trauma Principles

1. **Trauma Evaluation:**

   Evaluation and management of the trauma patient includes a primary survey followed by a detailed secondary survey. The ABCDEF approach provides a methodical approach to fully assess and treat a trauma patient.

1.1. Primary Survey: The goal is to identify and treat immediate life threats.

A. Airway:

- Assess with C-spine precaution.
- Establish patency by checking gag reflex, pooling of secretions, and sonorous respirations.
- Management:
  - ☐ Clear airway and give O_2.
  - ☐ Place in a cervical collar if not already on.
  - ☐ Perform chin lift or jaw thrust, and consider an oro or nasopharyngeal airway.
  - ☐ Intubate with C-spine precaution for AMS, GCS ≤ 8, severe face or neck injury, airway obstruction, class III/IV shock, severe flail chest, severe pulmonary contusion, head injury, and airway burns.

B. Breathing:

- Expose the chest and neck and inspect for external signs of injury.
- Determine the rate and depth of respirations
- Palpate and inspect for tracheal deviation, JVD, use of accessory muscles, subcutaneous emphysema, and crepitus.
- Listen for bilateral breath sounds.
- Management:
  - ☐ Identify and immediately treat any immediate life-threatening injury (tension pneumothorax, open pneumothorax, flail chest).
  - ☐ Order a CXR.

C. Circulation:

- Check pulse rate and rhythm, blood pressure, mental status, skin color, and capillary refill (peds).
- Identify any external sources of bleeding.
- Management:
  - ☐ Two large bore IVs with a bolus of LR or NS 1 to 2 L (20 mL/kg peds).
  - ☐ Direct pressure or tourniquet to bleeding sites.
  - ☐ If hypotensive after 2 L of crystalloid start blood. O^- for females and O^+ or O^- for males. Blood dose is 10 mL/kg in children.
  - ☐ Perform a FAST examination (**F**ocused **A**ssessment with **S**onography for **T**rauma).
  - ☐ Place pregnant patient in left lateral decubitus position to relieve uterine pressure on the IVC.

D. Disability:

- Check pupils for size, equality, and reaction.
- GCS

Eye Opening	Best Verbal	Best Motor Response
4: Open spontaneously	5: Oriented	6: Obeys verbal commands
3: Open to verbal	4: Disoriented	5: Localizes to pain
2: Open to pain	3: Inappropriate	4: Flex/withdrawal to pain
1: No response	2: Incomprehensible	3: Decorticate /flex
	1: No response	2: Decerebrate/extend
		1: No response

E. Exposure:

- Undress the patient looking for additional injuries to the torso and extremities.
- Look for medic-alert tags.
- Cover the patient with warm blankets to prevent hypothermia.
- Obtain a temperature.

F. Finger/Foley:

- While maintaining C-spine immobilization, roll patient off backboard as soon as possible.
- Perform a rectal examination assessing for gross blood, tone, and an abnormal prostate.

- Examine the pelvis for stability.
- Check the genitalia and perineum for discoloration or blood at urethral meatus.
- Management:
  - ☐ Consider a Foley catheter. Contraindications include scrotal hematoma, blood at the urethral meatus, high-riding prostate, known or suspected fracture of the pelvic ring, perineal hematoma.

1.2. **AMPLE FRIENDS**/Orders:

A. **A**llergies, **M**edications, **P**MH/pregnancy, **L**ast meal, **E**vents (HPI), **F**amily history, **R**ecords, **I**mmunizations, **E**MT (EMS field report), **N**arcotics, **D**octor (private doctor), **S**ocial history.
B. Laboratory work: CBC, BMP, finger stick glucose, T&S, UA, CPK, ETOH, urine drug screen, pregnancy test, cardiac enzymes, ABG.
C. Radiology: Basic x-rays include a CXR and AP pelvis. Order further tests based on the results of the history and physical examination.

1.3. Secondary Survey:

A. Detailed head-to-toe survey, rechecking VS and ABCs.
B. Tetanus prophylaxis and antibiotics for open fractures.
C. Splint fractures and reduce dislocations.
D. Obtain appropriate consults (trauma, orthopedics, neurosurgery, vascular surgery, obstetrics).
E. Arrange for transfer if required.

Trauma Cases

2. Trauma in Pregnancy:

MVCs account for 50% of trauma in pregnancy. Failure to wear a seatbelt and placement of the lap belt over the pregnant abdomen, increase the risk of fetal death. Intimate partner violence is also common with the abdomen being the most common site of injury. Normal changes in physiology, vital signs, and laboratory values complicate the trauma evaluation.

- Heart rate increase 10 to 15 bpm.
- Baseline BP decreases during the second and third trimesters.
- During the third trimester, supine hypotension may occur due to uterine compression of the IVC. Must position in the left lateral decubitus position.
- Normal fetal heart rate 120 to 160 bpm.
- Baseline Hgb/Hct is decreased.
- Tidal volume and respiratory rate are increased.
- Gastric tone and emptying time increases.

2.1. Clinical Evaluation:

A. **Pearls:**
- High aspiration risk.
- Patient may loose 1,500 to 2,000 mL of blood before BP decreases.
- Chest tubes should be inserted 1 to 2 intercostal spaces higher.
- Keep maternal PaO_2 >60 mm Hg. Fetal O_2 remains stable until this point.
- Peritoneum becomes desensitized and may not show guarding or rebound.
- No digital cervical examination (possible placenta previa).
- Resuscitation of mom is the priority, and this gives the fetus a better chance at survival.

B. **Physical examination:** Fundal height, gestational age, FHTs, sterile speculum examination (bleeding present possible abruption or uterine rupture), abdominal palpation.
C. **Workup:** CBC, BMP, PT/PTT/INR, fibrinogen, FDP, UA, T&S, T&Rh, US, Kleihauer–Betke (quantifies volume of fetomaternal hemorrhage), FAST examination, nitrazine vaginal fluid

(blue color change). If x-rays are needed then do them. CT/MRI, if US is equivocal and there is concern for significant injury.

2.2. RX:

A. Support ABCs, IV, O_2, pulse oximeter, monitor, and maintain spinal immobilization.
B. Put patient in left lateral decubitus position.
C. Give 1 to 2 L of NS or LR if hypotensive.
D. Give tetanus prophylaxis, treat pain and vomiting.
E. Consult OB/GYN for cardiotocographic monitoring and evaluation.
- A minimum of 4 hours of monitoring is required.
- Fetal distress (late decelerations), may be the first sign of maternal hemodynamic compromise.

F. Emergent c-section is indicated if the fetus is viable (>24 weeks), and shows signs of distress, uterine rupture, placental abruption, or premature labor with malpresentation.
G. Disposition: Admit and monitor all patients for at least 4 hours.

3. Hemorrhagic Shock:

Hemorrhagic shock is a condition of decreased tissue perfusion, resulting in the inadequate delivery of oxygen and nutrients that are necessary for cellular function. This is the most common type of shock seen in trauma.

3.1. ATLS classification of shock:

	Class I	Class II	Class III	Class IV
Blood loss (mL, %)	<750, <15%	750–1,500, 15–30%	1,500–2,000, 30–40%	>2,000, >40%
Pulse	<100	>100	>120	>140
BP	Normal	Normal	Decreased	Decreased
Cap refill	Normal	>3 s	>3 s	>3 s
UO (mL/h)	>30	20–30	5–15	<5
Mental status	Slight anxiety	Some more anxiety	Anxious and confused	Confused—lethargic
Treatment	Crystalloid	Crystalloid	Crystalloid and blood	Crystalloid and blood

3.2. RX:

A. Support ABCs, two large bore IVs, O_2, pulse oximeter, and monitor.
B. Control further blood loss by splinting fractures, applying direct pressure, and apply a tourniquet.
C. Give NS or LR, 1 to 2 L bolus. Assess patient status after infusion.
D. If blood is required, give 1 to 2 units PRBCs IV.
E. If more than 2 units are required, consider a massive transfusion protocol consisting of a ratio of PRBCs/platelets/FFP.
F. Based on the CRASH-2 trial, consider tranexamic acid, 1 g IV over 10 minutes followed by a 1 g infusion over 8 hours.

4. Spinal/Neurogenic Shock:

Spinal shock is a complete loss of all neurologic function, including reflexes and rectal tone, below a specific level of injury. That is a state of transient physiologic (rather than anatomic) reflex depression of cord function in injuries at or above T6. Reflex function below the level of injury spontaneously returns (24–48 hours), at which time the degree of cord injury can be fully determined.

Neurogenic shock refers to the hemodynamic triad of hypotension, bradycardia, and peripheral vasodilation resulting from severe autonomic dysfunction and the interruption of sympathetic nervous system control in acute spinal cord injury. The loss of sympathetic outflow leads to unopposed vagal tone. This condition does not occur with a spinal cord injury below the level of T6.

4.1. Clinical Evaluation:

A. Spinal shock: Flaccid paralysis, bowel and bladder incontinence, sensory loss, palor, parasthesias, loss of DTRs, sustained priapism, ileus.
- Symptoms tend to last 24 to 48 hours where flaccid quadriplegia changes to spastic paralysis. Return of the bulbocavernosus reflex heralds resolution of spinal shock.

B. Neurogenic shock: Hypotension, paradoxical bradycardia, flushed warm peripheral skin.
- The anatomic level of the injury impacts the likelihood and severity of neurogenic shock. Injuries above T1 disrupt the spinal cord tracts that control the entire sympathetic system. Injuries from T1 to L3 may only partially interrupt sympathetic outflow.

C. **Workup:** CBC, BMP, ETOH, urine drug screen, CXR, C-spine x-ray (not required if obtaining CT), CT (cervical, chest, abdomen, pelvis), MRI spine.

4.2. RX:

A. Support ABCs, IV, O_2, pulse oximeter, monitor, and maintain spinal immobilization.

B. Give 1 to 2 L of NS or LR if hypotensive.
- Systolic BP 90 to 1 mm Hg, MAP >70 mm Hg.
- Max of 2 L of crystalloid, more increases risk of pulmonary edema.
- If hypotension persists, use dopamine, phenylephrine or norepinephrine.
- If bradycardic, give atropine, 0.5 to 1.0 mg IV q 5 minutes (max 3 mg).
- At present there is no evidence to support the routine use of corticosteroids for spinal cord injury. If decide to use, give methylprednisolone 30 mg/kg IV over 15 minutes, followed by a 5.4 mg/kg/h infusion over 23 hours.

C. **Disposition:** Admit all patients to the ICU with a neurosurgery consult.

5. Spinal Trauma:

Always assume a spinal cord injury or vertebral fracture until proven otherwise. Maintain spinal immobilization until physical examination or x-rays have eliminated the possibility of a fracture or dislocation. The National Emergency X-Radiography Utilization Study (NEXUS) has identified five criteria that when present rule out the need for x-rays. The five criteria are no posterior midline C-spine tenderness, no focal neuro deficit, no evidence of intoxication, normal mental status, and no distracting injuries. A standard C-spine series includes an AP, lateral, and open mouth views. This is unnecessary if the patient is stable and can be taken to the CT scanner.

5.1. Clinical Evaluation:

A. **History:** Mechanism of injury, motor/sensory complaints, pain.

B. **Physical examination:** Motor and sensory examination, bony tenderness, DTRs, clonus, bulbocavernosus reflex, rectal examination.

C. **DDX:** Incomplete spinal cord injuries:
- Central cord syndrome: The most common incomplete spinal cord lesion. Caused by a hyperextension injury resulting in weakness and numbness greater in the arms than legs. Bowel and bladder function is not affected, and function usually returns over time.
- Anterior cord syndrome: Caused by a flexion or extension with vascular injury of the anterior spinal artery. Paraplegia occurs with loss of pain and temperature sensation. Dorsal column function is preserved (position sense, vibration, deep pressure). This has a poor prognosis for return of function.
- Brown–Sequard syndrome: Hemisection of the spinal cord, which results in ipsilateral motor paralysis, loss of position, and vibratory sensation, with contralateral loss of pain and temperature.

D. **Workup:** CBC, BMP, ETOH, urine drug screen, CXR, C-spine x-ray, T-L spine x-rays, CT C-spine, MRI as needed.

5.2. RX:

A. Support ABCs, IV, O_2, pulse oximeter, monitor, and maintain spinal immobilization.

B. Consult neurosurgery and trauma. Arrange transfer if resources not available.

C. Give 1 to 2 L of NS or LR if hypotensive.
- Systolic BP 90 to 100 mm Hg, MAP >70 mm Hg.
- Max of 2 L of crystalloid, more increases risk of pulmonary edema.
- If hypotension persists, use dopamine, phenylephrine or norepinephrine.
- If bradycardic, give atropine, 0.5 to 1.0 mg IV q 5 minutes (max 3 mg).
- At present there is no evidence to support the routine use of corticosteroids for spinal cord injury. If decide to use, give methylprednisolone 30 mg/kg IV over 15 minutes, followed by a 5.4 mg/kg/h infusion over 23 hours.

D. **Disposition:** Admit all patients with a spinal cord injury to the ICU with a neurosurgery consult. Patients with a stable cervical, thoracic, and/or lumbar fracture can be admitted to a non-ICU bed.

6. Neck Trauma:

Any injury above the clavicles requires a search for a C-spine injury. Blunt and penetrating injuries to the neck may damage major vascular and aerodigestive structures.

- Zone I: Clavicles to cricoid cartilage.
- Zone II: Cricoid cartilage to angle of mandible.
- Zone III: Angle of mandible to base of skull.

6.1. Clinical Evaluation:

A. **Symptoms:** Hoarseness, dyspnea, hemoptysis, odynophagia, dysphonia, subcutaneous air, stridor.

B. **Signs:** Pulsatile hematoma, bruit, Horner's syndrome (ptosis, miosis, anhydrosis), motor/sensory deficit, pulse deficit, tenderness, blood in oropharynx.

C. **DDX:** C-spine injury, vascular dissection, vascular thrombosis, esophageal injury, trachea injury, basilar skull fracture, laryngeal fracture.

D. **Workup:** CBC, BMP, T&S, PT/PTT/INR, C-spine x-ray, Lat soft tissue x-ray neck, CXR, CT neck.

6.2. RX:

A. Support ABCs, IV, O_2, pulse oximeter, and monitor.

B. Consult vascular surgery and trauma. Arrange transfer if resources not available.

C. Give NS or LR if hypotensive.

D. Treat pain and vomiting.

E. Treatment:
- Go directly to OR with the following hard signs; expanding hematoma, severe active bleeding, palpable thrill, bruit, stridor, subcutaneous emphysema, air bubbling from wound, cerebral ischemia, airway obstruction, violation of platysma.
- Zone I: CT angiography, esophagoscopy or esophagram, and bronchoscopy.
- Zone II: Immediate surgical exploration if hard signs are present, otherwise CT angiography, esophagoscopy or esophagram, and bronchoscopy.
- Zone III: CT angiography, CT head, and oropharyngeal examination.

F. **Disposition:** Admit all patients with significant injuries to the ICU or go directly to the OR. Penetrating injuries that do not violate the platysma may be repaired and observed.

7. Burns:

Burns are described according to depth, with first degree (superficial burns) involving the epidermis, second degree (partial-thickness) involving the epidermis and dermis, and third degree (full-thickness) involving the epidermis/entire dermis/dermal appendages.

7.1. Clinical Evaluation:

A. **Symptoms:** Time and duration of contact, heat source, closed or open space, associated trauma, toxic inhalation, stridor, hoarseness, pain.

B. Signs: Facial burns, singed nasal hair, carbonaceous sputum, soot in mouth/nose, wheezing, AMS.
- First degree: Blanching erythema, painful, edematous, indurated skin.
- Second degree: Red or mottled, swelling, blister formation, painful skin.
- Third degree: Translucent, waxy, mottled, leathery, chaired, painless, pale or white skin.

C. Rule of 9s: Adult Body Surface Area (BSA)—9% head, 9% each upper extremity, 9% back, 9% buttocks, 9% chest, 9% abdomen, 18% each lower extremity, and 1% perineum. A modified Lund/Browder chart may be used for peds.

D. Workup: ABG, CBC, BMP, COHb, CPK, UA, urine myoglobin, cardiac enzymes, ECG, CXR.

7.2. RX:

A. Support ABCs, two IVs, O_2, pulse oximeter, and monitor.

B. Treat pain with morphine, fentanyl, or hydromorphone IV.

C. Start fluids as described below.
- Parkland Formula: 4 mL × body weight (kg) ×% BSA burn = total fluid requirement for first 24 hours.
- Administer half over the first 8 hours and final half over the next 16 hours. Timing begins at time of injury.
- Consider a Foley catheter and monitor urine output, 50 to 75 mL/h in adults, and 1 mL/kg/h in children.
- Do not forget maintenance fluid (4–2–1).

D. Give tetanus prophylaxis.

E. Clean affected area with sterile saline. Avoid vigorous scrubbing. Remove charred epithelium, surface debris, and excise ruptured blisters. Apply sterile sheets for transfer and antibiotic dressings (silver sulfadiazine impregnated, mafenide acetate, bacitracin, xeroform), for patients not being transferred.

F. Escharotomy if neurovascular compromise is present.

G. Disposition:
- Discharge patients with second degree burns <15% of TBSA in adults and <10% in children.
- Admit patients with second degree burns >10% TBSA, extremes in age, burns involving the face, hands, feet, and those with significant comorbid factors.
- Transfer patients to a burn unit with the following conditions: (1) Burns that involve >25% TBSA, or 20% in children <10 y/o, (2) third-degree burns involving <10% of TBSA and second-degree burns that exceed 20% of TBSA, (3) burns involving the eyes, face, ears, hands, feet, or perineum, (4) third-degree burns in any age group, (5) electrical burns including lightening injuries, (6) burns associated with significant trauma.

8. Abdominal Trauma:

Blunt trauma may cause crushing or compression of the abdominal viscera with the spleen being the most common organ injured, followed by the liver. MVAs are a common cause and you need to determine the speed, type of collision, restraint usage, air bag deployment, and status of passengers. Penetrating injuries from GSWs and stabbings result in laceration of different organs. Determine the type of weapon used, time of injury, distance from assailant, number of shots or stab wounds, and amount of blood as the scene. Stab wounds to the abdomen require laparotomy in 1 of every 4 cases. With GSWs a laparotomy is required except in certain cases of tangential penetration. Wounds to the lower chest and back (nipple line anteriorly and the tip of the scapulae posteriorly) often involve the abdomen.

8.1. Clinical Evaluation:

A. Symptoms: Abdominal pain, right or left shoulder pain (referred), shortness of breath, AMS.

B. Signs: Abdominal pain to palpation, rebound, guarding, contusions, distention, abrasions, lacerations, bullet wounds, absent or decreased bowel sounds, tachycardia, tachypnea, hypotension, AMS, gross blood on rectal examination.

C. **Workup:** CBC, BMP, amylase, lipase, T&C, UA, PT/PTT/INR, ABG as needed, ETOH, urine drug screen, CPK, pregnancy test, CXR (free air, PTX), pelvis x-ray, C-spine x-ray series as needed, CT chest/abd/pelvis with IV contrast, as needed.

8.2. RX:

A. Support ABCs, two large IVs, O_2, pulse oximeter, and monitor.
B. If hypotensive give 1 to 2 L NS or RL in adults and 20 mL/kg in children. If there is no response, administer O^- blood in females and O^+/O^- in males.
C. Consider tranexamic acid 1000 mg IV over 10 minutes, followed by 1000 mg over 8 hours.
D. Consult a general or trauma surgeon and arrange transfer if not immediately available.
E. Perform FAST examination, insert a Foley catheter and NG/OG tube as needed.
F. Give tetanus prophylaxis.
G. GSWs go directly to the OR (90% have intra-abdominal injuries), start antibiotics.
H. Stab wounds to abdomen may be locally explored by a surgeon but should go to OR if peritoneal findings are present, blood per NG or rectum, free air on CXR, persistent shock, positive CT or FAST examination.
I. Consider a DPL (diagnostic peritoneal lavage) in a patient with AMS and in immediate need of neurologic operation.
   - It is the opinion of the authors and editors of this text that the DPL is an unnecessary and time-consuming test. With ease of ultrasound and CT scanning, there is no reason to obtain this test.
   - It will be described only for completeness.
J. Do not allow unstable patients to go to radiology.
K. **Disposition:** Admit patients with stable isolated solid-organ injuries for observation.

9. Urethral Injury:

Posterior urethral injuries are due to a pelvic fracture while anterior ones are due to a direct force. Urethral injuries are very rare and often missed in females. A vaginal examination is required and it is often associated with a vaginal laceration. What is important is to have a high index of suspicion and evaluate the urethra before inserting a catheter. Placing a Foley catheter in a patient with a partial tear could result in a complete tear and severe long-term complications.

9.1. Clinical Evaluation:

A. **Symptoms:** Perineal pain, hematuria, inability to void.
B. **Signs:** Perineal hematoma, blood at urethral meatus, distended bladder, abdominal pain to palpation, elevated/displaced bladder on rectal examination, vaginal laceration.
C. **Workup:** CBC, BMP, UA, PT/PTT/INR, T&S, pelvis x-ray, retrograde urethrogram, retrograde cystogram (bladder injury), CT abd/pelvis as needed.

9.2. RX:

A. Support ABCs, IV, O_2, pulse oximeter, and monitor.
B. Consult urology for endoscopic examination, suprapubic catheter insertion, or operative repair.
C. **Disposition:** Admit all patients with urethral injuries.

10. Pericardial Tamponade:

Pericardial tamponade is due to fluid accumulating in the pericardial space, most commonly the result of penetrating injuries. With increasing fluid there is a decrease in diastolic filling, a decrease in venous return and hemodynamic compromise. Rapid accumulation of as little as 150 mL can decrease cardiac output. Physical findings include JVD, hypotension, muffled heart tones (Beck's triad), and a pulses paradoxus (decrease in SBP >10 mm Hg on inspiration).

10.1. Clinical Evaluation:

- **A. Symptoms:** Chest pain, dyspnea, AMS.
- **B. Signs:** JVD, hypotension, muffled heart sounds, Kussmaul's sign (JVD during inspiration), pulsus paradoxus, tachycardia, tachypnea.
- **C. Workup:** CBC, BMP, T&C, PT/PTT/INR, cardiac enzymes, FAST examination, CXR (water bottle heart), ECG (electrical alternans, sinus tach, low QRS voltage).

10.2. RX:

- **A.** Support ABCs, IV, O_2, pulse oximeter, and monitor.
- **B.** Consult cardiothoracic and trauma surgery.
- **C.** Give NS or LR IV to increase right ventricular volume.
- **D.** Ultrasound guided pericardiocentesis is indicated if the patient is unresponsive to temporizing resuscitation measures, and cardiovascular collapse is imminent.
- **E. Disposition:** Admit to the ICU or OR.

11. Flail Chest:

Flail chest is a fracture in two or more ribs in two or more places. This causes a disruption of the normal chest wall movement during inspiration and expiration (paradoxical motion). The major problems are pain and the underlying lung damage (pulmonary contusion), which leads to hypoxia.

11.1. Clinical Evaluation:

- **A. Symptoms:** Severe chest wall pain, dyspnea, AMS.
- **B. Signs:** Freely movable rib segment, paradoxical chest wall motion, tachypnea, tachycardia, diminished breath sounds.
- **C. Workup:** CBC, BMP, T&S, PT/PTT/INR, LFTs, ABG, UA, ETOH, urine drug screen, cardiac enzymes, CPK, amylase/lipase as needed, FAST examination, CXR, CT chest/abd/pelvis as needed.

11.2. RX:

- **A.** Support ABCs, IV, O_2, pulse oximeter, and monitor.
- **B.** Consider early intubation (decreases mortality). Indications:
  - Clinical fatigue, labored breathing, accessory muscle use.
  - Saturation $<90\%$ on supplemental O_2.
  - $PaCO_2$ >55 mm Hg.
  - Shock.
  - Severe head injury or other associated injuries.
  - Age >65 y/o.
- **C.** Give NS or LR IV with caution, injured lung is sensitive to fluid overload.
- **D.** Control pain with morphine and/or intercostal nerve blocks.
- **E.** Consult trauma for care and possible operative rib fixation.
- **F. Disposition:** Admit to the ICU or OR.

12. Hemothorax:

A hemothorax is the result of a traumatic injury to the chest with bleeding from the lung parenchyma, intercostal arteries, internal mammary artery or hilar vessels. A massive hemothorax is defined as >1500 mL of blood in the thoracic cavity.

12.1. Clinical Evaluation:

- **A. Symptoms:** Chest pain, dyspnea, AMS, fatigue.
- **B. Signs:** Absent or diminished breath sounds, flat neck veins, dullness to percussion, hypotension, tachycardia, tachypnea, trachea midline, AMS.

C. **DDX:** Flail chest, pulmonary contusion, liver/spleen injury, pneumothorax, cardiac tamponade, tracheobronchial tree injury, aortic injury, diaphragmatic injury.

D. **Workup:** CBC, BMP, T&C, PT/PTT/INR, LFTs, ABG, UA, ETOH, urine drug screen, cardiac enzymes, CPK, amylase/lipase as needed, MTP as needed, FAST examination, CXR, CT chest/abd/pelvis as needed.

12.2. RX:

A. Support ABCs, two large bore IVs, O_2, pulse oximeter, and monitor.

B. Insert a large bore chest tube (36–40 Fr).

C. Indication for thoracotomy:
- >1500 mL initial chest tube output.
- >200 mL/h for 3 hours.
- Persistent hypotension regardless of the chest tube output.

D. Give 1- to 2-L bolus of NS or LR IV. If persistent hypotension give blood.

E. Consider tranexamic acid 1000 mg IV over 10 minutes, followed by 1000 mg IV over the next 8 hours.

F. Control pain and give tetanus prophylaxis.

G. Consult trauma.

H. **Disposition:** Admit to ICU or OR.

13. Tension Pneumothorax (TPTX):

A tension pneumothorax is caused by a one way communication from the lung parenchyma into the pleural space, allowing air into the space but not out. As air fills the pleural space the mediastinum is shifted, venous return decreases, the lung collapses, and cardiac output decreases. This results in hypoxia, shock, and death. TPTX is the most common complication of a pneumothorax and should never be diagnosed radiographically.

13.1. Clinical Evaluation:

A. **Symptoms:** Chest pain, dyspnea, AMS.

B. **Signs:** Tachypnea, tachycardia, hypotension, AMS, JVD, chest/neck crepitus, tympany on percussion, tracheal deviation, decreased breath sounds.

C. **DDX:** Flail chest, pulmonary contusion, liver/spleen injury, pneumothorax, cardiac tamponade, tracheobronchial tree injury, aortic injury, diaphragmatic injury.

D. **Workup:** CBC, BMP, T&S, PT/PTT/INR, LFTs, ABG, UA, ETOH, urine drug screen, cardiac enzymes, CPK, amylase/lipase as needed, FAST examination, CXR, CT chest/abd/pelvis as needed.

13.2. RX:

A. Perform immediate needle decompression followed by a chest tube.

B. Support ABCs, two large bore IVs, O_2, pulse oximeter, and monitor.

C. Trauma or thoracic surgery consult.

D. Give tetanus prophylaxis and treat pain.

E. **Disposition:** Admit to the ICU.

14. Head Injuries:

Bleeding and swelling within the skull can cause an increase in ICP. This can lead to herniation of the brain, most commonly along the falx cerebelli (uncal herniation). The goals of treatment are to diagnose injuries requiring intervention and minimizing secondary brain injury. Always assume a C-spine injury in any patient with a head injury until proven otherwise.

14.1. Clinical Evaluation:

A. **Symptoms:** Headache, N/V, LOC, AMS, visual complaints, confusion, sleepiness, vertigo, amnesia, strange behavior.

B. **Signs:** Pupillary defect, battle signs, raccoon eyes, CSF rhinorrhea/otorrhea, hemotympanum, scalp laceration/contusion, facial trauma, CN defects, nystagmus, tachycardia/bradycardia, tachypnea, periodic breathing,

- GCS: Eye opening response (4, spontaneous; 3, voice; 2, pain; 1, none), verbal (5, oriented; 4, confused; 3, inappropriate words; 2, incomprehensible words; 1, none), motor (6, obeys commands; 5, localizes pain; 4, withdraws pain; 3, flexion pain; 2, extension pain; 1, one).
- <8 severe head injuries, 9 to 12 moderate head injuries, 13 to 15 minor head injuries.

C. DDX: Concussion, epidural hematoma, subdural hematoma, traumatic SAH, cerebral contusion, diffuse axonal injury, alcohol intoxication, hypoglycemia, opioid overdose.

D. Workup: CBC, BMP, T&S, PT/PTT/INR, ABG, UA, ETOH, urine drug screen, cardiac enzymes, FAST examination, CXR, pelvis x-ray as needed, CT head and C-spine, CT chest/abd/pelvis as needed.

14.2. RX:

A. General Management Considerations:
- Support ABCs, IV, O_2, pulse oximeter, and monitor.
- IV fluid should be LR or NS.
- Give antiemetics for N/V.
- Aggressively resuscitate shock, and search for underlying causes (head injuries do not cause shock except in terminal stages).

B. General Management Considerations for Severe Head Injury (GCS <8).
- Perform RSI. Consider pretreatment with lidocaine 1.5 mg/kg IV, vecuronium 0.01 mg/kg IV, and fentanyl 3 μg/kg IV. Induction with etomidate 0.3 mg/kg IV and succinylcholine 1 to 2 mg/kg IV.
- Prevent early hypotension (SBP <90 mm Hg), increases morbidity/mortality.
- Maintain a $PaCO_2$ to 35 mm Hg. May go lower (30 mm Hg) in severe cases but only for a short time.
- Elevate head of bed to 30 degrees.
- Maintain normovolemia:
  - Keep the cerebral perfusion pressure (CPP) at 60 to 70 mm Hg.
  - Keep the mean arterial pressure (MAP) >90 mm Hg.
- Keep the ICP <20 mm Hg.
- Treat and prevent seizures with lorazepam, 2 to 4 mg IVP, repeat until seizures are controlled, followed by phenytoin, 10 to 15 mg/kg IV loading at a rate of 50 mg/min.
- Consider hyperosmolar therapy, with mannitol 0.5 to 2 g/kg IVP.

C. Maintain normothermia.

D. Clean and repair open head wounds.

E. Give tetanus prophylaxis.

F. Disposition: Mild head injuries with a normal CT but are intoxicated, have a skull fracture, or no reliable companion should be admitted. Moderate head injuries should be admitted for at least 1 day. Severe head injuries require a neurosurgery consult and an ICU admission. Consider admitting all patients who sustain a head injury while on anticoagulation for observation.

15. Epidural Hematoma:

Usually associated with a skull fracture in the temporoparietal region after blunt trauma. This fracture cuts through the middle meningeal artery causing blood under high pressure to accumulate between the skull table and the dural membrane.

15.1. Clinical Evaluation:

A. Symptoms: Clinical course is biphasic: injury + loss of consciousness + lucid interval + secondary depression in consciousness. Severe headache, AMS, dizziness, sleepiness, N/V, lethargy, confusion.

B. Signs: Hypertension, tachycardia, AMS, papilledema, nuchal rigidity, cerebellar signs, CN abnormalities.

C. DDX: Concussion, subdural hematoma, traumatic SAH, cerebral contusion, diffuse axonal injury, alcohol intoxication, hypoglycemia, opioid overdose.

D. Workup: CBC, BMP, T&S, PT/PTT/INR, LFTs, ABG, UA, ETOH, urine drug screen, cardiac enzymes, FAST examination, CXR, pelvis x-ray as needed, CT head (biconvex opacity) and C-spine, CT chest/abd/pelvis as needed.

15.2. RX:

A. Support ABCs, IV, O_2, pulse oximeter, and monitor.
- Perform RSI. Consider pretreatment with lidocaine 1.5 mg/kg IV, vecuronium 0.01 mg/kg IV, and fentanyl 3 μg/kg IV. Induction with etomidate 0.3 mg/kg IV and succinylcholine 1 to 2 mg/kg IV.
- Prevent early hypotension (SBP <90 mm Hg), increases morbidity/mortality.
- Maintain a $PaCO_2$ to 35 mm Hg. May go lower (30 mm Hg) in severe cases but only for a short time.
- Elevate head of bed to 30 degrees.
- Maintain normovolemia:
  - Keep the cerebral perfusion pressure (CPP) at 60 to 70 mm Hg.
  - Keep the mean arterial pressure (MAP) >90 mm Hg.
  - Keep the ICP <20 mm Hg.
- Treat and prevent seizures with lorazepam, 2 to 4 mg IVP, repeat until seizures are controlled, followed by phenytoin, 10 to 15 mg/kg IV loading at a rate of 50 mg/min.
- Consider hyperosmolar therapy, with mannitol 0.5 to 2 g/kg IVP.

B. Maintain normothermia.
C. Give tetanus prophylaxis.
D. Obtain a neurosurgical consultation STAT for evacuation in the OR.
E. If patient is in a frank coma or shows signs of increased intracranial pressure, neurosurgeon may consider emergency burr hole placement and evacuation of clot. Consider intracranial pressure monitoring, if indicated.
F. Disposition: Admit to the ICU or OR.

16. Acute Subdural Hematoma:

Subdural hematomas are a blood clot that forms between the dura and the brain. It is usually caused by the movement of the brain relative to the skull tearing bridging veins. Since the low pressure venous system is bleeding slowly, the signs/symptoms will not present as impressive as that seen in an epidural.

16.1. Clinical Evaluation:

A. History/Signs: Headache, AMS, dizziness, vertigo, N/V, lethargy, decreased concentration, seizures, subtle personality changes.
B. Workup: Papilledema, pupillary defects, hypertension, tachycardia/bradycardia, tachypnea, unilateral weakness, paralysis, motor/sensory deficits.
C. DDX: Concussion, epidural hematoma, traumatic SAH, cerebral contusion, diffuse axonal injury, alcohol intoxication, hypoglycemia, opioid overdose.
D. Workup: CBC, BMP, T&S, PT/PTT/INR, LFTs, ABG, UA, ETOH, urine drug screen, cardiac enzymes, FAST examination, CXR, pelvis x-ray as needed, CT head (crescent-shaped) and C-spine, CT chest/abd/pelvis as needed.

16.2. RX:

A. Support ABCs, IV, O_2, pulse oximeter, and monitor.
- Perform RSI. Consider pretreatment with lidocaine 1.5 mg/kg IV, vecuronium 0.01 mg/kg IV, and fentanyl 3 μg/kg IV. Induction with etomidate 0.3 mg/kg IV and succinylcholine 1 to 2 mg/kg IV.
- Prevent early hypotension (SBP <90 mm Hg), increases morbidity/mortality.
- Maintain a $PaCO_2$ to 35 mm Hg. May go lower (30 mm Hg) in severe cases but only for a short time.
- Elevate head of bed to 30 degrees.

- Maintain normovolemia:
  - Keep the cerebral perfusion pressure (CPP) at 60 to 70 mm Hg.
  - Keep the mean arterial pressure (MAP) >90 mm Hg.
  - Keep the ICP <20 mm Hg.
- Treat and prevent seizures with lorazepam, 2 to 4 mg IVP, repeat until seizures are controlled, followed by phenytoin, 10 to 15 mg/kg IV loading at a rate of 50 mg/min.
- Consider hyperosmolar therapy, with mannitol 0.5 to 2 g/kg IVP.

B. If patient on warfarin consider FFP, vitamin K, and/or prothrombin-complex concentrate.
C. Give tetanus prophylaxis.
D. Obtain a neurosurgical consultation STAT.
E. If patient is in a frank coma or shows signs of increased intracranial pressure, neurosurgeon may consider emergency burr hole placement and evacuation of clot. Consider intracranial pressure monitoring, if indicated.
F. **Disposition:** Admit small stable subdurals to the ICU.

17. Compartment Syndrome:

Occurs when a compartment pressure gets high enough to prevent adequate perfusion. Due to cast or external wrapping, fracture (tibia, forearm, supracondylar), deep circumferential burn, crush injury, or prolonged compression. Most commonly seen in the lower leg, forearm, foot, hand, and gluteal region. Remember the 7 Ps: Pain (first finding), pallor, pulselessness, paresthesia, paralysis, poikilothermia (cold), pressure (>30 mm Hg).

17.1. Clinical Evaluation:

A. **Symptoms:** Pain is severe, constant, and out of proportion to physical findings, swelling, numbness, tingling.
B. **Signs:** Tenderness, swelling, pain on passive motion, sensory/motor deficits, diminished pulses, pallor.
C. **DDX:** DVT, fracture, cellulitis, necrotizing fasciitis, snake bite.
D. **Workup:** CBC, BMP, PT/PTT/INR, x-rays as needed, urine myoglobin, CPK, ETOH, urine drug screen. Measure compartment pressures, 0 to 10 mm Hg is normal. Capillary blood flow is compromised at 20 mm Hg. Nerves and muscles ischemia and damage occurs with a pressure >30 mm Hg.

17.2. RX:

A. Support ABCs, IV, O_2, pulse oximeter, and monitor.
B. Treat pain and give tetanus prophylaxis as needed.
C. Obtain an immediate surgical consult for possible fasciotomy.

UROGENITAL/RENAL

1. Dialysis-Related Emergencies:

Patients with chronic renal failure (CRF) have a surgically created arteriovenous fistula, artificial arteriovenous graft, a dialysis catheter, or peritoneal catheter. Dialysis is performed several times per week for several hours. These patients are at risk for problems related to chronic kidney disease (CKD), dialysis, and the absence of dialysis.

- CRF: Encephalopathy, pericarditis, cardiac tamponade, platelet dysfunction, anemia, pulmonary edema, hyperkalemia, ACS.
- Dialysis complications: Hypotension, disequilibrium syndrome, bleeding from vascular access.
- Missed dialysis: Hyperkalemia, volume overload, and pericardial tamponade.

1.1. Clinical Evaluation:

A. **Symptoms:** Weakness, dizziness, dyspnea, N/V, constipation, hematochezia, muscle cramps, chest pain.
B. **Signs:** Hypotension (after dialysis), hypertension, JVD, rales/rhonchi, AMS, friction rub, tachycardia, tachypnea, bruising, fever, cellulitis neuro deficits, absent thrill to palpation of graft/fistula.

C. **Workup:** CBC, BMP, PT/PTT/INR, calcium, magnesium, phosphorus, T&S, ABG/VBG, serum ketones, blood cultures as needed, hemoccult stool, ECG, CXR.

1.2. RX:

A. Support airway, IV, O_2, pulse oximeter, and monitor.
B. No IV, blood draw, or BP in an arm with a fistula/graft.
C. Hypotension is treated with 250 mL NS bolus.
D. Dialysis disequilibrium syndrome is due to rapid changes in body fluid composition and osmolality, immediately after dialysis. Patient has N/V, headache muscle cramps, and weakness. Symptoms resolve over several hours. Treat with mannitol for severe symptoms (coma, seizures, AMS).
E. Bleeding at the puncture site of a fistula/graft requires 15 to 20 minutes of nonocclusive pressure over the site.
F. Uremic coagulopathy causing severe bleeding (CNS, GI) is treated with FFP and desmopressin (DDAVP) sq/IV or intranasal.
G. Volume overload is treated based on the severity of symptoms. O_2, BiPAP/CPAP, or intubation may be used as a temporizing measure until dialysis is performed. May use nitro, lasix, and/or hydralazine to reduce preload and afterload.
H. Hypertension treated with NTG 10 to 20 μg/min IV, esmolol drip, labetalol 20 mg q 10 to 20 minutes IV (max 300 mg), or nitroprusside, 0.5 μg/kg/min, IV (caution due to CN^- accumulation).
I. Hyperkalemia is treated with calcium chloride/calcium gluconate, insulin, glucose, albuterol, Lasix (residual renal function present), kayexalate, and HCO_3^- if acidotic.
J. Pericardial tamponade can de diagnosed by bedside US. Consult CV surgery and cardiology for possible pericardiocentesis or pericardial window. Keep a pericardiocentesis tray at the bedside.
K. Treat infection of access site with vancomycin, 1 g IV as loading dose. Thrombosis of access site requires immediate surgical consultation.
L. **Disposition:** Admit and perform emergency dialysis for patients with volume overload, acidosis, hyperkalemia, and uremia (pericarditis, N/V, encephalopathy).

2. Epididymitis:

Epididymitis is an infection/inflammation of the epididymis from retrograde spread of organisms up the vas deferens. It is the most common cause of an acute scrotal mass in adults. This condition is usually due to an STD, chronic prostatitis, and urethral instrumentation. Males <35 y/o are typically infected with *C. trachomatis* and/or *N. gonorrhoeae* whereas males >35 y/o are infected due to *E. coli, Enterococci, Pseudomonas,* or *Proteus.*

2.1. Clinical Evaluation:

A. **Symptoms:** Scrotal pain and swelling, fever, chills, dysuria, urgency, frequency.
B. **Signs:** Fever, pain to palpation, positive Prehn's sign (pain relief with testicular elevation), + cremasteric reflex, swollen epididymis.
C. **DDX:** Testicular torsion, orchitis, torsion of appendix testis, tumor, hernia.
D. **Workup:** CBC, ESR, CRP, UA with culture, STD testing, color-flow Doppler ultrasound testicle as needed.

2.2. RX:

A. Treat fever and pain.
B. Scrotal support, ice packs, reduce physical activity, and sitz baths.
C. Males <35 y/o, rocephin 250 mg IM and doxycycline 100 mg po bid × 10 days.
D. Males >35 y/o, fluoroquinolone po.
E. If caused by STD, recommend treating the partner.
F. **Disposition:** Admit the febrile toxic patient.

3. Testicular Torsion:

Torsion is a twisting of the spermatic cord and testis, occluding the venous system and decreasing arterial flow. It commonly occurs during puberty and is bilateral in 40% of cases. It is due to an abnormal testicular fixation, resulting in it being freely suspended within the tunica vaginalis. Testicular salvage rates are 90% to 100% if detorsion is done within 6 hours of symptoms. If detorsion occurs >24 hours, the salvage rate is ≤10%.

3.1. Clinical Evaluation:

- **A. Symptoms:** Sudden onset of scrotal, N/V, dysuria, abdominal pain.
- **B. Signs:** High-riding, swollen, tender testicle. Horizontally lie, absent cremasteric reflex, negative Prehn's sign (pain relieved with elevation of testicle), scrotal swelling.
- **C. DDX:** Epididymitis, orchitis, torsion of appendix testis, tumor, hernia, hydrocele, hernia, scrotal trauma, hematocele, appendicitis.
- **D. Workup:** CBC, BMP, CRP, UA, testicular US.

3.2. RX:

- **A.** IV hydration and pain medication.
- **B.** If suspected, consult urology before any studies are ordered or performed.
- **C.** If time permits, order a color-flow Doppler ultrasound of the testicle.
- **D.** May attempt a manual detorsion by rotating the testicle lateral (open book).
- **E. Disposition:** Obtain a urology consult for immediate surgical detorsion.

4. Pyelonephritis:

Pyelonephritis is an infection of the renal parenchyma and collecting system due to ascending spread from the lower urinary tract or hematogenous spread. Eighty percent of uncomplicated pyelonephritis is caused by uropathogenic *E. coli*. Pyelonephritis is considered complicated when it is associated with an obstructing ureteral stone, sepsis, and immunocompromised state.

4.1. Clinical Evaluation:

- **A. Symptoms:** Fever, chills, dysuria, frequency, urgency, retention, suprapubic pain, hematuria, N/V, back/flank pain.
- **B. Signs:** Fever, tachycardia, tachypnea, dehydration, costovertebral-angle tenderness, AMS, hypotension.
- **C. DDX:** Cystitis, pyelonephritis, PID, vaginosis, urethritis, renal calculus, renal infarction, renal thrombosis, glomerulonephritis, pancreatitis, cholecystitis, splenic infarct, appendicitis, AAA.
- **D. Workup:** CBC, BMP, blood cultures as needed, UA, urine culture, KUB (kidney stone), US kidney/gallbladder, CT abd/pelvis (kidney stone).

4.2. RX:

- **A.** For uncomplicated pyelonephritis, such as cases not involving the debilitated, immune-suppressed, septic, or dehydrated, and patients able to tolerate po, treat for 14 days with TMP-SMX DS bid **or** a quinolone for 10 days. Rule out AAA as indicated.
- **B.** For pyelonephritis or UTI patients requiring admission, many IV regimens are available, including ampicillin, 1 g IV + gentamicin, 1 mg/kg IV **or** levofloxacin po/IV **or** ciprofloxacin po/IV, **or** ceftriaxone, 1 to 2 g IV.
- **C.** Replace or remove indwelling catheters.
- **D.** If a ureteral stone is present you must find it via CT or US or KUB. Consult urology stat.
- **E. Disposition:** Admit patients with complicated pyelonephritis who have persistent vomiting, unable to get there meds, poor follow-up. Consider admission for individuals with complicated UTI and those who are debilitated, dehydrated, unable to tolerate po, and appear toxic. Admit all infected ureteral stones (stone + pyelonephritis/cystitis).

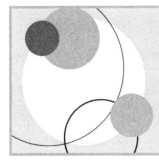

Procedure Pearls

PERICARDIOCENTESIS

1. Use ultrasound guidance when available to identify greatest fluid collection.
2. Monitor patient's vital signs during procedure.
3. Sedate as needed.
4. Surgically prepare the xiphoid and subxiphoid region.
5. Locally anesthetize the area being punctured.
6. Insert an 18 g to 16 g (15 cm) over-the-needle catheter attached to a 35-mL syringe with a three-way stopcock.
7. Insert the needle at a 45-degree angle, 1 to 2 cm inferior and to the left of the xiphochondral junction.
8. Advance the needle cephalad and toward the left shoulder. If advance too far PVCs will be seen on the monitor.
9. When in the pericardium aspirate as much nonclotted blood as possible and insert catheter.
10. Secure the catheter with stopcock closed.

NEEDLE THORACOSTOMY

1. Identify the anatomic landmarks and prep the skin.
2. Use a large-bore catheter over needle (16–14 g) that is >5 cm long.
3. Hold the catheter perpendicular to the chest and insert at the second intercostal space (just superior to the third rib), midclavicular line.
4. Once the needle is in the pleural space, listen for a rush of air. Remove the needle leaving the catheter in place.
5. Secure the catheter in place and attach a flutter valve.
6. Prepare for immediate chest tube insertion.

CHEST TUBE

1. Place patient in supine position with arm over the head.
2. Clean, drape, and anesthetize the site of insertion.
3. The usual site of insertion is the fourth or fifth intercostal space, at the midaxillary or anterior axillary line.
4. Make a 2- to 3-cm long incision over the rib just inferior to the interspace where the tube will penetrate the chest wall.
5. Using a Kelly clamp, bluntly dissect through the subcutaneous tissue, just over the top of the rib. Avoid the neurovascular bundle located at the inferior rib margin.

6. Penetrate the pleura with the clamp. Open the pleura 1 cm. With gloved finger, explore the subcutaneous tunnel and palpate the lung. Exclude possible abdominal penetration, adhesions, and ensure correct location within pleural space. With a clamp, grasp the tip of the chest tube and direct it into the pleural space in a posterior, superior direction. Guide the tube into the pleural space until the last hole is inside the pleural space.
7. Attach the tube to a Pleurovac or suction apparatus under a water seal of –20 cm H_2O.
8. Suture the tube to the skin of the chest wall by using O silk. Apply Vaseline gauze, 4 × 4 gauze sponges, and elastic tape. Obtain CXR to verify correct placement and evaluate re-expansion of lung.

CRICOTHYROIDOTOMY (CRICOTHYROTOMY)

1. Place the patient in a supine position with the neck in a neutral position.
2. Palpate the cricothyroid membrane between the thyroid and cricoid cartilage.
3. Prepare the area in a sterile fashion and anesthetize locally, if the patient is awake.
4. Stabilize the thyroid cartilage with the left hand and make a horizontal or transverse incision of the skin over the cricothyroid membrane.
5. Dissect down to the cricothyroid membrane and make a stab incision through it. Insert the blunt end of the scalpel through the incision and rotate 90 degrees to open the airway.
6. Insert a proper cuffed ETT or tracheostomy tube (#5 or #6) into the cricothyroid membrane incision, directing it distally into the trachea.
7. Inflate cuff, give breaths and observe chest movement.
8. Secure the tube in place.

INTERNAL JUGULAR CENTRAL LINE

1. Place patient in supine position, cleanse the skin around the venipuncture site and drape area.
2. Locate the site of entrance anteriorly: Locate the triangle formed by the sternal and clavicular heads of the sternocleidomastoid muscle superiorly and the clavicle inferiorly. The point of insertion is at the apex of this triangle.
3. Using an ultrasound as a guide insert a needle on a syringe, at a 30- to 40-degree angle at the apex of the triangle.
4. Direct the needle laterally and caudad toward the ipsilateral nipple, aspirating while advancing. The vein is only 1 to 2 cm below the skin.
5. When blood appears, remove syringe, occlude needle with finger, and insert the guidewire.
6. Remove the needle over the guidewire and insert and remove a dilator.
7. Start feeding the guidewire into the single or triple lumen, until it immerges from a port. Holding on to the wire with one hand, insert the line while removing the guidewire.
8. Aspirate and flush all ports, and secure the catheter in place.
9. Obtain a chest x-ray for placement and identify a possible a pneumothorax.

SUBCLAVIAN CENTRAL LINE

1. Place patient in 10- to 20-degree Trendelenburg. Cleanse the skin around the venipuncture site and drape area.
2. Keep one finger on the sternal notch and insert the needle on a syringe, to the inferior portion of the clavicle at the junction between the middle and lateral one-third of the clavicle. Ultrasound can be used as an adjunct for placement.

3. Walk the needle inferiorly under the clavicle, aspirating as you advance. When under the clavicle aim the needle toward the sternal notch.
4. When a free flow of blood appears in the syringe, remove it, occlude the needle with a finger, and insert the guidewire while monitoring the ECG for rhythm abnormalities.
5. Remove needle over the guidewire and insert and remove a dilator.
6. Start feeding the guidewire into the single or triple lumen, until it immerges from a port. Holding on to the wire with one hand, insert the line while removing the guidewire. The tip of the catheter should be above the right atrium.
7. Aspirate and flush all ports, and secure the catheter in place.
8. Obtain a chest x-ray for placement and identify a possible pneumothorax

FEMORAL CENTRAL LINE

1. Place patient in supine position, cleanse the skin around the venipuncture site and drape area.
2. Locate the femoral artery 2 to 3 cm below the inguinal ligament, and directly medial is the femoral vein. Remember the mnemonic NAVEL, from lateral to medial: nerve, artery, vein, empty space, lymphatic. US can be used as an adjunct for placement of the central line.
3. Keeping a finger on the femoral artery, insert the needle attached to a syringe, cephalad at a 45-degree angle, medial to the artery.
4. Advance the needle cephalad and posteriorly while gently withdrawing the plunger of the syringe.
5. When blood appears, remove syringe, occlude needle with finger, and insert the guidewire.
6. Remove the needle over the guidewire and insert and remove a dilator.
7. Start feeding the guidewire into the single or triple lumen, until it immerges from a port. Holding on to the wire with one hand, insert the line while removing the guidewire.
8. Aspirate and flush all ports, and secure the catheter in place.

FAST EXAMINATION

1. Start with the heart by using the subxiphoid and or parasternal view. Look for fluid in the pericardial space.
2. RUQ evaluation is a sagittal view in the midaxillary line, at the 10th or 11th rib space. Evaluate for fluid in the hepatorenal fossa (Morrison's pouch).
3. LUQ evaluation is a sagittal view in the midaxillary line at the eighth or ninth rib space. Evaluate for fluid in the splenorenal fossa.
4. Suprapubic evaluation is a transverse view over the bladder evaluating the bladder and the presence or absence of fluid posterior to this.

INTRAOSSEOUS PUNCTURE

1. Place the patient in the supine position and flex knee to 30 degrees.
2. Identify the puncture site at the anteromedial surface of the proximal tibia, one to two fingerbreadths below the tubercle. Clean and drape.
3. Insert the needle at a 90-degree angle, into the skin and periosteum. Advance through the cortex into the bone marrow.
4. Remove stylet or drill, and attach a fluid-filled syringe. Aspirate bone marrow and inject a few milliliters of saline.
5. Attach IV line, secure the IO in place, and dress.

❍ **What are the indications for intubation?**

Hypoventilation or hypoxia, decreased mental status from any cause, GCS <8, severe CNS injury, burns to face and upper airway, respiratory arrest, cardiopulmonary arrest, and severe chest injury (flail chest).

❍ **What are the contraindications for bag-valve-mask ventilation?**

Oral bleeding or vomiting, upper airway obstruction, and severe maxillofacial fractures.

❍ **What are the most common complications from bag-valve-mask ventilation?**

Inability to ventilate and gastric inflation.

❍ **What are the indications for laryngeal mask airway (LMA)?**

Inability to bag-mask ventilate or intubate.

❍ **What are the contraindications to insertion of an LMA?**

Less than 2 cm of mouth opening, an awake patient with a full stomach.

❍ **What are the most common complications of an LMA?**

Aspiration of gastric contents and hypoxia.

❍ **What are the predictors of a difficult intubation?**

History of previous difficult intubations, prominent upper incisors, limited neck mobility, poor visibility of pharyngeal structures, limited ability to open mouth, and a short thyromental distance.

❍ **What is the estimated ETT depth in a child, adult female, and adult male?**

Child: Tracheal tube depth (cm) = age (yr)/2 + 12

Adult female: 21 cm

Adult male 23 cm

❍ **What are the indications for performing a cricothyrotomy?**

Immediate airway management in a patient in whom oral or nasal intubation is either contraindicated or it cannot be established, massive oropharyngeal or nasopharyngeal bleeding, massive regurgitation, clenched teeth, and an upper airway obstruction.

❍ **What are the absolute contraindications to performing a cricothyrotomy?**

Children younger than 12 years, coagulopathy, transection of trachea with retraction of distal end into the mediastinum, a fractured larynx, and an easy endotracheal intubation in the absence of contraindications.

❍ **What are the potential complications of a cricothyrotomy?**

Hemorrhage, infection, subcutaneous, or mediastinal emphysema, pneumothorax, laceration of the trachea or esophagus, subglottic or laryngeal stenosis, prolonged hypoxia because of prolonged unsuccessful attempts, creation of a paratracheal tract, and right mainstem bronchus intubation.

What are the advantages of a cricothyrotomy compared to a tracheostomy?

A cricothyrotomy is easier and faster to perform, does not require the OR, and is associated with fewer early and late complications.

What is the complication rate of an emergency cricothyrotomy?

10% to 40%.

What are the most common complications of an emergency cricothyrotomy?

Bleeding, unsuccessful tube placement, and prolonged procedure time.

What is the most common cause of subglottic stenosis?

Endotracheal intubation; not cricothyrotomy or tracheostomy.

How is a needle cricothyrotomy performed?

Insert a large (14 g) intravenous cannula through the inferior part of the cricothyroid membrane, with the needle at a 45-degree angle to the skin, and oriented caudad. Once in the trachea, insert the catheter and confirm by aspirating air with a syringe. Ventilate for 1 second and allow exhalation for 4 seconds.

What are the indications for a needle cric?

(1) When orotracheal or nasotracheal intubation cannot be performed.

(2) When intubation cannot be performed in a timely manner.

(3) When intubation is contraindicated.

(4) When temporary relief of hypoxemia is required because of an airway obstruction.

What are the absolute contraindications to a needle cric?

(1) When endotracheal intubation is not contraindicated and can be accomplished easily and rapidly.

(2) When the trachea has been transected and retracted.

(3) When there is direct damage to the cricoid cartilage or larynx.

What is the most common complication of percutaneous transtracheal ventilation?

Subcutaneous emphysema.

What are the complications from a femoral venous line?

DVT, arterial injury, nerve injury, and arteriovenous fistula.

What are the benefits of the FAST examination?

Decrease the time to diagnosis for acute abdominal injury, accurately diagnose hemoperitoneum, assess the degree of hemoperitoneum, noninvasive, can be performed quickly, can be repeated easily, safe in pregnant patients and children, and can lead to fewer CT scans.

- **What are the complications of an oropharyngeal airway?**

Pushing the tongue posteriorly, thereby worsening the obstruction, incorrect size can be lost in oropharynx or obstruct the epiglottis, traumatize soft tissues, and vomiting.

- **What are the contraindications to using a nasopharyngeal airway?**

Severe nasal fracture, facial fractures, and the need for immediate intubation.

- **How is the appropriate endotracheal tube size in children determined?**

Tube diameter = (patients age + 16)4
= diameter of patient's fifth finger
= thumbnail width

- **What are the complications of endotracheal intubation?**

Esophageal intubation, right or left mainstem bronchus intubation, pharyngeal laceration, vocal cord damage, tracheal laceration, vomiting with aspiration, hypoxia from prolonged attempt times, dental fractures, transient increase in intracranial pressure, tachycardia, and bradycardia.

- **How is a patient with a possible C-spine injury intubated?**

Place the head and neck in a neutral position, and have an assistant provide in-line stabilization with or without the collar on.

- **What are the contraindications to nasotracheal intubation?**

Apnea, severe facial fractures, blunt laryngeal trauma with suspected tracheal disruption, and coagulopathy.

- **What are the advantages of a nasotracheal intubation over an orotracheal intubation?**

The tube can be passed with the patient sitting upright and with minimal neck manipulation. Tube fixation is more secure and the patient cannot bite down on the tube.

- **What is the most common complication of nasotracheal intubation?**

Epistaxis.

- **What are the complications of nasotracheal intubation?**

Epistaxis, turbinate fractures, nasal necrosis, intracranial placement through a basilar skull fracture, retropharyngeal laceration or dissection, and unsuccessful placement.

- **What is the contraindication to an oropharyngeal airway?**

A patient with an intact gag reflex.

- **What is the most common complication from inserting a nasopharyngeal airway?**

Nasal bleeding.

❍ **What percent of FiO_2 can be delivered by the bag-valve-mask system?**

If a tight seal is obtained, the bag-valve-mask system can deliver a 40% FiO_2 at 12 L/min. If an oxygen reservoir is attached, oxygen concentration approaches 90%.

❍ **What should be done if laryngospasm occurs while intubating?**

Hold constant pressure on the cords with the tip of the endotracheal tube or spray 1% lidocaine on them.

❍ **How is the correct positioning of an endotracheal tube determined?**

Auscultate in the anterior or midaxillary line bilaterally then over the stomach, check chest x-ray placement (tube 2 cm above the carina), and use a CO_2 detector.

❍ **What are the anatomic differences in children that make intubation more challenging?**

Small mandible, big tongue, large head, the larynx is more anterior and cephalad, and the angle between the laryngeal opening and the pharynx is more acute.

❍ **How should the head of a pediatric patient be positioned for intubation?**

Because of the large size of the head in relationship to the body, intubation should be performed with the head in the neutral position.

❍ **What are the indications for a pericardiocentesis?**

The diagnosis and relief of symptomatic cardiac tamponade, unresponsive to volume replacement.

❍ **How reliable is a pericardiocentesis?**

The false-negative rate is 20% to 40%.

❍ **What are the complications of a pericardiocentesis?**

Laceration of the myocardium or a coronary artery, pneumothorax, perforation of the right ventricle, dysrhythmias, venous embolism, hemopericardium, puncture/laceration of liver or diaphragm, and pneumopericardium.

❍ **What arrhythmias can occur from a pericardiocentesis?**

PVCs are the most common followed by asystole, V-Fib, and tachycardia.

❍ **What is the best sonographic view for diagnosing a pericardial effusion?**

The subxiphoid view.

❍ **What are the indications for chest tube insertion?**

Tension pneumothorax, simple pneumothorax of >20%, hemothorax, and hemopneumothorax.

❍ **What are the potential complications of inserting a chest tube too low, that is, below the fifth intercostal space?**

Perforation of the liver or spleen, insertion into the abdominal cavity, and diaphragmatic trauma.

❍ **What are the complications from a chest tube insertion?**

Bleeding from the chest wall, occlusion of the chest tube, continuing air leak, subcutaneous emphysema, persistent pneumothorax, laceration to the lung, liver or spleen, subcutaneous insertion, and intra-abdominal insertion.

❍ **What are the advantages of transcutaneous pacing?**

It can be instituted quickly, easy to use, and is noninvasive.

❍ **What conditions can render transcutaneous pacing ineffective?**

Dilated cardiomyopathy, obesity, emphysema, kyphoscoliosis, and a pericardial effusion.

❍ **What are the indications of transthoracic pacing?**

Unable to insert a transvenous pacemaker, early in asystole, bradycardia with altered hemodynamic state, Mobitz type II with symptoms, myocardial infarction with a type II second–degree heart block, third-degree heart block, symptomatic bundle branch blocks, and a malfunction of an implanted pacemaker.

❍ **What are the potential complications from a transthoracic pacemaker insertion?**

Coronary artery laceration, pericardial tamponade, laceration of the myocardium, and fracture of the pacing wire. Transthoracic pacemakers are no longer commonly used for these reasons.

❍ **How is a transvenous pacemaker blindly inserted?**

Cannulate a central vein (internal jugular, subclavian,) in the standard fashion. Insert the electrode catheter into the superior vena cava. Attach the pacemaker catheter to the generator and set the output to its maximum (mA) and a rate of 70/min. Turn the generator on and advance until ventricular pacing occurs. Confirm placement by chest x-ray.

❍ **What complications may occur from a transvenous pacemaker insertion?**

Myocardial perforation, perforation of the ventricular septum, malposition into the hepatic vein or inferior vena cava, failure to capture, arrhythmias, diaphragmatic pacing, and muscle spasm.

❍ **What findings indicate a possible interventricular septum perforation?**

Catheter tip in the left ventricle on a chest x-ray, increased pacing threshold, and the conversion of a left bundle branch block to a right bundle branch block.

❍ **What arrhythmias may occur with transvenous pacing?**

Ventricular fibrillation or ventricular tachycardia.

❍ **What are the indications for a lumbar puncture?**

Diagnosis of infections (meningitis, encephalitis, abscesses), cancer (metastatic carcinoma, leukemia), subarachnoid hemorrhage, and relief of intracranial pressure (pseudotumor cerebri).

❍ **What are the contraindications to performing a lumbar puncture?**

Coagulation defect, anticoagulation therapy, a history of progressively increasing headache (perform a CT scan first), the presence of localizing neurologic signs or symptoms (CT scan first), the presence of papilledema (CT scan first), and infection at the site of the puncture.

❍ **What are the complications associated with a lumbar puncture?**

Headache, epidermoid tumor, spinal subdural and epidural hematoma, infection, and herniation.

❍ **What are the indications for a culdocentesis?**

Identify the presence of peritoneal fluid, blood, or pus in the cul-de-sac.

❍ **How is a culdocentesis performed?**

Grasp the posterior lip of the cervix with a tenaculum, cleanse the posterior vaginal fornix, insert an 18-gauge spinal attached to a 20-cc syringe in the midline of the posterior fornix, aspirate as the needle is being inserted, and advance no further than 2 cm.

❍ **What constitutes a positive tap?**

The aspiration of 2 mL of blood.

❍ **How is a dislocated knee reduced?**

One person applies traction longitudinally in the line of the deformity to the involved extended knee while an assistant applies countertraction above the knee.

❍ **After the knee is reduced, what must be done?**

An arteriogram or CT angiogram should be performed to evaluate the popliteal artery. Duplex ultrasonography is an effective, low cost, noninvasive option.

❍ **What are the indications for bladder catheterization?**

Relief of acute urinary retention, the evaluation of urine output for the critically ill or for injured patients, neurogenic bladder, urethral or prostatic obstruction leading to hydronephrosis and decreased renal function, and a urologic study of the anatomy of the urinary tract.

❍ **What are the contraindications to bladder catheterization?**

Prostatic displacement or mobility on rectal examination, perineal hematoma, and blood at the urethral meatus.

❍ **What complication can occur from catheterizing a patient with pelvic trauma?**

A partial urethral disruption may be converted to a complete injury.

❍ **What are the complications of bladder catheterization?**

Creation of a false passage, cystitis, urethritis, pyelonephritis, hemorrhage, urethral trauma, and epididymitis.

❍ **What is the indication for suprapubic catheterization?**

Urinary obstruction in a patient where catheterization cannot be done.

❍ **What is the indication for suprapubic aspiration?**

For diagnostic purposes in pediatric patients.

❍ **What are the contraindications to the placement of a suprapubic catheter?**

Unable to define the bladder, lower abdominal scarring, a history of intraperitoneal surgery or irradiation, and bleeding disorders.

❍ **What complications are associated with suprapubic catheterization?**

Puncture of a large vessel, puncture of the large or small bowel, leakage around the catheter, hematuria, abdominal wall abscess, extraperitoneal extravasation, intraperitoneal extravasation, and ureteral catheterization.

❍ **How is a suprapubic aspiration performed?**

Percuss or use ultrasound to determine the level of the bladder. Insert a 22-gauge 1-in needle, 2 cm above the symphysis pubis at a 45- to 60-degree angle. Aspirate urine for analysis.

❍ **Describe the technique for a suprapubic catheter insertion.**

Percuss to determine the location of the bladder, prep and anesthetize the area, and insert the trocar-catheter system at a 30-degree angle 3 to 4 cm cephalad to the symphysis pubis. Insert the catheter 3 cm over the trocar and suture in place.

❍ **Describe how to detorse a testicle.**

Grasp the testicle and attempt to rotate laterally and superiorly (opening a book). If successful, the testicle will drop into a normal position.

❍ **What are the indications for insertion of a central venous catheter?**

Emergency IV route in a seriously ill or injured patient, transvenous pacemaker insertion, rapid administration of a large volume of fluid, infusion of concentrated hyperosmolar solutions, inability to obtain a peripheral IV, and central venous pressure monitoring.

❍ **What are the contraindications to subclavian venipuncture?**

Chest wall deformity, distorted local anatomy, extreme weight, radiation therapy to region, vasculitis, coagulopathy, agitated uncooperative patient, prior long-term subclavian cannulation, possible superior vena cava injury, and suspected subclavian vessel injury.

❍ **Why should a finger be placed over-the-needle hub once the syringe is removed?**

If the hub is left open, air may enter with each inspiration causing a potential air embolism.

❍ **When do most complications from a subclavian line occur?**

Forty percent of complications occur when the procedure is performed as an emergency.

❍ **What complications are associated with insertion of a subclavian line?**

Pneumothorax, hemothorax, tracheal perforation, catheter fragmentation, air embolus, thoracic duct laceration, pericardial tamponade, subclavian artery puncture, local hematoma, local cellulitis, generalized sepsis, phrenic nerve injury, dysrhythmias, catheter malposition, chest pain, and hydrothorax.

❍ **Which type of patient has a particular risk for a pneumothorax during a subclavian line insertion?**

A patient receiving mechanical ventilation, undergoing multiple attempts at cannulation, children (pleural reflection is higher), and emphysematous patients.

❍ **If a patient becomes cyanotic, tachypneic, hypotensive, with a new holosystolic murmur heard over the precordium during a subclavian line insertion, what complication must be considered?**

An air embolism.

❍ **Why should the right side be attempted first when inserting a subclavian line?**

There is a danger of injury to the thoracic duct on the left. In addition, the right subclavian has a straighter course in relation to the innominate and superior vena cava, resulting in a more successful cannulation when compared to the left side.

❍ **Why try a supraclavicular approach when cannulating the subclavian vein?**

The complication rate is lower because the needle is directed away from the pleural dome and subclavian artery.

❍ **What are the other advantages of the supraclavicular approach over the infraclavicular approach?**

The subclavian and internal jugular is the target used, it is less painful, the distance between the skin and vein is shorter, and the variability of the space between the first rib and the clavicle is avoided.

❍ **Describe the supraclavicular approach to subclavian vein cannulation?**

Place the patient in a Trendelenburg position, prep, drape, and anesthetize. Insert a 14-gauge needle, at a 45-degree angle to the sagittal plane, at the junction of the lateral aspect of the clavicular head of the sternocleidomastoid muscle with the superior border of the clavicle. Use the Seldinger technique to cannulate and secure the catheter in place.

❍ **What are the advantages of an internal jugular vein cannulation?**

There is a low risk of pleural puncture, hematomas are easier to compress, malpositioning is rare, may be used in a patient with a coagulopathy (only if absolutely necessary), and is useful in patients with a short, thick neck.

❍ **What are the disadvantages of an internal jugular line?**

Insertion failure rate is higher compared to infraclavicular attempts, more uncomfortable for the patient, easier to become dislodged and kinked, and is contraindicated with a C-spine injury.

❍ **What complications are associated with the insertion of an internal jugular line?**

Hematoma, thoracic duct injury, hemo/pneumothorax, air embolism, phlebitis, infection, nerve damage, and myocardial puncture.

❍ **What are the indications for femoral venous cannulation?**

Rapid volume replacement, unable to obtain peripheral access, and radiographic procedures.

❍ **What are the contraindications to femoral venous cannulation?**

Trauma to the inguinal region, possible injury to the inferior vena cava or iliacs, skin abnormalities such as burns, deep abrasions, or severe dermatitis.

❍ **What complications are associated with femoral venous cannulation?**

Femoral nerve injury, septic arthritis, hematoma, catheter insertion into the abdominal cavity, psoas abscess, thrombosis, and phlebitis.

❍ **What is the most common organism causing septic arthritis, as a result of a femoral line?**

Staphylococcus aureus.

❍ **Describe the procedure for performing a saphenous vein cutdown at the ankle.**

Prep, drape, and anesthetize an area two fingerbreadths above the medial malleolus. Make a transverse incision over the vein, dissect down to the vein with curved hemostats, isolate the vein between two ligatures tying off the distal portion, make a longitudinal incision between the two sutures, and insert a catheter into the vein. Secure the proximal ligature around the cannula, close the wound, and suture the cannula to the skin.

❍ **What are some advantages of a saphenous vein cutdown?**

Only vessel of significance in that area, always found just anterior to the medial malleolus, and easy to access.

❍ **What are the indications for a saphenous vein cutdown?**

Unable to insert a peripheral line or central line, the need for rapid volume replacement, and cardiac arrest in an infants or children.

❍ **What are the contraindications to a saphenous vein cutdown?**

When less invasive alternatives exist, when more rapid access is required, coagulation disorders, compromised host-defense mechanisms, or impaired healing.

❍ **What are the complications associated with a saphenous vein cutdown?**

Local hematoma, infection, sepsis, phlebitis, embolization, wound dehiscence, and injuries to associated arteries/nerves.

❍ **What are the complications from a thoracentesis?**

Pneumothorax, lung laceration, hemopneumothorax, diaphragmatic tear, intra-abdominal injuries, infection, hypoxia and pulmonary edema, hypotension, and chest wall bleeding.

❍ **What complications can occur if more than 1,500 to 2,000 mL are removed during a thoracentesis?**

Pulmonary edema and hypotension.

❍ **What are the indications for a thoracentesis?**

Evacuation of a large symptomatic pleural effusion, diagnostic analysis of a pleural effusion

❍ **What are the contraindications to performing a thoracentesis?**

Bleeding diathesis, anticoagulant use, rupture diaphragm, traumatic hemo/pneumothorax, and tension pneumothorax.

❍ **What are the indications for an intraosseous line?**

When fluids or drugs must be introduced into the circulation rapidly and when the venous access is not available. Other indications include cardiac arrest in an infant or child, shock, severe burns, dehydration, status epilepticus, or any condition requiring emergency administration of fluids and drugs.

❍ **What are the contraindications to the placement of an intraosseous line?**

Infection at the intended site and a fracture to the tibia.

❍ **What is the most common complication of intraosseous infusion?**

Subcutaneous and subperiosteal infiltration of fluid or leakage from the puncture site.

❍ **What are the indications for a nasogastric tube?**

To aspirate gastric contents for diagnostic or therapeutic reasons, the presence of an ileus or mechanical obstruction, to prevent gastric aspiration in a trauma patient before doing a peritoneal lavage, for feeding purposes, and for the administration of therapeutic substances such as charcoal.

❍ **What are the contraindications to nasogastric tube insertion?**

Facial fractures with possible cribriform plate fracture, esophageal perforation, strictures or a history of alkali ingestion, comatose state with an unprotected airway, and penetrating neck wounds in an awake trauma patient.

❍ **Describe the technique for inserting a nasogastric tube.**

Insert the tube along the floor of the nose directed posteriorly. After the tube passes the posterior pharynx continue inserting to the stomach.

❍ **What procedure(s) should be performed to ensure that a nasogastric tube is in place?**

Aspirate gastric contents, inject 20 to 30 cc of air while listening over the stomach, or obtain a chest x-ray for placement.

❍ **What are the indications that a nasogastric tube was inserted into the trachea?**

The patient will cough or is unable to speak.

❍ **What complications are the associated with nasogastric tube insertion?**

Epistaxis, rupture of the esophagus or stomach, perforation of the esophagus, intracranial insertion, insertion in the submucosa of the posterior pharynx, ulceration of the nasal mucosa, sinusitis, otitis media, and tracheal insertion.

❍ **Describe the procedure for performing a diagnostic peritoneal lavage.**

Insert a bladder catheter and nasogastric tube, prepare, drape, and anesthetize the area. Make a vertical incision one-third the distance from the umbilicus to the symphysis pubis, insert a peritoneal dialysis catheter, aspirate for blood and infuse 1 L of LR or NS, and allow the fluid to drain out.

❍ **What are the indications for a diagnostic peritoneal lavage (DPL)?**

To detect intra-abdominal injury in a patient with potential abdominal trauma requiring surgery, when a patient is unconscious because of a head injury or substance abuse, when there is a recent or pre-existing paraplegia, and when there is a penetrating injury to the thoracoabdominal, pelvic, back, and flank region.

❍ **What are the indications for a DPL in children?**

Unexplained shock following trauma, altered level of consciousness, major thoracic injury, multiple trauma, and major orthopedic injuries, such as a fractured pelvis, femur, or hip.

❍ **What are the absolute contraindications to a DPL?**

An unstable patient requiring immediate surgery is the only absolute contraindication. Previous surgeries to the abdomen, pregnant patient, and inability to catheterize the bladder are relative contraindications.

❍ **What approach should be used when performing a DPL on a pregnant patient?**

Supraumbilical approach.

❍ **What constitutes a positive DPL?**

Aspiration of >10 cc of blood, WBC >500, RBCs >100,000 (blunt), >10,000 (penetrating), elevated amylase, bile, or intestinal contents.

❍ **What are the indications for an ED thoracotomy?**

Control exsanguinating intrathoracic bleeding, manage cardiac tamponade not decompressed by needle aspiration, cross-clamp aorta to control intra-abdominal bleeding, perform open cardiac massage.

Random Pearls

❍ **What are the characteristics of an abusive relationship?**

The abusive relationship evolves over time usually escalating from jealousy and a desire to control a partner's behavior into humiliation, degradation, and use of the fear of physical violence. He may or may not have to actually hit her, if she knows that he is capable of hurting her or her children. The end result is low self-esteem, control, isolation, and entrapment.

❍ **How is a dystonic reaction treated?**

Diphenhydramine (Benadryl), 25 to 50 mg IM or IV, or benztropine (Cogentin), 1 to 2 mg IV or po.

❍ **Describe the symptoms of alcohol withdrawal.**

(1) Autonomic hyperactivity: tachycardia, hypertension, tremors, anxiety, agitation; 6 to 8 hours after drinking.

(2) Hallucinations: auditory, visual, tactile; 24 hours after drinking.

(3) Global confusion: 1 to 3 days after drinking.

❍ **List some life-threatening causes of acute psychosis.**

WHHHIMP: Wernicke's encephalopathy, hypoxia, hypoglycemia, hypertensive encephalopathy, intracerebral hemorrhage, meningitis/encephalitis, and poisoning.

❍ **What are the clinical findings that suggest acute glomerulonephritis (GN)?**

Oliguria, hypertension, pulmonary edema, and urine sediment containing red blood cells, white blood cells, protein, and red blood cell casts.

❍ **What is the most common presenting symptom of MS?**

Optic neuritis (about 25%).

❍ **Which three bacterial illnesses present with peripheral neurologic findings?**

Botulism, tetanus, and diphtheria.

❍ **What is the *most common* cause of intrinsic renal failure?**

Acute tubular necrosis (90% of cases), resulting from an ischemic injury (the most common cause of ATN), or a nephrotoxic agent. Less frequent causes of intrinsic renal failure (10–20% of cases) are vasculitis, malignant hypertension, acute GN, or allergic interstitial nephritis.

❍ **What is the eponym for idiopathic scrotal edema, and how is this disease treated?**

Fournier's gangrene is a polymicrobial infection of the subcutaneous tissue that is characterized by widespread tissue necrosis. Treatment consists of broad-spectrum parenteral antibiotics and immediate surgical debridement.

❍ **How does the pain associated with epididymitis differ from that of prostatitis?**

Epididymitis: The pain begins in the scrotum or groin and radiates along the spermatic cord. It intensifies rapidly, is associated with dysuria, and is relieved with scrotal elevation (Prehn's sign).

Prostatitis: Patients will have frequency, dysuria, urgency, bladder outlet obstruction, and retention. They may have low back pain, perineal pain associated with fever, chills, arthralgias, and myalgias.

❍ **Which are the causative organisms of prostatitis?**

Escherichia coli in 80% and Klebsiella, Enterobacter, Proteus, or Pseudomonas in 20%.

❍ **When are the two peaks in the incidence of testicular torsion?**

The first year of life and at puberty.

❍ **How does the treatment of epididymitis differ according to age?**

In patients younger than 40 years, the most common pathogens are *Chlamydia* and *gonorrhea*, treated with ceftriaxone IM and doxycycline po. In patients older than 40 years, the common causes are urinary pathogens such as *Escherichia coli* (*E. coli*) and *Klebsiella* that are treated with TMP-SMX or a quinolone.

❍ **What is the definitive diagnostic test for testicular torsion?**

Emergent surgical exploration. Although radionuclide imaging and Doppler ultrasonography may be helpful, they are time-consuming and their accuracy is operator dependent. The warm ischemia time for testicular salvage may be as short as 4 hours. Therefore, once the diagnosis is entertained, immediate urologic consultation and surgical exploration are necessary.

❍ **When is a retrograde urethrogram necessary in the evaluation of a patient with a penile fracture?**

A penile fracture is rupture of the corpus cavernosum with tearing of the tunica albuginea that results from blunt trauma to the erect penis. Urethral injury occurs in approximately 10% of patients with a penile fracture. Patients with hematuria, blood at the urethral meatus, or inability to void should undergo retrograde urethrography to rule out a urethral injury.

❍ **What is the treatment for priapism?**

(1) Pain control.

(2) Oral pseudoephedrine 30 to 60 mg po.

(3) Phenylephrine 250 to 500 μg every 5 minutes directly injected into the corpora cavernosa (may substitute epinephrine 10–20 μg).

(4) Consult urology for aspiration of the cavernous bodies.

❍ **Describe acute glomerulonephritis (GN).**

Hematuria, proteinuria, oliguria or anuria, edema, and hypertension.

❍ **What is the proper position to transport a pregnant trauma patient?**

With spinal backboard tilted 30 degrees to the left in order to prevent the supine hypotension syndrome.

❍ **What is the clinical significance of fixed and dilated pupils in a drowning victim?**

Don't give up the ship! Ten to twenty percent of patients presenting with coma and fixed and dilated pupils recover completely. Asymptomatic patients should be observed for a minimum of 4 to 6 hours.

❍ **What should be done if you suspect an air embolism has occurred while inserting a central line?**

Place the patient in the right lateral decubitus position trendelenburg and consult thoracic surgery.

❍ **What percentage of dog and cat bites become infected?**

About 10% of dog and 50% of cat bites become infected. *Pasteurella multocida* is the most common organism.

❍ **A 6-year-old child presents with headache, fever, malaise, and tender regional lymphadenopathy about a week after a cat bite. A tender papule develops at the site. What is the diagnosis?**

Cat-scratch disease. Usually develops from 3 days to 6 weeks following a cat bite or scratch. The papule typically blisters and heals with eschar formation or a transient macular or vesicular rash may develop.

❍ **A patient is brought to the ED from a local psychiatric facility, with a history of a bite wound. What bacterium is likely?**

Eikenella corrodens is more common in hospitalized and institutionalized patients. Most human bite infections are caused by *Staphylococcus aureus* or *Streptococcus*.

❍ **What is the frequency of eye injuries in lightning strike victims?**

Half develop structural eye lesions. Cataracts are the most common and develop within days to years. Unreactive dilated pupils may not equal death because transient autonomic instability may occur.

❍ **What is the most common otologic injury in a lightning strike victim?**

Fifty percent have tympanic membrane rupture. Hemotympanum, basilar skull fracture, and acoustic and vestibular deficits may also occur.

❍ **What is the most common arrhythmia found in a patient with hypothermia?**

Atrial fibrillation. Other ECG findings include PAT, prolongation of the P-R, QRS, or Q-T, decreased P-wave amplitude, T-wave changes, PVCs, or humped ST segment adjacent to the QRS complex (Osborn wave).

❍ **A 14-year-old football player presents to the ED with a history of light-headedness, headache, nausea, and vomiting. On examination, the patient has an HR of 110, RR 22, BP of 90/60, and is afebrile. Profuse sweating is noted. What is the diagnosis?**

Heat exhaustion. Treat with 0.9 NS IV fluid.

❍ **What is the treatment for heatstroke?**

Cool sponging, ice packs to groin and axilla, fanning, and/or mechanical cooling devices. Antipyretics are of no value.

❍ **An Osborn (J) wave displayed by an ECG is associated with what disorder?**

Hypothermia.

❍ **Compare the entrance and exit wounds of AC and DC.**

AC: Entrance and exit wounds are the same size.

DC: Small entrance and large exit.

❍ **What treatment options are available for patients who are bleeding and have liver disease?**

(1) Transfusion with PRBCs (maintains hemodynamic stability).

(2) Vitamin K.

(3) Fresh-frozen plasma.

(4) Platelet transfusion.

(5) DDAVP (desmopressin).

(6) Prothrombin complex concentrate.

❍ **What options are available for the treatment of patients with renal failure and coagulopathy?**

Dialysis.

Optimize hematocrit.

- Recombinant human erythropoietin.
- Transfusion with PRBCs.

Desmopressin.

Conjugated estrogens.

Cryoprecipitate and platelet transfusions, if hemorrhage is life-threatening.

❍ **What two conditions are associated with the most devastating form of DIC?**

Neisseria meningitidis sepsis and acute myelogenous leukemia (promyelocytic [M3] type).

❍ **What are the clinical complications of DIC?**

Bleeding, thrombosis, and purpura fulminans.

❍ **What three laboratory studies would be most helpful in establishing the diagnosis of DIC?**

Prothrombin time—prolonged.

Platelet count—usually low.

Fibrinogen level—low.

Fibrin split products—elevated.

D-dimer—elevated.

❍ **What are the most common hemostatic abnormalities in patients infected with HIV?**

Thrombocytopenia and acquired circulating anticoagulants, which causes prolongation of aPTT.

❍ **What is the pentad of thrombotic thrombocytopenic purpura (TTP)?**

Fever, thrombocytopenia, neurologic symptoms, renal insufficiency, and microangiopathic hemolytic anemia.

❍ **Which type of clinical crises are seen in patients with sickle cell disease?**

Vasoocclusive (thrombotic).

Hematologic.

- Sequestration.
- Aplastic.
- Infectious.

❍ **Which is the most common type of sickle cell crisis?**

Vasoocclusive, with an average of four attacks per year.

❍ **Which is the only type of vasoocclusive crisis that is painless?**

CNS crisis. Most commonly children are afflicted with cerebral infarction and cerebral hemorrhage develops in adults.

❍ **What are the major causes of GI bleeding in cancer patients?**

Hemorrhagic gastritis and peptic ulcer disease.

❍ **What are the mainstays of therapy for a patient with sickle cell crisis?**

Hydration, analgesia, and oxygen (only beneficial if patient is hypoxic).

❍ **What condition should be suspected in a patient with multiple myeloma who presents to the ED with paraparesis, paraplegia, and urinary incontinence?**

Acute spinal cord compression. This condition occurs primarily with multiple myeloma and lymphoma, but may be seen in cancer of the lung, breast, and prostate.

❍ **What are the laboratory abnormalities in DIC?**

Increased PT, elevated fibrin split products, decreased fibrinogen, and thrombocytopenia.

❍ **What is treatment for a life-threatening hypercalcemia?**

NS fluid infusion at 5 to 10 L/d, furosemide, glucocorticoids, calcitonin, and mithramycin and bisphosphonates.

❍ **Which blood product is given when the coagulation abnormality is unknown?**

FFP.

❍ **Which agent can be used for treating mild hemophilia A and von Willebrand's disease type 1?**

D-Amino-8. D-arginine vasopressin (DDAVP), induces a rapid rise in factor VIII levels.

❍ **What is the minimal β-hCG titer for which an experienced ultrasonographer should be able to visualize a viable intrauterine pregnancy?**

Transvaginal >1,500 hCG mIU/mL. Transabdominal, 6500.

❍ **What is the number one cause of maternal mortality?**

Thromboembolism. The risk progressively increases throughout pregnancy, peaking at >5 times nonpregnant controls during the postpartum period.

❍ **What is the indication for RhoGAM in the first trimester?**

An unsensitized Rh-negative woman with any vaginal bleeding.

❍ **What is the most common presentation of ectopic pregnancy?**

Amenorrhea followed by pain.

❍ **How does a spontaneous abortion most commonly present?**

Pain followed by bleeding.

❍ **What is the *most common* finding on pelvic examination in a patient with an ectopic pregnancy?**

Unilateral adnexal tenderness.

❍ **When can an intrauterine gestational sac be seen on US?**

Fifth week. Fetal pole, sixth week. Embryonic mass with cardiac motion, seventh week.

❍ **What is the most common cause of toxic shock syndrome?**

S. aureus. Other causes, which are clinically similar include group A Streptococci, *Pseudomonas aeruginosa*, and *Streptococcus pneumoniae.*

❍ **What criteria are necessary for the diagnosis of toxic shock syndrome?**

T >38.9°C (102°F), rash, systolic BP <90 and orthostasis, involvement of three organ systems (GI, renal, musculoskeletal, mucosal, hepatic, hematologic, or CNS), and negative serologic tests for such diseases as RMSF, hepatitis B, measles, leptospirosis, VDRL, etc.

❍ **Which type of rash develops with TSS?**

Blanching erythroderma, which resolves in 3 days and is then followed by a desquamation (full-thickness). This typically occurs between the sixth and fourteenth day with peeling prominent on the hands and feet.

How should a patient with toxic shock syndrome be treated?

FLUIDS, FFP or transfusions, vaginal irrigation with iodine or saline, and antistaphylococcal penicillin, or cephalosporin with anti—β-lactamase activity, such as nafcillin or oxacillin. Rifampin should be considered to eliminate the carrier state.

Define preeclampsia.

HTN after 20 weeks EGA with edema and proteinuria.

Define eclampsia.

Preeclampsia plus grand mal seizures or coma.

Why is Rh status important in a pregnant patient?

Rh-negative with Rh-positive fetus can result in fetal anemia, hydrops, and fetal loss. Rh immunoglobulin should be given to all Rh-negative patients.

When can a transvaginal and a transabdominal ultrasound identify an intrauterine gestational sac?

Transvaginal, 4 weeks. Transabdominal, 5 weeks.

A 24-year-old, 10-week pregnant patient presents with bleeding per vagina. She also complains of nausea, vomiting, and abdominal pain. The physical findings reveal a blood pressure of 150/100 and a uterus, which is larger than dates. The laboratory studies indicated proteinuria. What is the diagnosis?

Molar pregnancy. Uterus may be larger or smaller than expected dates.

What are the risk factors for placenta previa?

Previous cesarean section, previous placenta previa, multiparity, multiple induced abortions, and multiple gestations.

What are the risk factors for abruptio placenta?

Smoking, hypertension, multiparity, trauma, cocaine abuse and previous abruptio placenta.

What are the presenting signs and symptoms of abruptio placentae?

Placental separation before delivery is associated with vaginal bleeding (78%), abdominal pain (66%), as well as tetanic uterine contractions, uterine irritability, and fetal death.

Is life-threatening hemorrhage due to trauma during pregnancy most often intra- or retroperitoneal?

Retroperitoneal.

What are the two distinct causes of toxic epidermal necrolysis (scalded skin syndrome)?

Staphylococcal and drugs or chemicals. Both begin with the appearance of patches of tender erythema followed by loosening of the skin and denuding to glistening bases.

Staphylococcal scalded skin syndrome (SSSS) is commonly found in children younger than 5 years and is caused by toxin that cleaves within the epidermis under the stratum granulosum.

❍ **What is the treatment for SSSS?**

Oral or IV penicillinase-resistant penicillin, baths of potassium permanganate or dressings soaked in 0.5% silver nitrate, and fluids. Corticosteroids and silver sulfadine are contraindicated.

❍ **What is the mechanism of action of tetanospasmin?**

Enters peripheral nerve endings and ascends the axons to reach the brain and spinal cord. At this point it binds four areas of the nervous system:

- Anterior horn cells of the spinal cord: Impairs inhibitory interneurons resulting in neuromuscular irritability and generalized spasms.
- Sympathetic nervous system: Resulting in sweating, labile blood pressure, tachycardia, and peripheral vasoconstriction.
- Myoneural junction: Inhibits release of acetylcholine.
- Binds to cerebral gangliosides: Thought to cause seizures.

❍ **What is the most common cause of gas gangrene?**

Clostridium perfringens.

❍ **What is an ABI and what is its significance?**

(1) ABI = Ankle/brachial index. The ankle systolic pressure (numerator) is compared to the higher of the two brachial arterial pressures (denominator). It is used to determine if arterial obstruction or injury is present.

(2) Normal ABI = Greater than or equal to 1.

(3) ABI 0.5 to 0.9 = Obstructive disease of a single peripheral arterial segment, that is, claudication.

(4) ABI <0.5 indicates multiple arterial segments are obstructed.

(5) In trauma, <0.9 signifies an arterial injury.

❍ **Which is the diagnostic test of choice for documenting DVT?**

Duplex ultrasound. Although, it is highly operator dependent and not used in all centers, its sensitivity and specificity are virtually identical to venography. In addition, its benefits include being noninvasive and not utilizing contrast dye. The accuracy of physical examination for DVT is generally quoted to be approximately 50%.

❍ **Name some ultrasonographic abnormalities seen in patients with acute cholecystitis.**

Wall thickening, gallstones, surrounding fluid, US Murphy's sign, air in the biliary tree.

❍ **Where is the most common site for an ectopic implantation?**

The ampullae of the fallopian tube.

❍ **Name six risk factors for an ectopic pregnancy.**

Advanced maternal age, PID, prior ectopic, a history of pelvic surgery or tubal ligation, IUDs, in vitro fertilization.

❍ **What is the only true diagnostic sign of an ectopic pregnancy with ultrasound?**

A fetus with cardiac activity outside the uterus. Complex masses and fluid in the cul-de-sac can be seen in other conditions, that is, pelvic abscess, ruptured ovarian cyst.

❍ **What is the role of ultrasound in detecting placenta previa and abruption?**

Ultrasound is not sensitive for detecting placental abruption. However, in the patient with third-trimester vaginal bleeding, ultrasound is used primarily to rule out placenta previa.

❍ **List some of the advantages/disadvantages of CT scan, ultrasound, and DPL for assessing trauma patients.**

	Advantages	Disadvantages
DPL	Low complication rate done at bedside	Invasive, time consuming, can't ID retroperitoneal injury, significant false-positive rate
CT scan	IDs location/extent injury, including the retroperitoneum	Cost, time consuming, interpretation expertise, patient monitoring not optimal, requires travel
US	Cheap, noninvasive, done at bedside, good for hemoperitoneum, fast	Operator dependent, not good for diagnosing specific organ injury

❍ **Describe the typical shape and vessel origin of subdural hematomas (SDHs) and epidural hematomas (EDHs)?**

SDHs are typically crescent shaped and although can be arterial in origin are most often caused by the tearing of bridging veins. Acute SDHs are hyperdense relative to the brain and become isodense to the brain in 1 to 3 weeks. An EDH is biconvex (lenticular) in shape and usually arterial in origin. An EDH does not cross intact skull sutures but can cross the tentorium and the midline.

❍ **A laryngeal fracture is suggested by finding the hyoid bone elevated above what cervical level on x-ray?**

C3.

❍ **In children older than 1 year, where are foreign bodies in the airway usually located?**

In the trachea and mainstem bronchus.

❍ **Describe the presentation of SSSS.**

Disease begins after URI or purulent conjunctivitis. First lesions are tender, erythematous, and scarlatiniform, usually found on face, neck, axillae, and groin. Skin peels off in sheets with lateral pressure and a + Nikolsky's sign.

❍ **What is a positive Chvostek's sign?**

Twitch in the corner of the mouth occurring when the examiner taps over the facial nerve in front of the ear. It is present in approximately 10% to 30% of normal individuals. Eyelid muscle contraction with Chvostek's maneuver is generally considered to be diagnostic of hypocalcemia.

❍ **What is Trousseau's sign and when is it seen?**

Trousseau's sign is a carpal spasm–induced when a blood pressure cuff on the upper arm maintains a pressure above systolic for approximately 3 minutes. Fingers become spastically extended at the interphalangeal joints and flexed at the metacarpophalangeal joints. Trousseau's sign is generally a more reliable indicator of hypocalcemia than Chvostek's sign.

❍ **What is the *most common* rhythm disturbance in a pediatric arrest?**

Bradycardia.

❍ **Describe the common features of a slipped femoral capital epiphysis?**

Injury usually occurs in adolescence and typically presents with an insidious development of knee or thigh pain, and a painful limp. Frequently hip motion is limited, particularly that of internal rotation.

❍ **What are the common concerns with anterior dislocation of the shoulder?**

Axillary nerve injury, axillary artery injury in the elderly patients, compression fracture of the humeral head (Hillsack's deformity), a rotator cuff tear, fractures of the anterior glenoid lip, and fractures of the greater tuberosity.

❍ **Describe a Monteggia fracture/dislocation?**

A fracture of the proximal ulna with dislocation of the radial head.

❍ **Describe a Galeazzi's fracture/dislocation?**

A radial shaft fracture with dislocation of the distal radioulnar joint.

❍ **Describe botulism poisoning.**

Botulinum exotoxin is elaborated by *Clostridium botulinum.* It affects the myoneural junction and prevents the release of acetylcholine. In the United States, it is caused principally by ingestion of foods that have been inadequately prepared.

The most common neurologic complaints are related to the bulbar musculature. Neurologic symptoms usually occur within 24 to 48 hours of ingestion of contaminated foods. Muscle paralysis and weakness usually spread rapidly to involve all muscles of the trunk and extremities. It is important to distinguish between botulism poisoning and myasthenia gravis. This distinction can be made by using the edrophonium (Tensilon) test, usually performed by a neurologist.

❍ **Poor prognostic signs on admission of a patient with pancreatitis include?**

>55 year-old.

Glucose >200 mg/dL.

LDH >350 IU/L.

WBC count >16,000.

AST >250 U/L.

NOTICE: NO AMYLASE OR LIPASE INVOLVEMENT!

❍ **What test is best to confirm the diagnosis of Boerhaave's syndrome?**

An esophagram using a water soluble, contrast medium should be used in the place of barium to confirm the diagnosis.

❍ **What are the signs and symptoms of a patient with Boerhaave's syndrome?**

Substernal and left-sided chest pain with a history of forceful vomiting leading to spontaneous esophageal rupture.

❍ **What are Kanavel's four cardinal signs of infectious digital flexor tenosynovitis?**

Tenderness along the tendon sheath, finger held in flexion, pain on passive extension of the finger, and finger swelling.

❍ **A patient presents to your emergency department after being bitten by a wild raccoon. What treatment would you provide?**

Wound care, tetanus prophylaxis, RIG (rabies immune globulin), 20 IU/kg (half at bite site and half IM), and HDCV (human diploid cell culture rabies vaccine), 1 cc IM.

❍ **What is the appropriate treatment for cyanide poisoning?**

Amyl nitrite, sodium nitrite IV, followed by sodium thiosulfate IV.

❍ **Which animals are the most common vectors of rabies in the world? In the United States?**

Worldwide, the dog is the most common carrier of rabies.

In the United States, the skUnk has become the most common source of disease. Bats, raccoons, cows, dogs, foxes, and cats (descending order) are also sources.

Rodents like squirrels, chipmunks, and lagomorphs (rabbits) are NOT carriers of rabies.

❍ **A septic appearing adult has multiple 1 cm in skin lesions with a necrotic, ulcerated center, and an erythematous surrounding region. What is the likely pathogen?**

Pseudomonas aeruginosa.

❍ **Describe the signs and symptoms of spinal shock.**

Spinal shock represents complete loss of spinal cord function below the level of injury. Patients have flaccid paralysis, complete sensory loss, areflexia, and loss of autonomic function. Such patients are usually bradycardic, hypotensive, hypothermic, and vasodilated.

❍ **Describe the chest x-ray of Mycoplasma pneumonia.**

Bilateral patchy densities involving the all lobes are most common. Pneumatoceles, cavities, abscesses, and pleural effusions can occur, but are uncommon. Macrolides are the treatment of choice.

❍ **Where is the most likely location of a Boerhaave's tear?**

Left posterolateral region of the midthoracic esophagus.

❍ **How does a coin appear on AP view of the trachea?**

On its side.

❍ **How does a coin in the esophagus appear on AP?**

Like a solid circle.

❍ **What are the principal signs and symptoms of ulcerative colitis?**

Fever, weight loss, tachycardia, pancolitis, and six bloody bowel movements per day.

❍ **What are two fairly common conditions in pediatrics that produce cardiac syncope?**

Aortic stenosis, which is not cyanotic; tetralogy of Fallot, which is cyanotic.

❍ **What are the signs of left-sided heart failure in an infant?**

Increased respiratory rate, shortness of breath, and sweating during feeding.

❍ **What is the single most common cause of CHF in the second week of life?**

Coarctation of the aorta.

❍ **What is the drug of choice for treating a febrile seizure?**

Benzodiazepines if needed. Most seizures are self-limiting.

❍ **What is the most common cause of painless lower GI bleeding in an infant or child?**

Meckel's diverticulum.

❍ **A 16-month-old child presents with bilious vomiting, a distended abdomen, and blood in the stool. What is the diagnosis?**

Midgut volvulus.

❍ **What are some possible complications of sodium bicarbonate therapy?**

Hypokalemia, paradoxical CSF acidosis, impaired O_2 dissociation, and sodium overload.

❍ **Differentiate between nonketotic hyperosmolar coma and DKA.**

In nonketotic hyperosmolar coma, glucose is very high, often >800. The serum osmolality is also very high, with average about 380. A nitroprusside test is negative.

In DKA, glucose is more often in the range of 600, the serum osmolality is approximately 350, and the nitroprusside test is positive.

❍ **What focal signs may be present in a patient with nonketotic hyperosmolar coma?**

Hemisensory deficits or hemiparesis. Ten to fifteen percent of these patients have a seizure.

❍ **What is the most common cause of hyperthyroidism?**

Grave's disease (toxic-diffused goiter).

❍ **What is the most common precipitating cause of thyroid storm?**

Pulmonary infection.

❍ **What is another name for life-threatening hypothyroidism?**

Myxedema coma. Commonly occurs in elderly women during the winter months and is stimulated by infection and stress.

❍ **What is the most common cause of hypothyroidism?**

Overtreatment of Grave's disease with iodine or subtotal thyroidectomy.

❍ **What ECG finding would you expect in myxedema coma?**

Bradycardia.

❍ **What is a common "surgical problem" in myxedema that should be treated conservatively?**

Acquired megacolon.

❍ **What is primary adrenal insufficiency?**

Addison's disease, that is, failure of the adrenal cortex.

❍ **What is Waterhouse–Fredrickson syndrome?**

Septicemia secondary to meningococcemia with associated bilateral adrenal gland hemorrhage. The patient will have a petechial rash, purpura, shaking chills, and severe headache.

❍ **What effect does Addison's disease have on cortisol and aldosterone levels?**

Cortisol and aldosterone levels are low. Low cortisol levels lead to nausea, vomiting, anorexia, lethargy, hypoglycemia, and an inability to withstand even minor stress without shock. Low aldosterone levels mean sodium depletion, dehydration, hypotension, and syncope.

❍ **What are the principal signs and symptoms in adrenal crisis?**

Abdominal pain, hypotension, and shock. The common cause is the withdrawal of steroids. Treatment of adrenal crisis is hydrocortisone (Solu-Cortef), 100 mg IV bolus, and 100 mg added to the first liter of D_5 NS.

❍ **In the pediatric esophagus, where is the most common site of a foreign body?**

Cricopharyngeal narrowing.

❍ **Thyrotoxicosis may be treated with?**

Support and hydration, IV propylthiouracil, 1 g, sodium iodine, IV 1 g q 12 hours, and IV propanolol, 1 mg/min up to 10 mg.

❍ **A fracture of the proximal fibular shaft is commonly associated with?**

Medial ankle fracture or sprain. This is a Maisonneuve fx, it may be present with a widened mortise and no fx seen in the ankle.

❍ **What is the best x-ray view for diagnosing lunate and perilunate dislocations?**

Lateral x-ray views of the wrist.

❍ **What is the most common cause of periorbital cellulitis in a 2-year-old child?**

Hemophilus influenzae. The second most common cause is *S. aureus.*

❍ **In a humeral shaft fracture, which nerve is most commonly injured?**

Radial nerve.

❍ **What is the most common dysrhythmia in a child?**

Paroxysmal atrial tachycardia.

❍ **What are some common causes of increased anion gap?**

Aspirin, methanol, uremia, diabetes, idiopathic (lactic), ethylene glycol, and alcohol are reasonably common.

Numerous etiologies may produce the entity above listed demurely as "lactic." Lactic acidosis may be the result of shock, seizures, acute hypoxemia, INH, cyanide, ritodrine, inhaled acetylene, carbon monoxide, and ethanol. Sodium nitroprusside, povidone-iodine ointment, sorbitol, and xylitol can cause an anion gap acidosis.

Other causes of anion gap acidosis include toluene intoxication, iron intoxication, sulfuric acidosis, short bowel syndrome (D-lactic acidosis), formaldehyde, nalidixic acid, methenamine, and rhubarb (oxalic acid). Inborn errors of metabolism, such as methylmalonic acidemia and isovaleric acidemia may also cause a gap acidosis.

Recall some pearls for sorting out the differential diagnosis:

Methanol: Visual disturbances and headache common. Can produce quite wide gaps as each 2.6 mg/dL of methanol contributes 1 mOsm/L to gap. Compare this with alcohol, each 4.3 mg/dL adds 1 mOsm/L to gap.

Uremia: Is quite advanced before it causes an anion gap.

Diabetic ketoacidosis: Usually has both hyperglycemia and glucosuria; alcoholic ketoacidosis (AKA) often has a lower blood sugar and mild or absent glucosuria.

Salicylates: High levels contribute to gap.

Lactic acidosis: Can check serum level. Itself has broad differential as above.

Ethylene glycol: Causes calcium oxalate or hippurate crystals in urine. Each 5.0 mg/dL contributes 1 mOsm/L to gap.

A reasonably comprehensive mnemonic device for recalling causes of anion gap acidosis is A MUDPILE CAT.

A MUDPILE CAT

A = alcohol,

M = methanol,

U = uremia,

D = DKA,

P = paraldehyde,

I = iron and isoniazid,

L = lactic acidosis,

E = ethylene glycol,

C = carbon monoxide,

A = ASA (aspirin),

T = toluene.

❍ **What are the causes of normal anion gap metabolic acidosis?**

Causes include diarrhea, ammonium chloride, renal tubular acidosis, renal interstitial disease, hypoadrenalism, ureterosigmoidostomy, and acetazolamide.

❍ **What are some common causes of respiratory alkalosis?**

Respiratory alkalosis is defined as a pH above 7.45, and a pCO_2 less than 35. Common causes of respiratory alkalosis include any process that may cause hyperventilation, such as shock, sepsis, trauma, asthma, PE, anemia, hepatic failure, heat stroke and exhaustion, emotion, salicylate poisoning, hypoxemia, pregnancy, and inappropriate mechanical ventilation. Alkalosis shifts the O_2 disassociation curve to the left. It also causes cerebrovascular constriction. Kidneys compensate for respiratory alkalosis by excreting HCO_3^-.

❍ **How should a patient with hypertrophic cardiomyopathy be treated who presents with chest pain and a heart rate of 140?**

β-blockers are the primary treatment for hypertrophic cardiomyopathy. Calcium channel blocking drugs are second-line therapeutics.

❍ **What is the preferred management of neurogenic shock?**

Volume replacement with crystalloid followed by vasopressors.

❍ **An elderly male presents to your emergency department with ataxia, confusion, amnesia, and ocular paralysis. The patient is apathetic to his situation and has an otherwise normal neurologic examination. What is the likely cause of the patient's problem?**

Vitamin B deficiency associated with Wernicke–Korsakoff syndrome.

❍ **What are the classic ECG findings of a patient with a posterior MI.**

A large R-wave and ST depression in V1 and V2.

❍ **What is the classic ECG finding in Wolff–Parkinson–White syndrome?**

A shortened PR interval forming a delta wave.

❍ **What is the best treatment for an unstable patient with Wolff–Parkinson–White syndrome presenting with rapid atrial fibrillation?**

Electrical cardioversion.

❍ **What is the best treatment for a verapamil-induced bradycardia?**

Calcium chloride 10%, 10 to 20 mL IV (10–30 mg/kg in children).

❍ **What is the most common cause of valvular-induced syncope in the elderly patients?**

Aortic stenosis. Vasovagal mechanisms are the most common mechanism overall.

❍ **Describe the signs, symptoms, and ECG finding associated with lithium toxicity.**

Tremor, weakness, and flattening of the T-waves.

❍ **A patient has an orbital floor fracture. What are associated symptoms and signs?**

The most common symptom would be diplopia caused by entrapment of the inferior rectus and inferior oblique muscles and resultant paralysis of upward gaze. In addition, one would worry that the inferior orbital nerve could be damaged with paresthesia resulting to the lower lid, infraorbital area, and side of the nose (infraorbital hypesthesia).

❍ **What are the signs of an upper motor neuron lesion?**

Upper motor neuron lesion involves the corticospinal tract. The lesion usually gives paralysis with:

(1) Initial loss of muscle tone and then increased tone, resulting in spasticity;

(2) Babinski;

(3) Loss of superficial reflexes;

(4) Increased deep tendon reflexes.

A lower motor neuron lesion is associated with the anterior horn cells' axons. The lesion gives paralysis with decreased muscle tone and prompt atrophy.

❍ **Which condition commonly presents with ocular bulbar deficits?**

Botulism poisoning. Patients with myasthenia gravis may present similarly. Diphtheria toxin may rarely produce similar deficits.

❍ **Describe the symptoms and signs of myasthenia gravis.**

Weakness and fatigability with ptosis, diplopia, and blurred vision are the initial symptoms in 40% to 70% of patients. Bulbar muscle weakness is also common with dysarthria and dysphagia.

❍ **Describe the key features of vertebrobasilar insufficiency.**

Vertigo is nearly always positional, provoked by certain head positions. Nystagmus accompanies the vertigo. Other signs of arteriosclerosis may be found.

Vertebrobasilar insufficiency is usually seen in older persons and may occur with other symptoms of brainstem ischemia, visual symptoms being the most common.

❍ **What disease would you expect in a patient with a 2-week history of lower limb weakness?**

Guillain-Barré is usually an ascending weakness which begins in the lower extremities.

With botulism poisoning, the weakness is descending. Cranial nerves are typically affected first with myasthenia gravis.

❍ **What is the mortality rate of Wernicke's encephalopathy?**

10% to 20%. Treat with thiamine IV. Symptoms include ocular palsies, nystagmus, confusion, and ataxia.

❍ **What therapy should be used for a patient with hemophilia A who suffers a head injury?**

To raise factor VIII levels from 0 to 100%, administer 50 IU/kg, IV.

❍ **Describe a patient with a sigmoid volvulus.**

Patients are typically either psychiatric patients or elderly patients who suffer from severe chronic constipation. Symptoms include intermittent cramping, lower abdominal pain, and progressive abdominal distention.

❍ **Describe a typical patient with intussusception.**

Occurs in children age 3 months to 2 years. The majority are in the 5 to 10 months age group. It is more common in boys. The area of the ileocecal valve is usually the source of the problem.

❍ **What are the common symptoms and signs of hyperthyroidism?**

Weight loss, palpitations, dyspnea, edema, chest pain, nervousness, weakness, tremor, psychosis, diarrhea, hyperdefecation, abdominal pain, myalgias, and disorientation. Signs include fever, tachycardia, wide pulse pressure, CHF, shock, thyromegaly, tremor, weakness, liver tenderness, jaundice, and stare. Mental status changes include somnolence, obtundation, coma, or psychosis.

❍ **What is the current therapeutic regimen for the treatment of meningitis in a neonate?**

Ampicillin + gentamicin or ampicillin + cefotaxime ± acyclovir.

❍ **What is the formula for calculating a change in potassium with changes in pH?**

For each pH increase of 0.1, expect the potassium to drop by 0.5 mmol/L.

❍ **A patient has alcoholic ketoacidosis (AKA), what is the appropriate treatment?**

IV fluids, glucose, multivitamin with thiamine, and food. $NaHCO_3$ should not be given unless pH drops below 7.1. AKA presents with nausea, vomiting, and abdominal pain occurring 24 to 72 hours after cessation of drinking. No specific physical findings are typical, though abdominal pain is a common complaint. AKA is thought to be secondary to an increased mobilization of free fatty acids with lipolysis to acetoacetate and β-hydroxybutyrate.

❍ **Describe the symptoms of optic neuritis.**

The patient suffers a variable loss of central visual acuity with a central scotoma and change in color perception. The patient also has eye pain. The disk margins are blurred from hemorrhage and the blind spot is increased.

❍ **What is the antidote for ethylene glycol?**

Ethanol, dialysis, and fomepizole (Antizol).

❍ **What is the antidote for iron toxicity?**

Deferoxamine.

❍ **What are the signs and symptoms of acute pericardial tamponade?**

Triad of hypotension, JVD, and, muffled heart tones.

❍ **What ECG findings are pathognomonic for pericardial tamponade?**

Electrical alternans and low voltage in all leads.

❍ **How does a chronic pericardial effusion appear on chest x-ray?**

Gradual pericardial sac distention results in a "water bottle" appearance of the heart.

❍ **The treatment for myxedema coma includes?**

IV thyroxine, glucose, hydrocortisone, and water restriction.

❍ **What are the symptoms and signs of thyrotoxicosis?**

Weight loss, tachycardia, fever, hypotension, mental status changes, decreased consciousness, psychosis, CHF, thyromegaly, tremor, eye lid lag, and proptosis.

❍ **What is the standard dose of atropine in a child?**

0.2 mg/kg.

❍ **What are the signs and symptoms in a patient with acute narrow–angle closure glaucoma.**

N/V, headache, abdominal pain, diminished visual acuity, semidilated and nonreactive pupil. The eye is red and painful with a glassy haze over the cornea. IOP may be as high as 50 or 60 mm Hg.

❍ **Describe the treatment of acute narrow–angle glaucoma.**

(1) Mannitol to decrease intraocular pressure.

(2) Miotics, such as pilocarpine, to open the angle.

(3) Carbonic anhydrase inhibitor to minimize aqueous humor production.

(4) An iridectomy is eventually performed to provide aqueous outflow.

❍ **What is the appropriate treatment for a hyphema?**

Elevate the head. Other treatments are controversial; however, most ophthalmologists believe patients should be hospitalized. Treatment may include double eye patch, topical steroid, and cycloplegics.

❍ **Describe the classic symptoms and signs of a retinal detachment.**

The patient is myopic and will complain of seeing a curtain coming down across the eye. This is accompanied by flashes of light but no discomfort. On funduscopic examination, the detached areas will appear gray in comparison to the normal pink retina. Treatment includes bilateral eye patch, strict bed rest, and an STAT ophthalmology consult.

❍ **What is the initial dose of sodium bicarbonate for children during a cardiopulmonary arrest?**

1 mEq/kg.

❍ **How is the expected normal systolic blood pressure (SBP) for a pediatric patient calculated?**

Average SBP (mm Hg) = (Age × 2) + 90

Low normal limit SBP (mm Hg) = (Age × 2) + 70.

SBP for a term newborn is about 60 mm Hg.

❍ **What is the correct dose of epinephrine and atropine during a pediatric code?**

Epinephrine, 0.01 mg/kg/dose. Atropine, 0.02 mg/kg/dose.

❍ **What are the signs and symptoms of Kawasaki's disease?**

High fever, conjunctivitis, morbilliform rash, strawberry tongue, erythema of the distal extremities and cervical adenopathy. Patients should be hospitalized to rule out myocarditis, pericarditis, and coronary aneurysms. Aspirin is therapeutic.

❍ **Which antibiotic is used in the treatment of epiglottitis in a child?**

The most likely cause is *H. influenzae*, so a second- or third-generation cephalosporin is indicated.

❍ **What are the characteristics of a posterior hip dislocation?**

Posterior hip dislocations are typically caused by posteriorly directed force applied to the flexed knee. The extremity is shortened, internally rotated, and adducted. Acetabular fractures are associated with this injury. Ninety percent of hip dislocations are posterior.

❍ **Describe the key features of central cord syndrome.**

Central cord syndrome is due to a hyperextension injury, usually in older patients with spondylosis, degenerative changes, or stenosis in the cervical spine. Symptoms include weakness that is more pronounced in the arms than the legs.

❍ **What are the key features of anterior spinal cord syndrome?**

The anterior cord syndrome involves compression of the anterior cord causing complete motor paralysis and loss of pain and temperature sensation distal to the lesion. Posterior columns are spared—light touch and proprioception are preserved.

❍ **How does myasthenia gravis typically present?**

Weakness of voluntary muscles, usually the extraocular muscles. Diagnostic confirmation relies on the edrophonium (Tensilon) test. Treatment includes neurologic consultation, anticholinesterases, steroids, and thymectomy.

❍ **What are the signs and symptoms of posterior inferior cerebellar artery syndrome?**

Cerebellar dysfunction, such as vertigo, ataxia, and dizziness.

❍ **Describe the signs and symptoms of neuroleptic malignant syndrome.**

Muscle rigidity, autonomic disturbances, elevated blood pressure and pulse, fever as high as 42°C (108°F), and myoglobinuria. Mortality ranges as high as 20%.

❍ **Describe the presentation of placenta previa.**

Painless, bright red vaginal bleeding.

❍ **Describe the presentation of abruptio placentae.**

Dark red, painful, vaginal bleeding.

❍ **Signs of tension pneumothorax on physical examination include?**

Tachypnea, unilateral absent breath sounds, tachycardia, pallor, diaphoresis, cyanosis, tracheal deviation, hypotension, and neck vein distention.

❍ **Which medications should be used to treat preeclampsia and eclampsia?**

Magnesium and hydralazine or labetalol.

❍ **How much fluid in the pericardial sac is needed to increase the cardiac silhouette on chest x-ray?**

About 250 mL.

❍ **What is the most common dysrhythmia associated with Wolff–Parkinson–White syndrome?**

Paroxysmal atrial tachycardia.

❍ **What are the symptoms and signs of aortic stenosis?**

Exertional dyspnea, angina, and syncope, narrowed pulse pressure with decreased SBP, prominent S_4.

❍ **What is the best method to open an airway while maintaining C-spine precautions?**

Jaw-thrust.

❍ **What is the treatment for multifocal atrial tachycardia?**

Treat the underlying disorder. Administer magnesium sulfate, 2 g over 60 seconds with supplemental potassium to maintain serum K^+ above 4 mEq/L.

❍ **What is the treatment for ectopic SVT caused by digitalis toxicity?**

Stop digitalis, correct hypokalemia, consider digoxin specific Fab, magnesium IV, lidocaine IV, or phenytoin IV.

❍ **What is the treatment for SVT not caused by digitalis toxicity?**

Adenosine, verapamil, cardizem, β-blockers, or cardioversion.

❍ **What is the treatment for verapamil-induced hypotension?**

Calcium gluconate, 1 g IV over several minutes.

❍ **Which drugs are contraindicated in the treatment of Torsade de pointes?**

Drugs which prolong repolarization (QT interval). For example, class Ia antiarrhythmics, such as quinidine and procainamide. Other drugs that share this effect include TCAs, disopyramide, and phenothiazines.

❍ **What is the treatment for Torsade de pointes?**

(1) Magnesium sulfate, 2 g IV.

(2) Pacemaker at 90 to 120 bpm to "overdrive" pace.

(3) Isoproterenol.

❍ **Discuss the treatment for digitalis toxicity.**

(1) Charcoal.

(2) Phenytoin (Dilantin) for ventricular arrhythmias (increases AV node conduction) or lidocaine.

(3) Atropine or cardiac pacing for bradyarrthymias.

(4) Digoxin specific Fab (Digibind).

❍ **Which drug should be used to treat a patient in cardiac arrest secondary to hyperkalemia?**

Calcium chloride IV acts the fastest.

❍ **Which is the drug of choice for digitalis toxicity resulting in a ventricular arrhythmia?**

Phenytoin and digoxin specific Fab (Dilantin and Digibind).

❍ **For each 100 increase in glucose, what is the effect on serum sodium?**

Each 100 increase in glucose decreases the serum sodium by 1.6 to 1.8 mEq/L.

❍ **In a patient with tachycardia from cocaine abuse, which medications are appropriate?**

Sedation with benzodiazepines may calm the patient and decrease the heart rate. Nitroprusside may be used to treat hypertension. Caution must be used with β-adrenergic antagonist agents alone as they may leave α-adrenergic stimulation unopposed, increasing the patient's risk for intracranial hemorrhage, or aortic dissection.

❍ **What are the common presentations of a transfusion reaction?**

Myalgia, dyspnea, and fever associated with hypocalcemia, hemolysis, allergic reactions, hyperkalemia, citrate toxicity, hypothermia, coagulopathies, and altered hemoglobin function.

❍ **What are the signs of the Cushing reflex?**

Increased systolic blood pressure and bradycardia.

❍ **In testing a patient's oculovestibular reflex, what is the direction of nystagmus anticipated in response to cold-water irrigation; toward or away from the irrigated ear?**

Recall that nystagmus is defined as the direction of the fast component of saccadic eye movement. Emergency physicians will commonly perform a crude but secure test of the oculovestibular reflex using ice water. After irrigation, nystagmus should be away from the irrigated ear. Try the mnemonic COWS—Cold Opposite, Warm Same.

❍ **What three toxicologic ingestions require immediate dialysis?**

Ethylene glycol, methanol, and Amanita phalloides (mushroom).

❍ **Signs and symptoms of an uncal herniation include?**

Coma, ipsilateral pupillary dilation, either ipsilateral or contralateral hemiparesis, and blunting of the corneal reflex.

❍ **What is the antidote for organophosphates poisoning?**

Atropine and pralidoxime (2-PAM).

❍ **For which drugs may hemoperfusion be indicated?**

Salicylates, theophylline, and long-acting barbiturates.

❍ **For which drugs may dialysis be used?**

Salicylates, theophylline, long-acting barbiturates, methanol, ethylene glycol, amphetamines, lithium, and thiocyanate.

❍ **What are the four stages of acetaminophen toxicity?**

I. (Within an hour): Anorexia, nausea, vomiting, and diaphoresis.
II. (24–48 hours): Liver function test abnormalities and right upper quadrant pain.
III. (72–96 hours): Jaundice, return of GI symptoms, peak of liver function abnormalities, coagulation defects.
IV. (4 days–2 weeks): Get better or die.

❍ **When does acetaminophen become toxic?**

When there is no glutathione to detoxify its toxic intermediate.

❍ **How does N-acetylcysteine act to interrupt acetaminophen toxicity?**

Exact mechanism unknown, likely that NAC enters cells, and is metabolized to cysteine, which is a precursor for glutathione. Thus it may increase glutathione stores.

❍ **What is the early acid–base disturbance seen in salicylate overdose?**

Respiratory alkalosis. Approximately 12 hours later, one might see an anion gap metabolic acidosis or mixed acid–base picture.

❍ **What are the common symptoms and signs of chronic salicylism?**

Fever, tachypnea, CNS alterations, acid–base abnormalities, electrolyte abnormalities, chronic pain, ketonuria, and noncardiogenic pulmonary edema.

❍ **What is the treatment of salicylate overdose?**

Lavage, charcoal, fluid replacement, potassium supplementation, alkalinize the urine with use of bicarbonate, cooling for hyperthermia, glucose for hypoglycemia, oxygen and PEEP for pulmonary edema, multiple dose activated charcoal, and dialysis.

❍ **A child presents with vomiting, hematemesis, diarrhea, lethargy, coma, and shock after eating an entire bottle of children's vitamins. What toxic ingestion is suspected?**

Iron intoxication. Order a flat plate of the abdomen to look for concretions.

❍ **What is the treatment for iron ingestion?**

If there are no symptoms for 6 hours and the examination is normal, discharge home. If the patient has minimal symptoms and appears fine and has iron level close to maximum normal level (150 μg/dL) measured 4 hours after ingestion, discharge home. Hydrate, and support the ABCs.

Give deferoxamine (10–15 mg/kg/h IV) if:

- Moderate or severely symptomatic,
- Serum iron level > TIBC,
- Serum iron level >350 μg/dL.

❍ **What are the symptoms and signs of cyanide overdose?**

Dryness and burning in the throat, air hunger, and hyperventilation, loss of consciousness, seizures, bradycardia, and apnea.

❍ **What is the treatment for cyanide overdose?**

(1) Oxygen, CPR prn.

(2) Amyl nitrite perle inhaled.

(3) Sodium nitrite, 10 cc of 3% solution in an adult, which is 300 mg, or 0.2 to 0.33 mL/kg.

(4) Sodium thiosulfate, 12.5 mg, in an adult, which is 50 cc of a 25% solution or 1.0 to 1.5 mL/kg in a child (five times the volume of sodium nitrite).

(5) Hydroxocobalamin 70 mg/kg IV (5 g is standard dose).

❍ **Where do endoscopic perforations of the esophagus typically occur?**

They usually occur near the distal esophagus or at the site of pre-existing disease, such as a caustic burn.

❍ **How may a posterior urethral tear be diagnosed in a male?**

A high riding, free-floating, boggy prostate.

❍ **Describe the signs and symptoms associated with an anterior urethral tear?**

Perineal pain and bruising, blood at the meatus, and good urinary stream is maintained.

❍ **What is the mechanism of a posterior urethral tear?**

Straddle or crush injury associated with a pelvic fracture.

Urethral stricture, impotence, and incontinence.

❍ **How is an acute hemorrhagic from an overdose of Coumadin best treated?**

Fresh-frozen plasma, prothrombin complex concentrate, and vitamin K.

❍ **A patient has a pelvic fracture with suspected bladder or ureteral injury. Which test should be performed first, a cystogram or a CT with IV contrast?**

When a pelvic fracture is present or suspected, the cystogram is usually performed first so that distal ureteral dye from the CT will not mimic extravasation from the bladder.

❍ **What is the most common cause of immediate postpartum hemorrhage?**

Uterine atony, followed by vaginal/cervical lacerations, and retained placenta or placental fragments.

❍ **Describe a patient with tick paralysis.**

A rapid progressive ascending paralysis that develops over 1 to 2 days. First symptoms occur in the extremities and trunk and move to bulbar musculature. It is almost identical to Guillain-Barré syndrome.

❍ **What is the pathophysiology of myasthenia gravis?**

Circulatory antibody against ACh receptor, which binds at the motor end plate. In myasthenics, ACh receptors are in short supply resulting in fatigable weakness.

❍ **What are some factors commonly associated with meningitis?**

Age should be younger than 5 years or older than 60 years; low socioeconomic status; male sex; crowding; black race; sickle cell disease; splenectomy; alcoholism; diabetes and cirrhosis; immunologic defects; dural defect from congenital, surgical or traumatic source; contiguous infections, such as sinusitis, household contacts, malignancy, bacterial endocarditis, intravenous drug abuse; and thalassemia major.

❍ **How much elemental iron will 100 mg of deferoxamine bind?**

About 8.5 mg of elemental iron is bound by 100 mg of deferoxamine.

❍ **Explain how methylene blue functions as an antidote for methemoglobinemia.**

A normal level of 3% methemoglobin is usually maintained by an NADPH-dependent enzyme. This enzyme capacity can be exceeded with oxidant poisoning. Methylene blue enhances NADPH-dependent hemoglobin reduction by acting as a cofactor.

Methylene blue is usually only needed for metHb levels >30%; its dose is 1 to 2 mg/kg IV over 5 minutes.

❍ **What is a potential side effect of the use of Kayexalate?**

Bowel necrosis.

❍ **ECG changes associated with tricyclic antidepressant overdose?**

Prolongation of the PR, QRS, and QT interval, as well as conduction defects such as bundle branch block.

❍ **What dose of ASA will cause mild-to-moderate toxicity?**

200 to 300 mg/kg. Greater than 500 mg/kg is potentially lethal.

❍ **What is the treatment for lithium overdose?**

Saline diuresis and hemodialysis.

❍ **Which electrolyte abnormality commonly occurs with salicylate toxicity?**

Hypokalemia.

❍ **How does a patient present with Boerhaave's syndrome?**

Boerhaave's syndrome is spontaneous esophageal perforation. It usually occurs after forceful vomiting. The patient suffers an acute collapse, chest, and abdominal pain. A left pleural effusion is seen in 90% of patients on chest x-ray and most have mediastinal emphysema.

❍ **What are the classic findings of shaken baby syndrome?**

Failure to thrive, lethargy, seizures, and retinal hemorrhages. A CT scan may show subarachnoid hemorrhage or subdural hematoma from torn bridging veins.

❍ **What is the immediate treatment for cord prolapse?**

Displace the head cephalad.

❍ **Which nerve may be injured in a distal femoral fracture?**

Peroneal nerve.

❍ **Describe the signs and symptoms and x-ray tests for diagnosing a slipped capital femoral epiphysis.**

Gradual onset of hip pain and stiffness with restriction of internal rotation. Patient may walk with a limp. X-ray analysis should include both the anterior–posterior and lateral views of both hips. The slip of the epiphyseal plate posteriorly is best seen on the lateral view.

❍ **How does a patient present with a retropharyngeal abscess?**

Patients typically prefer a supine position. Retropharyngeal abscesses are common in patients younger than 3 years. On examination, the uvula and tonsil are displaced away from the abscess. Soft tissue swelling and forward displacement of the larynx are present.

❍ **How does an adult with epiglottitis present?**

Pharyngitis and dysphagia, muffled voice, and pain out of proportion to objective findings are prominent symptoms. Adenopathy is uncommon.

❍ **In a patient with acute testicular pain, relief of pain with elevation of the scrotum (Prehn's sign) is classically associated with?**

Epididymitis.

❍ **How much protamine is required to neutralize 100 units of heparin?**

1 mg of protamine will neutralize ~100 units of heparin. The maximum dose of protamine is 100 mg.

❍ **You see a patient with a severe high concentration burn from hydrofluoric acid. How do you treat this patient?**

In addition to topical jelly and cutaneous injections of calcium gluconate, provide IV treatment with 10 cc of 10% calcium gluconate (not calcium chloride), diluted in 50 cc of D_5W over 4 hours.

❍ **How should an ocular burn secondary to hydrofluoric acid be treated?**

Use calcium gluconate in a 1% solution mixed with saline and irrigate the eyes with this solution.

❍ **Which electrolyte is depleted when a victim is burned by hydrofluoric acid?**

Hydrofluoric acid results in hypocalcemia. Patients may require calcium replacement. Keep in mind that normal signs and symptoms of hypocalcemia, such as Chvostek's sign do not typically appear with hypocalcemia secondary to HF.

❍ **How should a patient with neuroleptic malignant syndrome be treated?**

Ice packs to the groin and axilla or a cooling blankets, fan, water mist evaporation, mechanical cooling device, and dantrolene 0.8 to 3 mg/kg IV q 6 hours to a total of 10 mg/kg.

❍ **A patient presents with back pain and complaints of incontinence. On examination, loss of anal reflex and decreased sphincter tone is noted. What is the diagnosis?**

Cauda equina syndrome. The most consistent finding is urinary retention and saddle anesthesia (numbness over the posterior superior thighs, buttocks, and perineum).

❍ **A trauma patient has a closed head injury with suspected elevated intracranial pressure. What treatments should be considered?**

(1) Paralyze the patient and ventilate to a PCO_2 of 32 to 35 mm Hg.

(2) Maintain hypovolemia (fluid restrict).

(3) Elevate the head of the bed to 30 degrees.

(4) Consider mannitol, 500 mL of a 20% solution over 20 minutes for a 70 kg adult.

❍ **When monitoring a pregnant female trauma victim, which vital signs are more appropriate to follow—the mother's or those of the fetus?**

It is probably best to consider monitoring the fetal heart rate because it is more sensitive to inadequate resuscitation. Remember that the mother may lose 10% to 20% of her blood volume without change in vital signs whereas the fetal heart rate may increase or decrease above 160 or below 120 indicating fetal distress.

❍ **What two findings on physical examination are indicative of uterine rupture?**

Loss of uterine contour and palpable fetal part.

❍ **What are the indications for administering digitalis specific Fab?**

Ventricular arrhythmias, K^+ >5.5 mEq/L, and unresponsive bradyarrhythmias.

Some authors refer to an ingestion of more than 0.3 mg/kg as requiring Fab (Digibind).

❍ **What distinguishes heat stroke from heat exhaustion?**

Heat exhaustion is body fluid depletion due to heat stress. Heat stroke is defined as hyperthermia (>41°C), anhydrosis, and an altered sensorium. Heat stroke requires much more aggressive treatment as compared to simple fluid rehydration.

❍ **How should a patient with heat stroke be treated?**

Cool water and fans or pack the axillae, neck, and groin with ice or use a mechanical cooling device. Hydrate maintaining good perfusion.

❍ **What complications can result from heat stroke?**

Renal failure, rhabdomyolysis, DIC, and seizures.

❍ **For which types of overdoses is activated charcoal not indicated?**

Alcohol ingestion, heavy metals, lithium, hydrocarbons, and caustic ingestions.

❍ **Which type of blood test is used to determine if a patient needs RhoGAM therapy?**

A Kleihauer–Betke checks for fetomaternal bleeding.

❍ **A young patient has a threatened abortion in the first trimester. Laboratory studies reveal she is Rh-negative and her husband is Rh-positive. What is the treatment?**

The patient will need 50 μg of Rh immunoglobulin (RhoGAM) IM. After the first trimester, the dose is increased to 300 μg IM.

❍ **What are the signs and symptoms of preeclampsia?**

Upper abdominal pain, headache, visual complaints, edema, and hypertension.

❍ **Which type of rattlesnake bite causes most deaths?**

Diamond back rattlesnake is the cause of nearly all lethal snake bites in the United States. However, the diamond back accounts for only 3% of the total incidences of snake bites. Treat with 10 to 20 vials of antivenin.

❍ **Which drugs most commonly induce toxic epidermal necrolysis?**

Phenylbutazone, barbiturates, sulfa drugs, antiepileptics, and antibiotics.

❍ **How is a retropharyngeal abscess diagnosed on a lateral plain films of a 1-year-old child?**

Look for prevertebral thickening of the soft tissues. More than 3 mm suggests the possibility of a retropharyngeal abscess. Air/fluid level may be present. If still unsure, order a CT scan of the neck. On CT scan, they are just anterior to the vertebral column, will appear in only a few cuts, and appear as a gray area of about the same density as the spinal canal.

❍ **How is a laryngeal fracture diagnosed on plain films?**

On a lateral soft tissue x-ray of the neck, check for retropharyngeal air, and elevation of the hyoid bone. The hyoid bone is normally at the level of C3. Elevation above C3 suggests a laryngeal fracture.

❍ **What is the Parkland formula for treating a pediatric burn victim?**

Ringer's lactate 4 mL ×%BSA × wt kg over 24 hours with half given in first 8 hours.

○ **Differentiate between a hypertensive emergency and a hypertensive urgency.**

Elevated BP + end organ damage = hypertensive emergency.

Elevated BP + no symptoms or signs of end organ damage = hypertensive urgency; usually DBP >115 mm Hg. Requires acute treatment.

○ **A patient presents with fever, neck pain or neck stiffness, and trismus. Examination reveals pharyngeal edema with tonsil displacement and edema in the area of the parotid gland. What is the diagnosis?**

Parapharyngeal abscess.

○ **What arrhythmia is frequently encountered during renal dialysis.**

Hypokalemia-induced ventricular fibrillation.

○ **A patient presents with hearing loss, nystagmus, complaint of facial weakness, and diplopia. Vertigo is provoked with sudden movement. A lumbar puncture reveals elevated CNS protein. What diagnosis is suspected?**

An acoustic neuroma.

○ **What are some of the common causes of prerenal acute renal failure?**

Volume depletion and decreased effective volume (CHF, sepsis, cirrhosis).

○ **What are the causes of acute renal failure, which are renal in nature?**

Acute tubular necrosis, acute interstitial nephritis, acute glomerulonephritis, and vascular disease.

○ **When can one auscultate the fetal heart?**

(1) Ultrasound: 6 weeks.

(2) Doppler: 10 to 12 weeks.

(3) Stethoscope: 18 to 20 weeks.

○ **Describe a Brudzinski sign.**

Flexion of the neck produces flexion of the knees.

○ **Describe Kernig's sign.**

Extension of the knees from the flexed thigh position results in strong passive resistance.

○ **A heroin addict presents with pulmonary edema. What is the best treatment?**

Naloxone, O_2, and ventilatory support.

○ **What is the initial drug of choice to treat SVT in a pediatric patient.**

Adenosine, 0.1 mg/kg is drug of choice.

❍ **What opening pressure and protein levels are expected with bacterial meningitis?**

Opening pressure of near 30 cm H_2O and a protein level of >150 mg/dL. Glucose level will drop with bacterial, TB, and fungal meningitis.

❍ **An alcoholic patient presents with complaints of abdominal pain and blurred vision. The patient is very photophobic and blood gases reveal a metabolic acidosis. What is the diagnosis?**

Methanol poisoning. These patients may describe seeing something resembling a snowstorm.

❍ **What are the signs and symptoms of ethylene glycol poisoning?**

Hallucinations, nystagmus, ataxia, papilledema, and a large anion gap.

❍ **What are the major laboratory findings in a patient with isopropanol poisoning?**

Elevated osmolal gap, acetone, and no anion gap.

❍ **What are the signs and symptoms of isopropanol poisoning?**

Sweet odor to breath (acetone), hypotension, hemorrhagic gastritis, abdominal pain, and CNS depression.

❍ **For which drugs will alkalinization of the urine increase excretion?**

TCAs, salicylates, and long-acting barbiturates. May be of some use to enhance lithium excretion.

❍ **Inferior wall MIs commonly lead to what type of heart blocks (via mechanism of damage to autonomic fibers in the atrial septum giving increased vagal tone impairing AV node conduction)?**

First-degree AV block, Mobitz type I (Wenckebach) second-degree AV block, and complete third-degree heart block.

❍ **Anterior wall MIs may directly damage intracardiac conduction. This may lead to which type of arrhythmias?**

Mobitz II second-degree AV block that can suddenly progress to complete AV block.

❍ **After the first month of life, what is the number one cause of pneumonia in children?**

S. pneumoniae with *H. influenzae* the second most common cause.

❍ **Which type of alcohol ingestion is associated with hypocalcemia?**

Ethylene glycol.

❍ **For what disorder is vigorous digital massage of the orbit indicated?**

Central retinal artery occlusion. DO NOT do this in central vein occlusion!

❍ **What is the initial dose of blood to be given in children?**

10 mL/kg of packed RBCs.

❍ **Who should receive prophylaxis after exposure to Neisseria meningitidis?**

People living with the patient or having close intimate contact.

❍ **What is the difference between carbamates and organophosphates?**

Carbamates produce similar symptoms as organophosphates, however, the bonds in carbamate toxicity are reversible.

❍ **What are key signs and symptoms of organophosphate poisoning?**

Ataxia, abdominal pain and cramping, blurred vision, seizures, diarrhea, diaphoresis, vomiting, sweating, and miosis.

❍ **What ECG changes may be associated with organophosphate poisoning?**

Prolongation of the QT interval, and ST- and T-wave abnormalities.

❍ **A patient presents with miotic pupils, muscle fasciculations, diaphoresis, and copious oral and bronchial secretions. The patient has an odor of garlic on his breath. What is the diagnosis?**

Organophosphate poisoning.

❍ **What is the key laboratory finding in the diagnosis of organophosphate poisoning?**

Decreased red blood cell cholinesterase activity. The serum cholinesterase level (pseudocholinesterase) is more sensitive but less specific. RBC cholinesterase is regenerated slowly and can take months to approach normal levels.

❍ **What is the treatment for organophosphate poisoning?**

Decontaminate, charcoal, large doses of atropine, and pralidoxime prn.

❍ **Which type of arrhythmia does lightning produce?**

It is a DC and produces asystole.

❍ **Which type of arrhythmia does AC tend to produce?**

Ventricular fibrillation.

❍ **What is a serious complication of ethmoid sinusitis?**

Orbital cellulitis.

❍ **What is the most accurate x-ray finding in traumatic rupture of the aorta?**

Rightward deviation of the esophagus more than 1 to 2 cm.

❍ **What ECG change is associated with hypocalcemia?**

Prolonged T-waves.

❍ **A patient is digitalis toxic. Which electrolytes will need to be replaced?**

It is important to replace potassium and magnesium.

❍ **Third-degree heart block is often seen in which type of myocardial infarction?**

Acute anterior wall myocardial infarction.

❍ **Which is the most common arrhythmia associated with Wolff–Parkinson–White syndrome?**

PAT. The patient presents with angina, syncope, and shortness of breath.

❍ **Name the drug of choice for Wolff–Parkinson–White with atrial flutter or fibrillation?**

Procainamide.

❍ **What laboratory findings are expected in a child with pyloric stenosis?**

Hypokalemia, hypochloremia, and metabolic alkalosis.

❍ **What is the most common cause of tricuspid regurgitation?**

Right heart failure secondary to left heart failure, typically caused by mitral stenosis.

❍ **What is the treatment for a β-blocker overdose?**

Glucagon, activated charcoal, consider atropine, hemodialysis, and consider insulin.

❍ **What are the x-ray findings in ischemic bowel disease?**

"Thumb" printing on the plain film and a ground glass appearance with the absence of bowel gas.

❍ **A patient with currant jelly sputum is likely to have which type of pneumonia?**

Klebsiella or Type 3 pneumococcus.

❍ **How do patients present with Babesia infection?**

Intermittent fever, splenomegaly, jaundice, and hemolysis. The disease may be fatal in patients without spleens. The disease can simulate rickettsial diseases like Rocky Mountain spotted fever (RMSF). Treatment is with clindamycin and quinine.

❍ **Which is the most frequently transmitted tick-borne disease?**

Lyme disease. The causative agent is spirochete *Borrelia burgdorferi*. The vector is *Ixodes dammini* (deer tick) also *I. pacificus*, *Amblyomma americanum*, and *Dermacentor variabilis*.

❍ **When is dobutamine used in CHF?**

Potent inotrope with some vasodilation activity used when heart failure is not accompanied by severe hypotension.

❍ **How is atrial flutter treated?**

Initiate A-V nodal blockade with β-adrenergic or calcium channel blockers or with digoxin. If necessary, in a stable patient, attempt chemical cardioversion with a class IA agent such as procainamide or quinidine after digitalization. If such treatment fails, or if patient is unstable and requires immediate electrocardioversion with 50 to 100 J.

❍ **What are the causes of atrial fibrillation?**

Hypertension, rheumatic heart disease, pneumonia, thyrotoxicosis, ischemic heart disease, pericarditis, ethanol intoxication, PE, CHF, and COPD.

❍ **How is atrial fibrillation treated?**

Control rate with β-blockade or calcium channel blocker, then convert with procainamide, amiodarone, or a calcium channel blocker. Digoxin may be considered, although its effect will be delayed. Use synchronized cardioversion at 120 to 200 J (biphasic) in an unstable patient. In a stable patient with a-fib of unclear duration, anticoagulation should be considered prior to chemical or electrical cardioversion.

❍ **What are the contraindications to β-blockers?**

CHF, variant angina, AV block, COPD, asthma (relative), bradycardia, hypotension, and IDDM.

❍ **What are the causes of SVT?**

Ectopic SVT may be because of digitalis toxicity (25% of digitalis induced arrhythmias), pericarditis, MI, COPD, pre-excitation syndromes, mitral valve prolapse, rheumatic heart disease, pneumonia, and ethanol.

❍ **Describe the key features of Mobitz I (Wenckebach) second-degree AV block.**

Progressive prolongation of the PR interval until atrial impulse is not conducted. If symptomatic, administer atropine and transcutaneous/transvenous pacing.

❍ **Describe the features and treatment of Mobitz II second-degree AV block.**

Constant PR interval. One or more beats fail to conduct. Treat with atropine and transcutaneous/transvenous pacing.

❍ **Name five causes of mesenteric ischemia.**

Arterial thrombosis at sites of atherosclerotic plaques, emboli from left atrium in patients with a-fib or rheumatic heart disease, arterial embolism most commonly to the superior mesenteric artery, insufficient arterial flow, and venous thrombosis.

❍ **What laboratory abnormalities are expected in a patient with mesenteric ischemia?**

Leukocytosis >15,000, metabolic acidosis, hemoconcentration, and elevation of phosphate, amylase and lactate.

❍ **What can a new systolic murmur indicate in a patient with an AMI?**

Ventriculoseptal rupture or mitral regurgitation as a result of papillary muscle rupture or dysfunction.

❍ **What ECG changes are seen in a true posterior infarction?**

Large R-wave and ST depression in V1 and V2.

❍ **Why do T-waves invert in an AMI?**

Infarction or ischemia causes a reversal of the sequence of repolarization (endocardial-to-epicardial as opposed to normal epicardial-to-endocardial).

❍ **How should PSVT be treated during an AMI?**

Vagal maneuvers, adenosine, or cardioversion.

❍ **A patient presents 1 day after discharge for an AMI with a new harsh systolic murmur along the left sternal border and pulmonary edema. What is the diagnosis?**

Ventricular septal rupture. Diagnosis is confirmed with an echo. Treatment includes nitroprusside for afterload reduction and possible intra-aortic balloon pump followed by surgical repair.

❍ **Which type of infarct commonly leads to papillary muscle dysfunction?**

Inferior MI. Signs and symptoms include a mild transient systolic murmur and pulmonary edema.

❍ **A patient presents 2 weeks after an AMI with chest pain, fever, and shortness of breath. A pleural effusion is detected on CXR. What is the diagnosis?**

Dressler's (postmyocardial infarction) syndrome, which is caused by an immunologic reaction to myocardial antigens.

❍ **What is the most common symptom of acute pericarditis?**

Sharp or stabbing retrosternal or precordial chest pain. Pain increases when supine and decreases when sitting-up and leaning forward.

❍ **What is the most important cause of hypoxia in a patient with a flail chest?**

The underlying lung contusion.

❍ **What physical findings are associated with acute pericarditis?**

Pericardial friction rub is the most common. Rub is heard best at the left sternal border or apex in a sitting leaning forward position. Other findings include fever and tachycardia.

❍ **What ECG changes occur with acute pericarditis?**

ST-segment elevation in the precordial leads, especially V5 and V6 and in lead I. PR depression occurs in leads II, aVF, V4 to V6.

❍ **What are the most common symptoms and signs of a PE?**

CP (88%), tachypnea (92%), dyspnea (84%), anxiety (59%), fever (43%), tachycardia (44%), DVT (32%), hypotension (25%), and syncope (13%).

❍ **What is the most common CXR finding in PE?**

Elevated hemidiaphragm as a result of decreased lung volume observed in 50% of PEs. Other common findings include pleural effusions, atelectasis, and pulmonary infiltrates.

❍ **What are two relatively specific findings in PE on CXR?**

(1) Hampton's hump: Area of lung consolidation with a rounded border facing the hilus.

(2) Westermark's sign: Dilated pulmonary outflow tract ipsilateral to the emboli with decreased perfusion distal to the lesion.

❍ **What does a normal perfusion scan rule out?**

A PE. An abnormal scan can be caused by PE, asthma, emphysema, bronchitis, pneumonia, pleural effusion, carcinoma, CHF, and atelectasis.

❍ **What does normal ventilation with decreased perfusion suggest?**

PE.

❍ **What physical findings may be found with mitral stenosis?**

Prominent a-wave, early-systolic left parasternal-lift, first heart sound is loud and snapping, and early-diastolic opening snap with a low-pitched, mid-diastolic rumble that crescendos into S1.

❍ **What triad of symptoms is characteristic of aortic stenosis?**

Syncope, angina, and left heart failure. As the disease progresses, systolic BP decreases and pulse pressure narrows.

❍ **What are the signs and symptoms of acute aortic regurgitation?**

Dyspnea, tachycardia, tachypnea, and chest pain.

❍ **What are the causes of acute aortic regurgitation?**

Infectious endocarditis, acute rheumatic fever, trauma, spontaneous rupture of valve leaflets, or aortic dissection.

❍ **What are the signs and symptoms of hypertensive encephalopathy?**

Nausea, vomiting, headache, lethargy, coma, blindness, nerve palsies, hemiparesis, aphasia, retinal hemorrhage, cotton wool spots, exudates, sausage linking, and papilledema.

❍ **Which drugs are used to treat eclampsia?**

Magnesium sulfate, 4 to 6 g bolus IV followed by a 2 g/h infusion, as well as hydralazine, 10 to 20 mg IV or labetalol.

❍ **What physical findings are suspicious for an acute aortic dissection?**

BP differences between arms, neuro deficits, new murmur, an aortic insufficiency murmur. bruits, hypertension, JVD, and muffled heart tones.

❍ **What CXR findings occur with a thoracic aortic aneurysm?**

Change in the appearance of aorta, mediastinal widening, hump in the aortic arch, pleural effusion (most common on the left), and extension of the aortic shadow.

❍ **How are Stanford type A and B aortic dissections defined and treated?**

Type A: Ascending, proximal to left subclavian (DeBakey I and II)—surgery.

Type B: Descending, distal to left subclavian (DeBakey III)—usually medical treatment.

❍ **What is the initial fluid bolus that should be given to a child in shock?**

20 mL/kg.

❍ **What is the initial treatment of a tension pneumothorax?**

Large bore IV catheter placed in the second intercostal space, midclavicular line.

❍ **What is Hamman's sign?**

Also called Hamman's crunch. Crunching sound over the heart during systole secondary to pneumomediastinum.

❍ **What is the most common complaint in a patient with a traumatic aortic injury?**

Retrosternal or intrascapular pain.

❍ **Name five clinical signs of a basilar skull fracture.**

Periorbital ecchymosis (raccoon's eyes), retroauricular ecchymosis (Battle's sign), CSF otorrhea or rhinorrhea, hemotympanum or bloody ear discharge, and first, second, seventh, and eighth CN deficits.

❍ **What is the most common cause of shock in patients with blunt chest trauma?**

Pelvic or extremity fractures.

❍ **What is the differential diagnosis of distended neck veins in a trauma patient?**

Tension pneumothorax, pericardial tamponade, air embolism, and cardiac failure. Neck vein distention may not be present until hypovolemia has been treated.

❍ **A trauma patient presents with a "rocking-horse" type of ventilation. What is the diagnosis?**

Probable high spinal cord injury with intercostal muscle paralysis.

❍ **A trauma patient presents with subcutaneous emphysema. What is the differential diagnosis?**

Pneumothorax, laryngeal injury, pneumomediastinum, or bronchial injury.

❍ **A pneumothorax is suspected but does not show up on a CXR. What other x-rays should be considered?**

Expiratory AP/PA CXR.

❍ **A fracture of what rib has the worst prognosis?**

The first rib. First and second rib fractures are associated with bronchial tears, vascular injury, and myocardial contusions.

❍ **What cardiovascular injury is commonly associated with a sternal fracture?**

Myocardial contusions.

❍ **Describe Beck's triad.**

Muffled heart tones, hypotension, and distended neck veins. Causes include: myocardial contusion, AMI, pericardial tamponade, and tension pneumothorax.

❍ **What is the most likely cause of a new systolic murmur and ECG infarct pattern observed in a patient with chest trauma?**

Ventricular septal defect.

❍ **What is the pathophysiology of compartment syndrome?**

Increased pressure within closed tissue spaces compromising blood flow to muscle and nerve tissue. There are three prerequisites to the development of compartment syndrome:

(1) Limiting space.

(2) Increased tissue pressure.

(3) Decreased tissue perfusion.

❍ **What are the two basic mechanisms for elevated compartment pressure?**

(1) External compression: By burn eschar, circumferential casts, dressings, or pneumatic pressure garments.

(2) Volume increase within the compartment: Hemorrhage into the compartment, IV infiltration, or edema secondary to direct injury or postischemic reperfusion.

❍ **What are the early signs and symptoms of compartment syndrome?**

Early findings: (1) Tenderness and pain out of proportion to the injury, (2) pain with active and passive motion, (3) hypesthesia (paresthesia)—abnormal 2-point discrimination. Late findings: (1) Compartment tense, indurated, and erythematous, (2) slow capillary refill, (3) pallor and pulselessness.

❍ **Define increased intracranial pressure.**

ICP >than 15 mm Hg.

❍ **What intracompartmental pressure is of concern?**

Normal pressure is less than 10 mm Hg. It is generally agreed that >30 mm Hg mandates an emergent fasciotomy. The treatment for compartment pressures between 20 and 30 mm Hg is controversial and requires a surgical consult.

❍ **Where is the most common site of a basilar skull fracture?**

Petrous portion of the temporal bone.

❍ **Which is the most common artery involved with an epidural hematoma?**

The meningeal artery, specifically the middle.

❍ **Where are epidural hematomas located?**

Between the dura and inner table of the skull.

❍ **Where are subdural hematomas located?**

Beneath the dura and over the brain and arachnoid. Caused by tears of pial arteries or of bridging veins.

❍ **What clues are evident with a duodenal injury?**

Increased serum amylase and retroperitoneal free air.

❍ **What is Kehr's sign?**

Left shoulder pain due to blood irritating the diaphragm from a splenic injury.

❍ **Which type of injury most commonly damages the pancreas?**

Penetrating.

❍ **Inability to pass a nasogastric tube in a trauma victim suggests damage to which organ?**

Diaphragm, usually on the left.

❍ **Describe the three zones of the neck and their evaluation?**

I. Below the cricoid cartilage—CT angiogram, esophagoscope, bronchoscopy.

II. Between the cricoid and the mandible—Surgery. "2 surgery!"

III. Above the angle of the mandible—CT angiogram.

❍ **On a lateral C-spine x-ray, how much soft tissue (prevertebral) swelling is normal from C1 to C4?**

Up to 4 mm is normal; >5 mm suggests a fracture.

❍ **How much anterior subluxation is normal on an adult lateral C-spine x-ray?**

3.5 mm.

❍ **On a lateral C-spine x-ray, what does "fanning" of the spinous processes suggest?**

Posterior ligamentous disruption.

❍ **What are the three most unstable cervical spine injuries?**

(1) Transverse atlantal ligament rupture.

(2) Dens fracture.

(3) Burst fracture with posterior ligament disruption.

❍ **Describe a Jefferson fracture.**

Burst of the ring of C1, usually from vertical compression force. Best detected on an odontoid view.

❍ **Describe a Hangman's fracture.**

C2 bilateral pedicle fracture. This fracture is usually caused by hyperextension.

❍ **Which are the two most commonly injured genitourinary organs?**

Kidney and bladder, associated with pelvic fracture.

❍ **What is a Clay-Shoveler fracture?**

In order of frequency, C7, C6, or T1 avulsion fracture of the spinous process, caused by forced flexion, or a direct blow.

❍ **Describe the key features of spinal shock.**

Sudden areflexia, which is transient and distal which lasts hours to weeks. Blood pressure is usually 80 to 100 mm Hg with paradoxical bradycardia.

❍ **A trauma patient has blood at the urethral meatus. What test should be ordered?**

A retrograde urethrogram. Ten milliliters of contrast solution is injected into the urinary meatus and an x-ray is performed.

❍ **Describe the leg position in a patient with a femoral neck fracture.**

Shortened, abducted, and slightly externally rotated.

❍ **Describe the leg position in a patient with an anterior dislocation.**

Hip is abducted and externally rotated. Mechanism is forced abduction.

❍ **Describe the leg position in a patient with a posterior hip dislocation.**

Shortened, adducted, and internally rotated. Force is applied to a flexed knee directed posteriorly. Associated with sciatic nerve injury (10%), and avascular necrosis of the femoral head.

❍ **What factors increase the probability of a wound infection?**

Dirty or contaminated wounds, stellate or crushing wounds, wounds longer than 5 cm, wounds older than 6 hours, and infection prone anatomic sites.

❍ **Which has greater resistance to infection, sutures, or staples?**

Staples.

❍ **Which type of wounds result in the majority of tetanus cases?**

Lacerations, punctures, and crush injuries.

❍ **What is the risk associated with not treating a septal hematoma of the nose?**

Aseptic necrosis, followed by absorption of the septal cartilage resulting in septal perforation.

❍ **Which are the three most common carpal fractures?**

The scaphoid, triquetrum, and lunate. All may be second-degree falls on an outstretched hand. Radiographs may initially be normal. The scaphoid is the most common.

❍ **What is Kienböck's disease?**

Avascular necrosis of the lunate with collapse of the lunate secondary to fracture. As with a navicular (scaphoid) fracture, initial wrist x-rays may not demonstrate the fracture. Therefore, tenderness over the lunate warrants immobilization.

❍ **Which tarsal bone is most commonly fractured?**

Calcaneus (60%). Calcaneal fractures are commonly associated with lumbar compression injuries (10%).

❍ **The second metatarsal is the locking mechanism of the midpart of the foot. A fracture at the base of the second metatarsal should raise suspicion of what?**

A disrupted joint—treatment may require ORIF.

❍ **Which patellar fracture requires orthopedic consultation?**

Displaced transverse fracture, comminuted fractures, and open fractures.

❍ **What is the most common mechanism for fractures of the femoral condyles?**

Direct trauma, fall, or blow to the distal femur.

❍ **Of tibial plateau fractures, where is the most common site?**

Lateral, more common in the older population, usually presenting with swollen painful knee and limited range of motion.

❍ **With complete rupture of medial or collateral ligaments, how much laxity is expected on examination?**

Greater than 1 cm without endpoint as compared to uninjured knee.

❍ **Which ligamentous injury to the knee is most common?**

Anterior cruciate ligament, usually from noncontact injury.

❍ **Why "tap" a knee with an acute hemarthrosis?**

To relieve pressure and pain and to determine whether fat globules are present indicating a fracture.

❍ **How is a "locked" knee "un-locked"?**

Hang leg over table at 90-degree flexion, allow relaxation, and apply a longitudinal traction with internal and external rotation.

❍ **Where is the most common site of compartment syndrome?**

Anterior compartment of the leg—contains tibialis anteriorus, extensor digitorum longus, extensor hallucis longus, and peroneus muscles, as well as anterior tibial artery and deep peroneal nerve.

❍ **Where is the most common site for a palpable defect of Achilles' tendon?**

2 to 6 cm proximal to its insertion.

❍ **What are the most common lower extremity fractures in children?**

Tibial and fibular shaft fractures, usually secondary to twist forces.

❍ **What is a toddler fracture?**

Common cause of limp or refusal to walk in this age group is a spiral fracture of the tibia without fibular involvement.

❍ **What is the most common cause of a painful hip joint in infants?**

Septic arthritis. *Staphylococcus* is the most common cause in infancy. The hip usually abducted, flexed, and externally rotated.

❍ **What is the most common cause of a painful hip in children 3- to 10-year olds?**

Transient synovitis. It can be difficult to distinguish from septic arthritis.

❍ **An 8-year-old child presents with a limp. On examination, hip range of motion is decreased. What rare disease should be considered?**

Children, 5 to 9 years, may acquire idiopathic avascular necrosis of the femoral heal, that is, Legg–Calvé–Perthes disease.

❍ **Describe a common patient with a slipped capital femoral epiphysis.**

Obese boy, aging from 10 years to 16 years. Groin or knee discomfort increases with activity; may have a limp. Often bilateral. The slip is best detected by a lateral view.

❍ **What is the most important complication of a proximal tibial metaphyseal fracture?**

Arterial involvement, especially when there is a valgus deformity.

❍ **What is unique about an avulsion fracture at the base of the fifth metatarsal?**

It is one of the most commonly missed fractures and usually due to plantar flexion and inversion of the ankle. It must be diagnosed because of the high risk for malunion if not treated appropriately.

❍ **A 21-year-old female complains of pain and a "clicking" sound located at the posterior lateral malleolus. You sense a fullness beneath the lateral malleolus. What is the diagnosis?**

Peroneal tendon subluxation with associated tenosynovitis.

❍ **A patient cannot actively abduct her shoulder. What injury do you suspect?**

Rotator cuff tear. The cuff is comprised of the supraspinatus, infraspinatus, subscapularis, and the teres minor muscles and tendons.

❍ **Why is the displaced supracondylar fracture (of distal humerus) in a child considered a true emergency?**

The injury often results in injury to brachial artery or median nerve. It can also cause a compartment syndrome.

❍ **What signs and symptoms develop from a compartment syndrome involving the anterior compartment of the leg?**

Pain on active and passive dorsi-flexion, plantar-flexion of the foot, and hypesthesia of the first web space of the foot.

❍ **How is a scaphoid fracture diagnosed?**

Frequently, the initial radiograph will appear normal. Therefore, if the patient has tenderness in the anatomical snuff box, a scaphoid (navicular) fracture is presumed and the hand splinted. A follow-up radiograph, 10 to 14 days following the injury, may then reveal the fracture. A CT, MRI, or bone scan can be used for difficult cases.

❍ **What metatarsal fracture is highly associated with a disrupted tarsal-metatarsal joint?**

Fracture to the base of the second metatarsal. Treatment may require ORIF.

❍ **What fracture is frequently missed when the patient complains of an ankle injury?**

Fracture at the base of the fifth metatarsal caused by plantar flexion and inversion. Radiographs of the ankle may not include the fifth metatarsal.

❍ **What life-threatening injury is associated with pelvic fractures?**

Severe hemorrhage. It is usually retroperitoneal. Up to 6 L of blood can be accommodated in this space.

❍ **Which fracture is associated with avascular necrosis of the femoral head?**

Femoral neck fractures. Avascular necrosis occurs with 15% of nondisplaced femoral neck fractures and with near 90% of displaced femoral neck fractures.

❍ **A child presents after falling and knocking out his front tooth. How would the management differ if the child was 3 years versus 13 years?**

With primary teeth, no reimplantation should be attempted because of the risk of ankylosis or fusion to the bone. However, with permanent teeth, reimplantation should occur as soon as possible. Remaining periodontal fibers are a key to success. Thus, the tooth should not be wiped dry because this may disrupt the periodontal ligament fibers still attached.

❍ **Why shouldn't topical analgesics be used for Ellis Class III tooth fractures?**

Severe tissue irritation or sterile abscesses may occur with their use. Treatment includes application of tinfoil, analgesics, and immediate dental referral.

❍ **A 3-year-old child presents with a unilateral purulent rhinorrhea. What is the probable diagnosis?**

Nasal foreign body.

❍ **A patient presents 3 days after tooth extraction with severe pain and a foul mouth odor and taste. What is the diagnosis? What is the treatment?**

Alveolar osteitis (dry socket) results from loss of the blood clot and local osteomyelitis. Treat by irrigation of the socket and application of a medicated dental packing or iodoform gauze moistened with Campho-Phenique or eugenol.

❍ **A patient presents with gingival pain and a foul mouth odor and taste. On examination, fever and lymphadenopathy are present. The gingiva is bright red and the papillae are ulcerated and covered with a gray membrane. What is the diagnosis? What is the treatment?**

Acute necrotizing ulcerative gingivitis (ANUG).

❍ **What is the most common oral manifestation of AIDS?**

Oropharyngeal thrush. Some other AIDS-related oropharyngeal diseases are Kaposi's sarcoma, hairy leukoplakia, and non-Hodgkin's lymphoma.

❍ **What potential complications of nasal fractures should always be considered on physical examination?**

Septal hematoma and cribriform plate fractures. A septal hematoma appears as a bluish mass on the nasal septum and, if not drained, aseptic necrosis of the septal cartilage and septal abnormalities may occur. A cribriform plate fracture should be considered in a patient who has a clear rhinorrhea after trauma.

❍ **A patient presents with a swollen, tender, red left auricle. What is the diagnosis?**

Perichondritis caused by *Pseudomonas.*

❍ **What physical examination findings suggest the diagnosis of posterior epistaxis rather than anterior epistaxis?**

(1) Inability to see the site of bleeding. Anterior nosebleeds usually originate at Kiesselbach's plexus, an area easily visualized on the nasal septum.

(2) Blood from both sides of the nose. In a posterior nosebleed the blood can more easily pass to the other side because of the proximity of the choanae.

(3) Blood trickling down the oropharynx.

(4) Inability to control bleeding by direct pressure.

❍ **A child with a sinus infection presents with proptosis, a red swollen eyelid, and an inferiolaterally displaced globe. What is the diagnosis?**

Orbital cellulitis and abscess associated with ethmoid sinusitis.

❍ **An ill-appearing patient presents with a fever of 103°F, bilateral chemosis, a third nerve palsy, and untreated sinusitis. What is the diagnosis?**

Cavernous sinus thrombosis. This life-threatening complication occurs from direct extension through the valveless veins. Complication of sinusitis may be local (osteomyetitis), orbital (cellulitis), or within the central nervous system (meningitis or brain abscess).

❍ **Retropharyngeal abscess is most common in which age group? Why?**

Six months to 3 years. This is because the retropharyngeal lymph nodes regress in size after the age of 3 years.

❍ **How does a patient with a retropharyngeal abscess appear?**

Ill appearing, febrile, stridorous, and drooling. Patients may complain of difficulty swallowing or may refuse to feed.

❍ **A 48-year-old male presents with a high fever, trismus, dysphagia, and swelling inferior to the mandible in the lateral neck. What is the diagnosis?**

Parapharyngeal abscess.

❍ **Peritonsillar abscesses are most common in which age group?**

Adolescents and young adults. Symptoms include ear pain, trismus, drooling, and an alteration of the voice.

❍ **What is the most common origin of Ludwig's angina?**

Infection to at the lower second and third molars. It is a swelling in the region of the submandibular, sublingual, and submental spaces causing displacement of the tongue upward and posteriorly. The most common organisms are hemolytic *Streptococci, Staphylococcus,* and mixed anaerobe and aerobes.

❍ **What are the signs and symptoms of a mandibular fracture?**

Malocclusion, pain, deviation or abnormal movement, decreased range of motion, bony deformity, swelling, ecchymosis, and lower lip (mental nerve) anesthesia.

❍ **Bilateral mental fractures may cause what acute complication?**

The tongue may cause acute airway obstruction because of loss of anterior support.

❍ **What are the two most common findings with an orbital floor fracture?**

Diplopia and globe lowering.

❍ **In which Le Fort fracture is CSF rhinorrhea most common?**

III.

❍ **What is the most common neuropathy associated with acoustic neuroma?**

Because of trigeminal nucleus involvement the corneal reflex may be lost.

❍ **Define a Le Fort I fracture.**

Fracture line runs from the nasal opening along the wall of the maxillary sinuses bilaterally, across the pterygomaxillary tissue to the lateral pterygoid plates. Also called a horizontal maxillary fracture. X-rays often do not detect this fracture. Mobility of the maxilla without movement at the nasal bridge or zygoma is noted on physical examination.

❍ **Describe a Le Fort II fracture.**

Fracture involves facial aspects of the maxillae extending to the nasal and ethmoid bones. The fracture also involves the maxillary sinuses and infraorbital rims bilaterally and cross the nasal bridge. This is also called a pyramidal fracture. Swelling of the nose, lips, and midface may be noted. Subconjunctival hemorrhage may present with blood in the nares. Suspect cerebrospinal involvement and check for CSF rhinorrhea. Diagnosis can be made clinically by crepitation or movement at the nasal bridge when the maxilla is moved.

❍ **Describe a Le Fort III fracture.**

The fracture line runs through the frontozygomatic suture lines bilaterally extending through the orbits, the base of the nose, and the ethmoid region. Movement of the zygoma and midface is suggestive. This is also called a complete craniofacial dysjunction.

❍ **A 16-year-old boxer presents with right ear pain and swelling after receiving a blow to the ear. What is the treatment?**

The ear should be aseptically drained by incision or aspiration and a mastoid conforming dressing should be applied. An ENT follow-up is mandatory. If the ear is not treated appropriately, a cauliflower deformity may result.

❍ **What would the physical finding be in unilateral sensory hearing loss?**

The patient will lateralize, have air conduction greater than bone conduction, that is, normal Rinne test indicating no conductive loss. The Weber test will lateralize to the normal ear. The most common cause of this is viral neuronitis.

❍ **If a patient has bilateral sensory hearing loss, what causes should be suspected?**

Noise or ototoxins such as certain antibiotics, loop diuretics, or antineoplastics.

❍ **Name some causes of tympanic membrane perforation.**

Blast injuries (water or air), foreign bodies in the ear (particularly Q-tips), lightning strikes, otitis media, and a temporal bone fracture.

❍ **What is the most common cause of laryngeal trauma?**

Blunt trauma secondary to motor vehicle accidents.

❍ **A patient presents with well-demarcated swelling of the lips and tongue. She was started on an antihypertensive agent 3 weeks ago. Which agent is most likely?**

Angiotensin-converting enzyme inhibitor. Although, angioedema may occur anytime during therapy with an ACE inhibitor, it is most likely in the first month of treatment.

❍ **A patient presents with the sensation of a foreign body in the eye. Slit-lamp reveals a dendritic figure that has a Christmas tree pattern. What is the treatment?**

Antiviral agents and cycloplegics are used to treat herpes simplex keratitis.

❍ **A patient presents with sudden vision loss in one eye which returns quickly. What is the diagnosis?**

Amaurosis fugax. This condition usually is caused by central retinal artery emboli from extracranial atherosclerosis.

❍ **When and where do retinal detachments occur after a blunt traumatic injury?**

There is a delay between the incident and detachment. Fifty percent occur in the first 8 months and 80% within 2 years. The detachment most commonly occurs in the inferotemporal quadrant.

❍ **A patient was hit in the eye during a fight last night while intoxicated. He presents 8 hours after the incident with proptosis and visual loss. The examination reveals an intact globe and an afferent pupillary defect. What is the problem?**

Retro-orbital hematoma with ischemia of the optic nerve or retina. The pressure of the blood in the orbit exceeds the perfusion pressure causing a decreased blood flow and loss of function. Treatment involves performing a lateral canthotomy.

❍ **What are complications of a hyphema?**

The four Ss:

(1) *Secondary rebleeds*, which usually occur between the second and fifth day postinjury since this is the time of clot retraction. Rebleeds tend to be worse than the initial bleed.

(2) *Significantly increased intraocular pressure*, which can lead to acute glaucoma, chronic late glaucoma, and optic atrophy.

(3) *Staining* of the cornea because of hemosiderin deposits.

(4) *Synechiae*, which interfere with iris function.

❍ **Why do patients with sickle-cell anemia and a hyphema require special consideration when presenting with ophthalmologic concerns?**

Increased intraocular pressure can occur, if the cells sickle in the trabecular meshwork preventing aqueous humor from leaving the anterior chamber. Medication, such as hyperosmotics and acetazolamide, which increase the likelihood of sickling, must be avoided.

❍ **What are the causes of a subluxed or dislocated lens?**

Trauma, Marfan's syndrome, homocystinuria, and Weill–Marchesani syndrome.

❍ **Which is worse, acid or alkali burns of the cornea?**

Alkali, because of deeper penetration than acid burns. A barrier is formed from precipitated proteins with acid burns. The exception is hydrofluoric acid and heavy metal containing acids, which can penetrate the cornea.

❍ **Three hours ago, a patient experienced sudden, painless visual loss in her right eye. Central retinal artery occlusion is suspected. What would be the expected finding on eye examination? What is the prognosis?**

Afferent pupillary defect, pale gray retina, and a small pink dot near the fovea. This cherry red spot is the choroidal vasculature being seen at the macula where the retina is the thinnest. After 2 hours, the prognosis is extremely poor for visual recovery. Digital massage or anterior chamber paracentesis may dislodge the clot.

❍ **What conditions have been associated with central retinal vein occlusion?**

Hyperviscosity syndromes, diabetes, and hypertension. Funduscopic examination shows a chaotically streaked retina with congested dilated veins. There are superficial and deep retinal hemorrhages, cotton wool spots, and macular edema.

❍ **A patient presents with atraumatic pain behind the left eye, a left pupil afferent defect, central visual loss, and a swollen optic disc? What is the diagnosis and potential causes?**

Optic neuritis. This may be idiopathic or may be associated with multiple sclerosis, Lyme's disease, neurosyphilis, lupus, sarcoid, alcoholism, toxins, or drug abuse.

❍ **After entering a dark bar, a patient developed eye pain, nausea, vomiting, blurred vision, and sees "halos" around lights. Why would this patient be given mannitol, pilocarpine, and acetazolamide?**

This patient has acute narrow–angle glaucoma. The goal of treatment is to decrease intraocular pressure. This can be done by:

(1) decreasing the production of aqueous (carbonic anhydrase inhibitor),

(2) decreasing the intraocular volume by making the plasma hypertonic to the aqueous humor (as with glycerol or mannitol),

(3) constricting the pupil, allowing increased flow of the aqueous through the previously blocked canal of Schlemm.

❍ **A patient felt something fly into his eye while mowing the lawn. On examination, there is a brown foreign body on the cornea and a teardrop iris pointing toward the foreign body. What is the diagnosis?**

Perforated cornea with extruded iris. A similar foreign body may appear black on the sclera with scleral perforation.

❍ **What is the risk of placing a patient with COPD on a high FiO_2?**

Suppression of the hypoxic ventilatory drive.

❍ **If a patient has patchy infiltrates on a chest x-ray and bullous myringitis, which antibiotic should be given?**

A macrolide for mycoplasma.

❍ **Describe the classic chest x-ray findings in Legionella pneumonia.**

Patchy non-segmental and unilateral infiltrates.

❍ **An older patient with GI symptoms, hyponatremia, and a relative bradycardia most likely has what type of pneumonia?**

Legionella.

❍ **What is the treatment for Legionella pneumonia?**

IV macrolide. Fluoroquinolones are an alternative.

❍ **Describe the classic lab findings seen with Legionella pneumonia.**

Leukocytosis, elevated liver enzymes, and hyponatremia.

❍ **What are the classic signs and symptoms of TB?**

Night sweats, fever, weight loss, malaise, cough, and a green/yellow sputum most commonly seen in the mornings.

❍ **Where are some common extrapulmonary TB sites?**

Lymph node, bone, GI tract, GU tract, meninges, liver, and the pericardium.

❍ **Right upper lobe cavitation with parenchymal involvement is classic for:**

TB. Lower lung infiltrates, hilar adenopathy, atelectasis, and pleural effusion are also common.

❍ **Which pneumonias are commonly associated with a pneumothorax?**

Staphylococcus, TB, Klebsiella, and PCP.

❍ **Which diagnostic test is helpful in subclinical PCP infection?**

Pulse oximetry decrease on exertion. If after 3 minutes of exercise the O_2 saturation decreases by 3% or the A-a gradient increases by 10 mm Hg from the resting value, consider PCP infection.

❍ **Which laboratory tests aid in the diagnosis of PCP?**

A rising LDH or LDH >450 and an ESR >50. A low albumin implies a worse prognosis.

❍ **The initial therapy for PCP includes which antibiotics?**

TMP-SMZ or pentamidine.

❍ **When are corticosteroids recommended for severe PCP?**

pO2 <70 mm Hg or an A-a gradient >35 mm Hg.

❍ **List two drugs that can cause ARDS.**

Heroin and aspirin.

❍ **How is the A-a gradient calculated for a patient breathing room air?**

A—a = $150 - Pa_{O2} - (Pa_{CO2} \times 1.25)$ or $4 + age/4$ or $140 - (Pa_{O2} + Pa_{CO2})$ Normal $\simeq$ 5 to 10 mm Hg.

❍ **A patient says food gets stuck in his midchest, then is regurgitated as a putrid, undigested mess. A barium study shows a dilated esophagus with a distal "beak." What is the diagnosis?**

Achalasia.

❍ **A woman with telangiectasias, "tight knuckles," and "acid indigestion" might have what findings on an upper GI series?**

Aperistalsis, characteristic of scleroderma.

❍ **A patient with an "acid stomach" develops melena and vomits bright red blood. Is esophagitis a probable cause?**

No. Capillary bleeding rarely causes impressive acute blood loss. Arterial bleeding, from a complicated ulcer, foreign body, or Mallory–Weiss tear, or variceal bleeding is much more likely.

❍ **A cirrhotic patient vomits bright red blood. He has a systolic blood pressure of 90 mm Hg. After an aggressive fluid resuscitation, 4 units of PRBC, and gastric lavage, his pressure is 90 mm Hg. What's next?**

Assume a coagulopathy and transfuse fresh-frozen plasma, start a vasopressin drip, and arrange for an emergent endoscopic intervention.

❍ **Repeated, violent bouts of vomiting can result in both Mallory–Weiss tears and Boerhaave's syndrome. Differentiate the two.**

Mallory–Weiss tears involve the submucosa and mucosa, typically in the right posterolateral wall of the GE junction. Boerhaave's is a full-thickness tear, usually in the unsupported left posterolateral wall of the abdominal esophagus.

❍ **After a high-speed MVA, an unrestrained driver develops abdominal and chest pain radiating to the neck. An upper chest film shows left pleural fluid. What gastroesophageal catastrophe might have occurred?**

Impact against a steering wheel can result in Boerhaave's syndrome with esophageal perforation and mediastinitis.

❍ **You suspect a perforated esophagus. Which test should be ordered next?**

A water-soluble contrast study. In the meantime, start broad-spectrum antibiotics and call the surgeons ASAP.

❍ **Pediatric foreign bodies lodge at which esophageal levels?**

Typically at levels of the cricopharyngeus muscles (most usual), thoracic inlet, aortic arch, tracheal bifurcation, and lower esophageal sphincter.

❍ **When is removing a button battery lodged in the esophagus indicated?**

Always.

❍ **X-rays are crucial in the search for a suspected swallowed foreign body. In kids, what physical findings can tip you off?**

Besides a child's distress, you may also find a red or scratched oropharynx, dysphagia, a high fever, or peritoneal signs. Subcutaneous air suggests perforation.

❍ **An obstructing meat bolus should be removed within 12 hours. What's the best approach?**

Endoscopy. May first try glucagon, 1 mg IV.

❍ **After fluid and blood resuscitation for a bleeding ulcer, what is the most useful diagnostic test?**

Endoscopy.

❍ **Are "stress ulcers" a surgical problem?**

Not usually. The diffused gastric bleeding that results from CNS tumors, head trauma, burns, sepsis, shock, steroids, aspirin, or alcohol is usually mucosal, can be life-threatening, and can most often be managed medically. Endoscopic diagnosis is key.

❍ **Burning epigastric pain shooting to the back, hypovolemic shock, and a high amylase suggests?**

Posterior perforation of a duodenal ulcer.

❍ **Who gets acalculous cholecystitis?**

Dehydrated postop, post-trauma, and burn patients, as well as those with transfusion-related hemolysis or narcotic use.

❍ **What is the most common cause of a lower GI perforation?**

Diverticulitis, followed by tumor, colitis, foreign bodies, and instrumentation.

❍ **A pregnant woman with right upper quadrant pain should be assumed to have what intra-abdominal pathology until proven otherwise?**

Acute appendicitis.

❍ **What does ultrasound show in an acute appendicitis?**

A fixed, tender, noncompressible mass (bagel sign), in 75% to 85% of cases.

❍ **What is the most common cause of a small bowel obstruction?**

Adhesions, followed by an incarcerated hernia. Gallstones and bezoars are the most common causes of an intraluminal obstruction.

❍ **Recurrent small bowel obstruction in an elderly woman associated with unilateral pain into one thigh suggests what occult process?**

Obturator hernia incarceration.

❍ **What are the most common causes of colonic obstruction?**

Cancer, then diverticulitis followed by volvulus.

❍ **A patient tells you that 2 days ago his groin bulged and he developed severe pain with progressive nausea and vomiting. He has a tender mass in his groin. What shouldn't he do?**

Don't try to reduce a long-standing, tender incarcerated hernia! The abdomen is no place for dead bowel.

❍ **A young man with atraumatic chronic back pain, eye trouble, and painful red lumps on his shins develops bloody diarrhea. What is the point of this question?**

To remind you of extraintestinal manifestations of inflammatory bowel disease, such as ankylosing spondylitis, uveitis, and erythema nodosum, and kidney stones.

❍ **At least a third of patients with Crohn's disease have kidney stones. Why?**

Dietary oxalate is usually bound to calcium and excreted. When terminal ileal disease leads to decreased bile salt absorption, the resulting fattier intestinal contents bind calcium by saponification. Free oxalate is "hyperabsorbed" in the colon, resulting in hyperoxaluria, and calcium oxalate nephrolithiasis.

❍ **A patient with new diarrhea and abdominal pain tells you she took antibiotics for sinusitis 2 weeks ago. Sigmoidoscopy might reveal what?**

Yellowish superficial plaques suggestive of pseudomembranous colitis. Stool studies would show *C. difficile* toxin.

❍ **What's the treatment?**

Oral vancomycin, 125 mg qid or oral metronidazole, 500 mg qid. Either regimen should be given for 7 to 10 days. Cholestyramine, which binds the toxin, can help limit the diarrhea. Follow-up stool studies should confirm clearance of the toxin.

❍ **What barium findings distinguish colonic obstruction caused by acute diverticulitis from that caused by colon cancer?**

Diverticulitis is extraluminal, so the mucosa appears intact and involved bowel segments are longer. Adenocarcinoma distorts the mucosa, involves a short segment of bowel, and has overhanging edges.

❍ **Which is more sensitive for locating the source of GI bleeding, a radioactive Tc-labeled red cell scan, or angiography?**

A bleeding scan can find a site bleeding at a rate as low as 0.12 mL/min, while angiography requires rapid bleeding greater than 0.5 mL/min.

❍ **A postsurgical patient develops right upper quadrant pain, nausea, and low-grade fevers. According to his surgeon, the gallbladder was normal intraoperatively. What's a probable diagnosis?**

Acalculous cholecystitis.

❍ **Eight years after her cholecystectomy, a woman develops right upper quadrant pain and jaundice. What's the chance of developing recurrent biliary tract stones after cholecystectomy?**

At least 10%, either because of retained stones or in situ formation by biliary epithelium.

❍ **List the ultrasound findings suggestive of acute cholecystitis.**

Presence of gall stones (or sludge, in acalculous cholecystitis), ultrasonographic Murphy's sign, gall bladder wall thickening >5 mm, and pericholecystic fluid. A dilated common bile duct (>10 mm) suggests common duct obstruction.

❍ **Name two findings in acute cholecystitis that mandate emergent laparotomy.**

Emphysematous cholecystitis and perforation. Otherwise, timing of surgery is somewhat institution- and surgeon-dependent.

❍ **What medical conditions are associated with an increase incidence of PUD?**

COPD, cirrhosis, and chronic renal failure.

❍ **A high fever and leukocytosis accompanying acute alcoholic hepatitis is worrisome. Why?**

Alcohol is marrow toxic, so leukocytosis often reflects serious associated infection. Obtain a chest x-ray, obtain blood cultures, a urinalysis, and collect ascitic fluid for cell count and culture.

❍ **A confused cirrhotic presents to the ED. She is afebrile and has asterixis. What should your examination consist of as you look for the precipitant of hepatic encephalopathy?**

Assess her mental status and search for localizing neurologic signs, such as an occult head injury; examination for dry mucous membranes and a low jugular venous pressure, including hypovolemia and azotemia; and check a stool Guaiac to determine GI bleeding.

❍ **An ascitic patient presents with fever but no localizing signs or symptoms of infection and a normal WBC. Because you know that spontaneous bacterial peritonitis can be an occult disease, you perform an abdominal paracentesis. What WBC in ascitic fluid suggests SBP?**

Greater than $250/mm^3$. You should also Gram stain the fluid and send at least 10 cc in blood culture bottles for aerobic and anaerobic culture.

❍ **Which two therapies can reduce the risk of recurrent SBP?**

Diuretics decrease ascitic fluid and nonabsorbable oral antibiotics decrease the gut bacterial load, limiting bacterial translocation. Both treatments have cut the risk of recurrence in compliant patients.

❍ **The most common causes of dysphagia in the elderly population include what?**

Hiatal hernia, reflux esophagitis, webs/rings, and cancer.

❍ **Which is a more sensitive test for pancreatitis, serum amylase, or lipase?**

Amylase elevation is 70% to 90% sensitive for pancreatitis; lipase is 75% to 100% sensitive; the combination is up to 95% to 97% sensitive. Remember that up to 10% of patients with severe acute pancreatitis may have a normal amylase. In chronic pancreatitis, up to 30% may have a normal amylase.

❍ **Symptoms that last longer than a week or the presence of an abdominal mass, hyperamylasemia, and leukocytosis suggest what potentially disastrous complications of pancreatitis?**

Pancreatic abscess or pseudocyst.

❍ **Distinguish, by location, the following: anal cryptitis, anal fissure, anorectal abscess, and fistula in ano.**

Cryptitis, fissures, and perianal abscess typically occur in the posterior midline; deep abscesses can point to areas far from the anus. Goodsall's rule on fistulas: those that open anteriorly go straight to the anal canal, while those that open posteriorly may follow a circuitous route.

❍ **True/False: Antibiotics are unnecessary after an uncomplicated perirectal abscess is incised and drained.**

True, assuming the patient has no underlying immunoincompetence, such as HIV, diabetes, malignancy. Sitz baths beginning the next day are the primary after care.

❍ **Procidentia in adults mandates what intervention?**

Rectal prolapse can be manually reduced in children with good results. Adults typically require proctosigmoidoscopy and surgical repair.

❍ **What is the management of button batteries that have passed the esophagus?**

In the asymptomatic patient—repeat radiographs. The symptomatic patient and those patients where the battery has not passed the pylorus after 48 hours require endoscopic retrieval.

❍ **Where is the most common location of a perforated peptic ulcer?**

Anterior surface of the duodenum or pylorus and the lesser curvature of the stomach.

❍ **Which types of patients are at risk for gallbladder perforation?**

Elderly, diabetics, and those with recurrent cholecystitis.

❍ **What percentage of patients with a perforated viscus have radiographic evidence of a pneumoperitoneum?**

60% to 70%. Therefore, one-third of patients will not have this sign. Keep the patient in either the upright or left lateral decubitus position for at least 10 minutes prior to performing x-rays.

❍ **What are the indications for the surgical removal of a GI foreign body?**

GI obstruction, GI perforation, toxic properties of the material, and length, size, and shape that will prevent the object from passing safely.

❍ **What size objects rarely pass the stomach?**

Objects longer than 5 cm and wider than 2 cm.

❍ **Are gastric and duodenal perforations more common in malignant or benign ulcers?**

Benign ulcerations.

❍ **What are the most common causes of nontraumatic perforations of the lower GI tract?**

Diverticulitis, carcinoma, colitis, foreign bodies, barium enemas, and endoscopy.

❍ **Which is one of the earliest signs of sepsis on an ABG?**

Respiratory alkalosis.

❍ **What conditions are associated with an atypical presentation of acute appendicitis?**

Situs inversus viscerum, malrotation, hypermobile cecum, long pelvic appendix, and pregnancy.

❍ **What are the most frequent symptoms of an acute appendicitis?**

Anorexia and pain. Anorexia and periumbilical pain with progression to constant RLQ pain is present in only 60% of cases.

❍ **What are the causes of pseudohyponatremia?**

Hyperglycemia, hyperlipidemia, or hyperproteinemia.

❍ **What are the ECG findings in a patient with hypokalemia?**

Flattened T-waves, depressed ST segments, prominent P- and U-waves, and prolonged QT and PR intervals.

❍ **What is the first ECG finding in a patient with hyperkalemia?**

At levels of 5.6 to 6.0 mEq/L, the development of tall, peaked T-waves, best seen in the precordial leads, occurs first.

❍ **What are the causes of hyperkalemia?**

Acidosis, tissue necrosis, hemolysis, blood transfusions, GI bleed, renal failure, Addison's disease, primary hypoaldosteronism, excess po K^+ intake, RTA IV, medication (succinylcholine, β-blockers, captopril, spironolactone, triamterene, amiloride, and high-dose penicillin).

❍ **What are the causes of hypocalcemia?**

Shock, sepsis, multiple blood transfusions, hypoparathyroidism, vitamin D deficiency, pancreatitis, hypomagnesemia, alkalosis, fat embolism syndrome, phosphate overload, chronic renal failure, loop diuretics, hypoalbuminemia, tumor lysis syndrome, and medication (Dilantin, phenobarbital, heparin, theophylline, cimetidine, and gentamicin).

❍ **What are the most common causes of hypercalcemia?**

(1) Malignancy.

(2) Primary hyperparathyroidism.

(3) Thiazide diuretics.

❍ **What are the signs and symptoms of hypercalcemia?**

A classic mnemonic can be used to remember these:

Stones	Renal calculi
Bones	Osteolysis
Abdominal groans	Peptic ulcer disease and pancreatitis
Psychic overtones	Psychiatric disorders

❍ **What are the most common GI symptoms in a patient with hypercalcemia?**

Anorexia and constipation.

❍ **What are the two primary causes of primary adrenal insufficiency?**

Tuberculosis and autoimmune destruction account for 90% of cases.

❍ **What are the signs and symptoms of primary adrenal insufficiency?**

Fatigue, weakness, weight loss, anorexia, hyperpigmentation, nausea, vomiting, abdominal pain, diarrhea, and orthostatic hypotension.

❍ **What are the characteristic laboratory findings associated with primary adrenal insufficiency?**

Hyperkalemia, hyponatremia, hypoglycemia, azotemia (if volume depletion is present), and a mild metabolic acidosis.

❍ **How should acute adrenal insufficiency be treated?**

Hydrocortisone, 100 mg IV, and crystalloid fluids containing dextrose.

❍ **What are the main causes of death during an adrenal crisis?**

Circulatory collapse and hyperkalemia-induced arrhythmias.

○ **What are the causes of acute adrenal crisis?**

It occurs secondary to a major stress such as surgery, severe injury, myocardial infarction, or any other illness in a patient with primary or secondary adrenal insufficiency.

○ **What is thyrotoxicosis and what are the causes?**

A hypermetabolic state that occurs secondary to excess circulating thyroid hormone caused by thyroid hormone overdose, thyroid hyperfunction, or thyroid inflammation.

○ **What are the hallmark clinical features of myxedema coma?**

Hypothermia (75%), and coma.

○ **What is the role of phosphate replacement during the treatment of DKA?**

Phosphate supplementation is not indicated until a serum concentration is below 1.0 mEq/dL.

○ **What is the most important initial step in the treatment of DKA?**

Rapid fluid administration with the first liter given over 30 minutes to 1 hour followed by 3 to 5 L over the next 3 hours.

○ **Why would the nitroprusside test be negative in a patient with alcoholic ketoacidosis?**

This test is used to detect the presence of ketones in the urine and serum. It does not detect β-hydroxybutyrate, which may be the predominant ketone in a patient with alcoholic ketoacidosis.

○ **In the first 2 years of life, what is the most common cause of drug-induced hypoglycemia?**

Salicylates. In the 2- to 8-year-old group, alcohol is the most likely cause, and in the 11- to 30-year-old group, insulin and sulfonylureas are the most probable culprits.

○ **How is sulfonylurea-induced hypoglycemia treated?**

IV glucose alone may be insufficient. It may require diazoxide, 300 mg slow IV over 30 minutes repeated every 4 hours octreotide 50 mcg SC/IV, glucagon (after dextrose) 1 to 2 mg IV/IM/SC (controversial).

○ **What is the most common cause of hypoglycemia in a child?**

Ketotic hypoglycemia. Attacks usually occur when the child is stressed with caloric deprivation. It is most common in boys typically between 18 months and 5 years. Attacks may be episodic, vomiting may occur, and are more frequent in the morning or during periods of illness.

○ **What are the neurologic signs and symptoms of hypoglycemia?**

Mental status changes, coma, paresthesias, cranial nerve palsies, transient hemiplegia, diplopia, decerebrate posturing, and clonus.

○ **What laboratory findings are expected with diabetic ketoacidosis?**

Elevated β-hydroxybutyrate, acetoacetate, acetone, and glucose. Ketonuria and glucosuria. Serum bicarbonate level, pCO_2, and pH are decreased. Potassium may be initially elevated but falls, if the acidosis is corrected.

❍ **What is the most common cause of neonatal stridor?**

Laryngotracheomalacia.

❍ **What is the most common precipitant of thyroid storm?**

Infections, typically pulmonary infections, are the most common precipitating event.

❍ **What is the treatment for DKA in an adult?**

(1) Fluids, approximately 5 to 10 L of normal saline alternating with half normal saline.
(2) Potassium, 100 to 200 mEq in the first 12 to 24 hours.
(3) Insulin, 0.1 U/kg bolus, followed by 0.1 U/kg/h infusion.
(4) Add glucose to the IV fluid when glucose levels fall below 250 mg/dL.
(5) Phosphate supplement when level drops below 1.0 mg/dL.
(6) For peds, NS, 20 mL/kg/h for 1 to 2 hours, and insulin, 0.1 U/kg drip.

❍ **What is the treatment for nonketotic hyperosmolar coma?**

Fluids (normal saline), potassium, 10 to 20 mEq/h, insulin, 5 to 10 U/h, and glucose should be added to the IV when the blood sugar drops below 250 mg/dL.

❍ **What are the pathognomonic findings as well as confirmatory laboratory tests diagnostic of thyroid storm?**

Trick question. Thyroid storm is based on clinical impression. There are no findings or confirmatory tests available.

❍ **What clinical clues might help in the diagnosis of thyroid storm?**

Eye signs of Graves' disease, a history of hyperthyroidism, widened pulse pressure, and a palpable goiter.

❍ **What are the signs and symptoms of thyroid storm?**

Tachycardia, fever, diaphoresis, increased CNS activity, emotional lability, heart failure, coma, and death.

❍ **What are the diagnostic criteria for thyroid storm?**

Tachycardia, CNS dysfunction, cardiovascular dysfunction, GI system dysfunction, and a temperature greater than 37.8°C (100°F).

❍ **What are the complications of bicarbonate therapy in DKA?**

Paradoxical CSF acidosis, hypokalemia, cardiac arrhythmias, decreased oxygen delivery to tissue, and fluid and sodium overload.

❍ **What is the most common cause of hypothyroidism?**

Primary thyroid failure. The most common etiology of hypothyroidism in adults is the use of radioactive iodine or subtotal thyroidectomy in the treatment of Graves' disease. The second most common cause is autoimmune thyroid disorders.

❍ **In a patient receiving anticoagulation therapy with heparin, when is adrenal hemorrhage most likely to strike?**

Typically between the third and eighteenth day of anticoagulation. Patients present with sudden hypotension and flank or epigastric pain. Nausea, vomiting, fever, and a change in sensorium may be associated.

❍ **What is the most common cause of secondary adrenal insufficiency and adrenal crisis?**

Iatrogenic adrenal suppression from prolonged steroid use. Rapid withdrawal of steroids may lead to collapse and death.

❍ **How is the anion gap calculated from electrolyte values?**

Anion gap = Na − Cl − CO_2. The normal gap is 12 +/− 4 mEq/L.

❍ **What are the two primary causes of metabolic alkalosis?**

(1) Loss of hydrogen and chloride from the stomach.

(2) Overzealous diuresis with loss of hydrogen, potassium, and chloride.

❍ **What is central pontine myelinolysis, a.k.a., osmotic demyelination syndrome?**

The complication of brain dehydration following too rapid correction of severe hyponatremia. Correct hyponatremia slowly, less than 12 mEq/d.

❍ **Tetralogy of Fallot (TOF) consists of VSD, an "overriding" aorta, pulmonary stenosis, and right ventricular hypertrophy. Which type of intracardiac shunting occurs?**

Right-to-left shunting whose severity is related to the degree of pulmonary stenosis.

❍ **Describe the murmurs of TOF.**

(1) Holosystolic of VSD—third ICS @ LSB.

(2) Crescendo–decrescendo murmur of pulmonary stenosis—second ICS @ LSB.

❍ **What common physical diagnostic sign can be detected in a childhood atrial septal defect?**

A fixed split of S-2 on deep inspiration.

❍ **What do x-ray findings often reveal in coarctation of the aorta?**

The "three" sign made up of the aortic knob and the dilated postcoarctation segment of the descending aorta. The "E" sign is the same thing seen in a negative image on barium esophagram.

❍ **Define apnea.**

No respiration for >20 seconds.

❍ **If cardioversion is necessary to treat an infant with unstable SVT, what is the appropriate energy to use?**

0.5 to 1 J/kg.

❍ **Can the type of stridor localize the level of the obstruction?**

Yes, inspiratory stridor points to a site of obstruction above the vocal folds while expiratory stridor points to obstruction below the vocal folds.

❍ **A neonate presents with a history of poor feeding, vomiting, and respiratory distress. He also has abdominal distention and is found to have hyperbilirubinemia. What is the probable cause of this complex?**

Sepsis.

❍ **Jaundice caused by breast feeding occurs after 7 days and can reach very high levels over weeks; how high?**

Levels of bilirubin near 25 mg/dL can be reached.

❍ **A septic pediatric patient is in shock. An initial bolus of normal saline at 20 mL/kg has been given. What urine output should be maintained by delivery of appropriate fluid?**

1 to 2 mL/kg/h.

❍ **Why is albuterol the usual agent of choice in treating bronchospasm?**

Of nebulized β-adrenergic agonists, it has the longest duration of action and the greatest degree of β_2-adrenergic selectivity.

❍ **If mechanical ventilation is required, what is an appropriate initial tidal volume?**

6 to 7 mL/kg.

❍ **Neonatal seizures have a broad range of presentations. What are the two frequent causes of myoclonic seizures?**

Metabolic disorders and hypoxia.

❍ **The spectrum of likely etiology of a pneumonia changes with patients age. Which are probable pneumonia-causing agents in neonates?**

Bacterial:

- Group B *Streptococci* (Lancefield Group B, mostly *S. agalactiae*).
- *Listeria monocytogenes*.
- Enteric gram-negative bacilli.
- *Chlamydia*.

Viral:

- Rubella, CMV, Herpes

❍ **SIDS is the most common cause of death of infants between 1 month and 1 year. The incidence is 2/1,000 = 10,000/y. What are the four risk factors that increase an infant's risk of SIDS?**

(1) Prematurity with low birth weight.

(2) Previous episode of apnea or apparent life-threatening event (ALTE).

(3) Mother is a substance abuser.

(4) Sibling of infant who died of SIDS.

❍ **Pyloric stenosis usually presents at about what age?**

4 weeks.

❍ **Among pediatric emergency patients, what is the most common skin infection?**

Nonbullous impetigo caused by Group A, *β-hemolytic Streptococcus.* Impetigo is a bacterial infection of the dermis, most commonly caused by group A *β-hemolytic Streptococcus.* It comes in two flavors—impetigo contagiosa and the bullous form.

❍ **"Strawberry tongue" is a physical finding associated with what systemic bacterial infection also caused primarily by Group A, *β-hemolytic Streptococci*?**

Scarlet fever. Also seek characteristic Pastia's lines found in the antecubital area. Recall the scarlet rash that spares the perioral area usually has onset 1 to 2 days after high fever, sore throat, headache, and occasional vomiting and abdominal pain. Mucocutaneous lymph node syndrome (Kawasaki disease), a disorder of unclear etiology, may also present with this finding.

❍ **Dermacentor andersoni is a vector for Rickettsia rickettsii, which causes RMSF. The rash of RMSF usually begins on the wrists and ankles and spreads centripetally. What is the underlying pathologic lesion that induces the serious sequelae of this disease, as well as the hemorrhagic rash?**

Vasculitis secondary to rickettsial invasion of endothelial cells in small blood vessels, including arterioles.

❍ **What are the characteristic findings in measles?**

The three "Cs," cough, coryza, and conjunctivitis, in addition to the characteristic morbilliform rash that begins on the head and spreads downward.

❍ **A child presents in DKA. On an average, how dehydrated is this patient likely to be, in mL/kg?**

125 mL/kg average fluid volume deficit.

❍ **What is the dose of insulin to be used for low-dose continuous infusion therapy?**

0.1 unit/kg/h of regular insulin.

❍ **Is intestinal intussusception associated with GI bleeding?**

Yes, though the classic history of a sudden onset of severe pain that often is relieved as quickly as it arose and is recurrent is more sensitive. The currant jelly stool associated with this disorder is present in about half of cases.

❍ **About how old is the average patient presenting with intussusception?**

1 year, +/−6 months.

❍ **What is the eponym for congenital aganglionic megacolon? (Remember, this disease involves a portion of the distal colon that lacks ganglion cells thereby impairing the normal inhibitory innervation in the myenteric plexus. As a result, coordinated relaxation is also impaired, which can in turn causes clinical symptoms of obstruction. Eighty-five percent of the time, this condition presents after the newborn period.)**

Hirschsprung's disease.

❍ **Acute enterocolitis with development of "toxic" megacolon is the life-threatening complication of Hirschsprung's disease. Between what range of ages does this complication most frequently present?**

2 to 3 months.

❍ **Describe stage I and stage II of Reye's syndrome.**

Stage I: Vomiting, lethargy, and liver dysfunction.

Stage II: Disorientation, combativeness, delirium, hyperventilation, increased deep tendon reflexes, liver dysfunction, hyperexcitable, tachypnea, fever, tachycardia, sweating, and papillary dilatation.

❍ **What is the treatment for stages I and II?**

Supportive.

❍ **Describe Stages III, IV, and V of Reye's syndrome.**

Stage III: Coma, decorticate rigidity, increased respiratory rate, mortality rate of 50%.

Stage IV: Coma, decerebrate posturing, no ocular reflexes, loss of corneal reflexes, and liver damage.

Stage V: Loss of DTRs, seizures, flaccid, respiratory arrest, 95% mortality.

❍ **What is the treatment for advanced stages of Reye's syndrome?**

Manage ICP—elevate HOB, paralyze, intubate and hyperventilate, furosemide, mannitol, dexamethasone, pentobarbital coma. Also consider hypertonic glucose and bowel sterilization.

❍ **Which motor deficit occurs with an anterior cerebral artery infarct?**

Leg weakness greater than arm weakness on the contralateral side.

❍ **What signs develop with a middle cerebral artery stroke?**

(1) Contralateral sensory/motor deficits.

(2) Arm/ face weakness greater than leg weakness.

❍ **What is the most common neurologic findings in adult botulism?**

Eye and bulbar muscle deficit.

❍ **What is the typical presentation of Guillain–Barré syndrome?**

Ascending motor neuron involvement.

❍ **What is the most common medication associated with neuroleptic malignant syndrome?**

Haloperidol. Other drugs antipsychotic medications are also causative.

❍ **What is the hallmark motor finding in neuroleptic malignant syndrome?**

"Lead-pipe" rigidity.

❍ **What neoplastic process is most commonly associated with myasthenia gravis?**

Thymoma.

❍ **What is the definition for status epilepticus?**

Continuous seizure activity for >5 minutes or more or two or more seizures, which occur without full recovery of consciousness between attacks.

❍ **What is the significance of bilateral nystagmus with cold caloric testing?**

It signifies that an intact cortex, midbrain, and brainstem are present.

❍ **How can upper motor neuron (UMN) lesions of CN VII (facial nerve) be distinguished from peripheral lesions?**

(1) UMN: Unilateral weakness of the lower half of the face.

(2) Peripheral: Involves entire half of the face.

❍ **A patient presents with facial droop on the left and weakness of the right leg. Where is the most likely site of the lesion?**

Brainstem, specifically the left pons.

❍ **A 30-year-old presents with progressively severe intermittent vertigo for 6 months and progressive unilateral hearing loss for 3 months. What is the diagnosis?**

Cerebellopontine angle tumor. Confirm diagnosis with MRI scan.

❍ **An observation period of what time length is required prior to medically clearing a TCA overdose?**

6 hours.

❍ **A 29-year-old intoxicated male presents after having his head driven into the concrete. The patient had a brief LOC, but was then ambulatory and alert. Now he appears drowsy and just threw up on you. What is the diagnosis?**

Epidural hematoma.

❍ **A 64-year-old female presents with a bilateral "burning" headache. She describes jabs of pain, which are worse at night. What is the treatment?**

Temporal arteritis is treated with long-term steroids. Treatment should begin immediately, do not wait for biopsy or ultrasound confirmation. ESR over 50 mm/h is highly suggestive.

❍ **A 53-year-old female presents with unilateral right sided sudden-onset lancinating pain in the distribution of the second and third branches of the fifth cranial nerve. What is the treatment?**

Carbamazepine treats trigeminal neuralgia.

❍ **A 50-year-old female presents with acute vertigo, nausea, and vomiting. She reports similar episodes over the last 20 years, sometimes but not always associated with hearing change and/or hearing loss and tinnitus. She has permanent right > left sensorineural hearing loss. What is the diagnosis?**

Ménière's disease.

❍ **The Nylen–Barany maneuver is performed as follows: the patient is rapidly brought from the sitting to supine position and the head is turned 45 degrees. Match the findings with peripheral and central vertigo:**

(1) Nystagmus is multi-directional, nonfatiguing, has no latent period, and lasts over a minute.

(2) Vertigo increased. Nystagmus is unidirectional, fatiguing, latent period is 2 to 20 seconds, with duration less than a minute.

(a) Central.

(b) Peripheral.

❍ **What is the dangerous diagnosis of a purpuric, petechial rash?**

Think meningococcemia. Other causes include *H. influenzae*, *S. pneumoniae*, and *S. aureus*.

❍ **A patient presents with acute meningitis; when should antibiotics be initiated?**

Immediately. Do not wait. Patients should receive a CT scan prior to LP only if papilledema or focal deficit is present.

❍ **What is the appropriate treatment for QRS widening in a TCA poisoning?**

Give $NaHCO_3$ IV, for patients with a QRS >100 ms, 1 to 2 mEq/kg are initially administered and repeated until the blood pH is between 7.50 and 7.55. A continuous infusion of $NaHCO_3$.

Three amp in 1 L of D_5W may then be initiated and run in over 4 to 6 hours titrating to maintain appropriate pH. Potassium levels are closely monitored and supplementation may be required to prevent hypokalemia.

❍ **What is the appropriate treatment of TCA-induced seizures?**

Benzodiazepines and barbiturates are the agents of choice; phenytoin is not generally effective. Bicarbonate and alkalosis are the mainstay of treatment.

❍ **Which TCA may induce seizures without concomitant cardiac toxicity?**

Amoxapine.

❍ **What is the treatment for TCA-induced hypotension?**

Isotonic saline is initially administered. If the patient is resistant to fluid resuscitation, a directly acting α-agonist should be started such as norepinephrine. Dopamine and dobutamine administration are contraindicated as these agents may increase hypotension through β-adrenergic stimulation. Further, dopamine acts in part by releasing norepinephrine; this agent may already be depleted by the reuptake inhibition of the TCA and by stress.

❍ **What is the clinical presentation of anticholinergic poisoning?**

Mydriasis, tachycardia, hypoactive bowel sounds, urinary retention, dry axilla, hyperthermia, and mental status changes.

❍ **What signs and symptoms are typical for the serotonin syndrome?**

Agitation, anxiety, sinus tachycardia, shivering, tremor, hyperreflexia, myoclonus, muscular rigidity, and diarrhea.

❍ **A 32-year-old female is given meperidine (Demerol) for an open fracture. The patient is chronically on fluoxetine (Prozac). What is a potential complication?**

The serotonin syndrome.

❍ **A patient presents to the ED status post Thorazine poisoning. You expect her pupils to be?**

Miotic. Thorazine is a potent α-antagonist resulting in miosis in overdose.

❍ **What constellation of findings occur with the neuroleptic malignant syndrome?**

Altered mental status, muscular rigidity, autonomic instability, hyperthermia, and rhabdomyolysis.

❍ **What are the signs and symptoms of lithium toxicity?**

(1) Neuro: Tremor, hyperreflexia, clonus, fasciculations, seizures, and coma.

(2) GI: Nausea, vomiting, and diarrhea.

(3) CV: ST-T-wave changes, bradycardia, conduction defects, and arrhythmias.

❍ **What is the treatment for lithium toxicity?**

Supportive care, normal saline diuresis, hemodialysis for patients with clinical signs of severe poisoning (seizures, arrhythmias etc.), renal failure, or decreasing urine output.

❍ **The administration of flumazenil to acutely poisoned patients has resulted in what adverse effect?**

Seizures. Flumazenil has induced seizures in patients status postingestion of potential seizure-inducing agents particularly TCAs. Flumazenil may induce withdrawal seizures in patients chronically on benzodiazepines.

❍ **What is the pharmacological treatment for alcohol withdrawal?**

Benzodiazepines.

❍ **Isopropanol is metabolized via which enzyme to which metabolite?**

Isopropanol is metabolized by alcohol dehydrogenase in the liver to acetone.

❍ **What methanol level warrants dialysis?**

50 mg/dL. Other indications include visual impairment, severe metabolic acidosis, and ingestion of greater than 30 cc.

❍ **What two cofactors are administered to the patient with ethylene glycol poisoning?**

Thiamine and pyridoxine. These cofactors will aid in transforming glyoxylic acid to nontoxic metabolites. Both are administered intravenously in 100 mg increments.

❍ **Isopropanol, ethylene glycol, and methanol are all metabolized by alcohol dehydrogenase. Is an alcohol drip beneficial to all of these poisonings?**

No. Isopropanol is converted via alcohol dehydrogenase to the nontoxic acetone.

❍ **What are the three clinical phases of ethylene glycol poisoning?**

Stage I. Neurologic symptomatology, that is, inebriation.

Stage II. Metabolic acidosis and cardiovascular instability.

Stage III. Renal failure.

❍ **When should dialysis be initiated for ethylene glycol poisoning?**

At a serum level greater than 25 mg/dL, renal insufficiency, or severe metabolic acidosis.

❍ **What is the toxic dose of naloxone?**

There is none. Narcan is a safe drug and may be given in large quantities. The usual adult dosage is 2 mg IV and 0.01 mg/kg for a child. Narcan may precipitate acute withdrawal and may therefore be titrated to effect.

❍ **How does treatment for a cocaine-induced MI differ from a typical MI?**

Both are treated the same with the exception that β-blockers are not used in a cocaine-induced MI secondary to unopposed α-adrenergic activity. The tachycardia of a cocaine-associated MI is first treated with benzodiazepine sedation.

❍ **Metabolic acidosis favors which form of salicylate, ionized or un-ionized?**

Unionized. Patients with salicylate poisoning should have arterial pH maintained at or greater than 7.4 so that salicylate is in the ionized form and therefore unable to cross the blood–brain barrier. Urinary alkalinization promotes the formation of the ionized form of salicylate, which is unable to be reabsorbed by the tubules thereby enhancing excretion.

❍ **What is the acid–base disturbance typical for salicylate poisoning?**

Mixed respiratory alkalosis (secondary to central respiratory center stimulation) and metabolic acidosis (secondary to uncoupling of oxidative phosphorylation).

❍ **Arterial pH is 7.5 through alkalinization but urine pH is still low. Which electrolyte is probably responsible?**

Potassium. When reabsorbing sodium, the renal tubules will preferentially excrete hydrogen ions into the tubular lumen rather than potassium ions thus, potassium should be maintained at 4.0 mmol/L.

❍ **What is the treatment for a prolonged prothrombin time in salicylate poisoning?**

Parenteral vitamin K administration. Salicylates inhibit vitamin K epoxide reductase in poisoning resulting in an ability for the inactive vitamin K epoxide to be regenerated into the active vitamin K.

❍ **What are the indications for dialysis in salicylate poisoning?**

(1) Persistent CNS involvement.

(2) ARDS.

(3) Renal failure.

(4) Severe acid–base disturbance despite appropriate care.

(5) Acute salicylate level >100 mg/dL.

❍ **Can a patient present with salicylate poisoning and a therapeutic level?**

Yes. Patients with chronic salicylate poisoning have a large Vd and thus may present with mental status changes and a therapeutic level.

❍ **What are the four stages of acetaminophen (APAP) poisoning?**

(1) 0.5 to 24 hours: Nausea, vomiting.

(2) 24 to 48 hours: Abdominal pain, elevated LFTs.

(3) 72 to 96 hours: LFTs peak, nausea, vomiting.

(4) 4 days to 2 weeks: Resolution or fulminant hepatic failure.

❍ **APAP poisoning produces which type of hepatic necrosis?**

Centrilobular necrosis. The toxic metabolite of APAP is generated in the liver via the P450 system, located in the centrilobular region.

❍ **Which is the toxic metabolite of APAP?**

NAPQI. When the glucuronidation and sulfation pathways are saturated, APAP is metabolized by the P450 system to the toxic metabolite N-acetyl-para-benzoquinoneimine (NAPQI).

❍ **What hepatic laboratory parameter is the first to become abnormal in APAP poisoning?**

The prothrombin time (PT).

❍ **Per the Rumack–Matthew nomogram, which 4 hours APAP level requires treatment?**

150 mg/mL.

❍ **How is the nomogram utilized in a patient who ingests an extended relief formulation of APAP?**

A 4-hour and an 8-hour level are obtained. If either level is in the "possible" hepatotoxic range, the patient should be treated.

❍ **What are absolute indications for Digibind administration in digoxin poisoning?**

Ventricular arrhythmias, hemodynamically significant bradyarrhythmias unresponsive to standard therapy, and a potassium level greater than 5.0 mEq/L.

❍ **Why is calcium chloride administration contraindicated in digoxin poisoning?**

Digoxin inhibits the Na-K-ATPase, resulting in an increased intracellular concentration of sodium. The sodium-calcium exchange pump is then activated leading to high intracellular concentrations of calcium. Calcium chloride administration would further increase intracellular calcium leading to increased myocardial irritability.

❍ **What is the appropriate treatment for hyperkalemia in digoxin poisoning?**

(1) Digibind.

(2) Insulin and glucose.

(3) Sodium bicarbonate.

(4) Potassium resin binder (Kayexalate).

(5) Hemodialysis.

❍ **A patient on Digoxin presents bradycardic and hypotensive with significantly peaked T-waves. What would be your initial line of treatment?**

Administer 10 vials of Digibind intravenously and simultaneously treat the presumed hyperkalemia with insulin and glucose, sodium bicarbonate, and Kayexalate. Once the Digibind is administered, hyperkalemic-induced arrhythmias may be safely treated with calcium chloride.

❍ **What is the antidote for β-blocker poisonings and what is the biochemical rational?**

Glucagon. Glucagon receptors, located on myocardial cells, are G protein–coupled receptors, which activate adenylate cyclase leading to increased levels of intracellular cAMP. Thus, glucagon administration leads to the same intracellular effect as β-agonism. Consider insulin, appears to improve inotropy by providing substrate for aerobic metabolism within the myocyte.

❍ **A child presents to the ED status postingestion of a sustained release calcium channel blocker. What is the disposition?**

Hospital admission to a monitored setting. Sustained release preparations have the capability of producing delayed toxicity.

❍ **What are potential treatment modalities for calcium channel blocker poisoning?**

Symptomatic patients are admitted to an intensive care unit and therapeutic interventions include intravenous calcium, isoproterenol, glucagon, transvenous pacer, atropine, and vasopressors, such as norepinephrine, epinephrine, or dopamine.

❍ **Chronic solvent abusers develop what metabolic complication?**

Renal tubular acidosis.

❍ **Oral hydrofluoric acid exposure may result in which life-threatening electrolyte abnormalities?**

Hyperkalemia and hypocalcemia.

❍ **What enzyme is inhibited by organophosphates?**

Cholinesterase.

❍ **Is pralidoxime administration beneficial in carbamate poisoning?**

No. Carbamates bind reversibly to cholinesterases whereas organophosphates bind irreversibly. Pralidoxime is used to reactivate cholinesterase molecules phosphorylated by an organophosphate molecule. Pralidoxime should be administered prior to the onset of irreversible aging of the enzyme.

❍ **What antihypertensive agent may induce cyanide poisoning?**

Nitroprusside. One molecule of sodium nitroprusside contains 5 molecules of cyanide. In order to prevent toxicity, sodium thiosulfate should be infused with sodium nitroprusside at a ratio of 10:1 (thiosulfate:nitroprusside). Beware of thiocyanate toxicity!

❍ **What order are the kinetics of elimination of ASA overdose?**

Zero-order elimination with hepatic enzymatic clearance saturated and renal clearance becoming important.

❍ **We all remember to think of ASA poisoning when a patient presents with mental status changes associated with respiratory alkalosis and metabolic acidosis. Many of us may recall that salicylate toxicity may be associated with elevated, normal, or decreased glucose levels. By what mechanisms are hyperglycemia and hypoglycemia caused?**

Hyperglycemia is caused by salicylate-induced mobilization of glycogen. Hypoglycemia is caused by salicylate inhibition of gluconeogenesis.

❍ **Is ARDS more likely to be a complication of acute or chronic ASA poisoning?**

Chronic.

❍ **What is the "magic number" for the dose of nonenteric–coated ASA which must be exceeded to cause toxicity, in mg/kg?**

150 mg/kg.

❍ **Can a patient, who is symptomatic with mental status changes from chronic salicylate poisoning have a level in the therapeutic range?**

Yes! Interestingly, patients taking acetazolamide are at particular risk for chronic salicylate poisoning because the carbonic anhydrase inhibitor results in acidified plasma (leading to increased Vd) and more alkalotic CSF, thereby encouraging salicylate concentration in the CNS.

❍ **Is hemodialysis used to treat salicylate toxicity?**

Yes, in severe poisoning (coma, ARDS, cardiac toxicity, serum level >100 mg/dL), and for patients who are unresponsive to maximal therapy.

❍ **Which measures of hepatic function are better indicators of prognosis, liver enzyme levels, or bilirubin level and prothrombin time?**

Bilirubin level and prothrombin time.

❍ **Aromatic hydrocarbons, such as toluene present in glue, may be sniffed. Resulting effects most closely resemble those of which other class of compounds?**

Effects are similar to those of inhalational anesthetic agents. Initial excitatory response gives way to CNS depression.

❍ **Is degree of toxicity in TCA overdose closely related to QRS duration?**

QRS >100 ms has a specificity of 75% and a sensitivity of 60% for serious complications. A normal ECG will not rule out a serious overdose! Of those with QRS >100 ms, 30% will seize; of those with QRS >160 ms, 50% will develop arrhythmias.

❍ **What is the most common cause of focal encephalitis in AIDS patients?**

Toxoplasmosis. Symptoms include focal neurologic deficits, headache, fever, altered mental status, and seizures. Ring enhancing lesions are seen on the CT scan.

❍ **The differential diagnosis of a ring enhancing lesions in an AIDS patient is?**

Lymphoma, cerebral tuberculosis, fungal infection, CMV, Kaposi's sarcoma, toxoplasmosis, and hemorrhage.

❍ **What are the signs and symptoms of CNS cryptococcal infection in an AIDS patient?**

Headache, depression, lightheadedness, seizures, and cranial nerve palsies. A diagnosis is made by India ink prep, fungal culture, or by the detection of the *Cryptococcal* antigen in the CSF.

❍ **An AIDS patient presents with complaints of decreased visual acuity, photophobia, redness, and eye pain. What is the diagnosis?**

Retinitis or malignant invasion of the periorbital tissue or eye.

❍ **What is the most common cause of retinitis in an AIDS patient?**

Cytomegalovirus. Findings include photophobia, redness, scotoma, pain, or change in visual acuity. On examination, findings include fluffy white retinal lesions.

❍ **What is the most common opportunistic infection in AIDS patients?**

Candidiasis.

❍ **What is the incubation period in tetanus?**

Hours to over 1 month. The shorter the incubation the more severe the disease. Most patients in the United States who contract the disease are older than 50 years.

❍ **What are the confirmatory tests for RMSF?**

Immunofluorescent antibody staining of skin biopsy or serologic fluorescent antibody titer. The Weil-Felix reaction and complement fixation tests are no longer recommended.

❍ **What antibiotics are used for RMSF?**

Tetracycline or chloramphenicol. Antibiotic therapy should not be withheld pending serologic confirmation.

❍ **Which type of paralysis does tick paralysis cause?**

Ascending paralysis. The venom which causes paralysis is probably a neurotoxin, which causes a conduction block at the peripheral motor nerve branches. This prevents acetylcholine release at the neuromuscular junction.

❍ **What is the treatment of choice for a patient in anaphylactic shock?**

Epinephrine, 0.3 to 0.5 mg IV of 1:10,000 solution IV or 0.3 mg 1:1,000 solution sq or IM.

❍ **What is the most common cause of anaphylactoid reactions?**

Radiographic contrast agents.

❍ **An RA patient presenting with painful speaking or swallowing, hoarseness, or stridor requires what type of diagnostic procedure?**

Urgent laryngoscopy to evaluate the involvement of the paired cricoarytenoid joints. These may become fixed in the closed position, resulting in airway compromise.

❍ **Myocardial infarction can be related to which two rheumatic diseases?**

Kawasaki disease and polyarteritis nodosa.

❍ **A patient presents with fever, acute polyarthritis, or migratory arthritis a few weeks after a bout of Streptococcal pharyngitis, they should be evaluated for which disease?**

Rheumatic fever. Approximately 30% will have subcutaneous nodules, erythema marginatum, or chorea.

❍ **What disease entity should be investigated in a child with joint swelling following minor trauma?**

JRA. Minor trauma may cause intra-articular bleeding. The joint should not be immobilized.

❍ **What is the appropriate management for a child with normal x-rays and tenderness over the end of a long bone after trauma.**

Immobilization and orthopedic evaluation for Salter–Harris type I fracture. These fractures may be occult.

❍ **What pathologic process must be considered in a patient with painless progressive weakness in a C-spine distribution?**

Cervical ventral root compromise by a degenerative disk. The dorsal and ventral nerve roots remain discrete in the C-spine in over half the population.

❍ **What constitutes admission criteria for a patient with acute low back pain?**

Paraparesis, bowel or bladder incontinence, intractable L-S pain and spasticity, inability to sit or stand, metastatic cancer, second ED visit, or x-ray film with defects.

❍ **What are the two most common causes of fatal anaphylaxis?**

#1 = Drug reactions, 95% to penicillin. Parenteral is the most dangerous with 300 deaths per year.

#2 = Hymenoptera stings with 100 deaths per year.

○ **What are characteristics of failure to thrive syndrome in infants?**

Body mass index (BMI) <5%, irritable, hard to console behavior, increased muscle tone in the lower extremities or hypotonia, and subsequent weight gain in the hospital.

○ **When considering failure to thrive syndrome, which historical features are important to assess?**

A history of prematurity, birth weight, maternal use of cigarettes, alcohol, and or drugs during the pregnancy, previous hospitalizations, and parental stature.

○ **In the case of child sexual assault, which laboratory tests should be performed?**

As indicated, oral, rectal, vaginal, or urethral swabs for GC, and *Chlamydia.* Serologic tests for syphilis or HIV testing should be done, if there is a history of or a clinical evidence of infection in the assailant or the victim. Urine or plasma β-HCG should be checked in girls beyond age of menarche.

○ **What is considered as a physical evidence of acute ano-genital trauma in the genital examination of a child?**

The presence of fissures, abrasions, hematomas, changes in tone (either dilation or spasm), or discharges, such as semen (fluoresces with a woods light), or examine under microscope. Erythema is a sign of inflammation, irritation, or manipulation, and is not specific for abuse.

○ **What is considered as a physical evidence of chronic ano-genital trauma in the genital examination of a child?**

Signs of an STD, such as vaginal or anal discharge, venereal warts or vesicles may be observed. Because injuries can heal without residual scarring, a lack of physical changes in no way rules out child sexual abuse.

○ **How soon does xanthochromia develop during a subarachnoid hemorrhage?**

6 to 12 hours.

○ **In addition to the history, physical, laboratory tests, and collection of physical evidence, what else needs to be done in the case of child sexual abuse?**

File a report with child protective services and law enforcement agencies. Provide emotional support for the child and family. Arrange a return appointment for follow-up of STD cultures and testing for pregnancy, HIV, and syphilis as indicated. Assure follow-up for psychologic counseling by connecting the family/child to the appropriate services in your area.

○ **In a patient with meningococcemia, what factors are associated with a poor prognosis?**

Petechia within 24 hours of admission, the presence of purpura, shock, coma, DIC, thrombocytopenia (<150,000), metabolic acidosis, and the absence of meningitis.

○ **How can a tension PTX lead to death?**

As air progressively collects in the pleural space, intrapleural pressure increases causing a decrease in functional lung volume leading to a ventilation–perfusion mismatch subsequent to hypoxia and acidosis.

The increasing intrapleural volume causes a mediastinal shift and a decreased systemic venous return because of a mechanical collapse of the venae cavae and increased intrathoracic pressure. The increased CO_2 and decreased O_2 lead to cardiovascular depression and collapse.

Sample Cases

"Two roads diverged in a wood and I took the one less traveled by, And that has made all the difference."
Robert Frost

CASE 1 (3 y/o Male with Weakness)

Examiner

This child has overdosed on iron. The candidate should be aggressive in rehydrating the patient. Vital signs will not normalize until packed RBCs are started. If therapy for iron toxicity is started prematurely, instruct a nurse to try to push activated charcoal. The patient's mother will probably be concerned, inquisitive, and demanding. The physician should appropriately calm her.

1.1. Introduction

A 3 y/o boy is brought to the ED by his mother with a complaint of weakness.

Vital signs: BP 82/50, P 135, R 24, T 98.6°F, Wt 18 kg.

1.2. Primary Survey:

- General impression: The patient is a WN/WD child who appears in distress. He is unable to provide a history, but responds to verbal stimuli with appropriate motor response and speech.
- Airway: No pooling of secretions and the patient can speak.
- Breathing: Lungs are clear, but the patient is tachypneic.
- Circulation: Tachycardia, capillary refill >4 seconds.
- Disability: GCS 14, the patient opens eyes to command, and pupils are equal and reactive.
- Exposure: No signs of trauma, no medic alert tags. No petechiae, ecchymoses, or rash. Diaphoretic and cool to the touch.
- Finger: Hemoccult positive stools.

1.3. Management:

- Intubation is not indicated at this time but ensure that the airway equipment is available.
- Start IV, O_2, place on a cardiac monitor, and pulse oximeter.
- Administer two 20 mL/kg fluid boluses of NS.
- Insert a Foley catheter.
- Order appropriate x-rays and laboratory studies, including type and cross for packed RBCs.
- Consult Poison Control.
- Apply warm blankets.

1.4. History: A 3 y/o male is brought in by mother with a possible vitamin overdose. When mom picked him up from the babysitter he seemed very sleepy. Upon questioning the 12 y/o babysitter via the phone, she noted the child ate a few "harmless" vitamins while she was not looking. After the remaining pills were counted, 25 tablets of ferrous sulfate 325 mg (20% elemental iron) were missing. Mom states no vomiting, diarrhea, abdominal, pain, fever, or recent trauma. The ingestion occurred 4 hours before arrival to the ED.

- Allergies: None.
- Medications: None.
- PMH: No significant illnesses or injuries.
- Last meal: 2 hours ago.
- Amount of iron ingested per kg

$$\frac{65 \text{ mg} \times 25 \text{ tablets}}{18} = 90 \text{ mg/kg}$$

- Family: Mother is present to answer questions. Family history is not applicable.
- Records: None.
- Immune: Up to date.
- Doctor: Dr. Pediatrician who is available.

1.5. Secondary Survey:
- General: If appropriate rehydration has occurred, the patient will be more awake and alert.
- Skin: Diaphoretic, decreased capillary refill, no bruises, abrasions, or petechiae.
- HEENT: Normocephalic and atraumatic, pupils equal, round, and reactive to light and accommodation (PERRL), conjunctiva normal, EOM-I, fundi normal, oropharynx moist, gag reflex is intact.
- Neck: Supple, no nodes.
- Chest: Normal.
- Lungs: Clear to auscultation.
- Heart: Tachycardia, no murmur.
- Abdomen: Diffusely tender with guarding. No masses or organomegaly, bowel sounds are hyperactive.
- Perineum/GU: Normal male genitalia, tanner stage I, both testes descended.
- Rectal: Loose stool, positive for occult blood.
- Back: Normal.
- Extremities: Normal and equal pulses without edema.
- Neuro: Moves all extremities, normal strength and sensation, symmetric deep-tendon reflexes. Cranial nerves intact.

1.6. Laboratory:
- CBC: WBC 20,000, Hgb 10, Hct 30%, Plt 178,000.
- Chemistry: Na 143, K 4, Cl 100, CO_2 17.
- BUN/Cr: 26/0.8.
- Glucose: 160.
- Ca/Mg: Normal.
- LFTs: Normal.
- PT/PTT: 14/24.
- ABG: pH 7.30, pO_2 95, pCO_2 40, HCO_3 23.
- U/A: Normal.
- Iron studies: Iron levels and TIBC are not available.
- Lactate 3.1.
- Acetaminophen/salicylate: Negative.

1.7. X-rays:
- KUB: Retained pills are present in the stomach.

1.8. Special Tests:
- ECG: Sinus tachycardia.

1.9. Critical Actions:
- Protect the airway and have intubation equipment present.
- No activated charcoal or gastric lavage.
- Monitor cardiac responses.
- Start IV fluids.
- Monitor urine output with a Foley catheter.

- Transfuse PRBCs.
- Contact Poison Control.
- Admit to the pediatric ICU.
- Start deferoxamine therapy.
- Consider whole bowel irrigation with polyethylene glycol 25 mL/kg/h for 6 to 10 hours

1.10. Pearls:

❍ **When should deferoxamine therapy be instituted?**

Patients who present with vomiting, diarrhea, and signs and symptoms of shock, peak iron levels >500 μg/dL, symptoms with iron levels >350 μg/dL and pills seen on KUB.

❍ **What are the stages of iron poisoning?**

Stage 1: Initial period (0.5–6 hours): Nausea, vomiting, abdominal pain, hematemesis, diarrhea, melena, and lethargy.
Stage 2: Latent period (6–24 hours): Improvement is seen, but the patient may be lethargic and hypotensive.
Stage 3: Systemic toxicity (4–40 hours): Cyanosis, lethargy, restlessness, disorientation, convulsions, coma, shock, and coagulopathy.
Stage 4: Late complications (2–8 weeks): Gastric outlet or small bowel obstruction.

CASE 2 (68 y/o Male with Inguinal Pain)

Examiner

The patient falls because of a leaking abdominal aortic aneurysm. He is vague about being light-headed, and passing out just prior to falling. The patient continually complains about his painful hip and groin. It is important for the physician to make this conclusion after obtaining a history and performing a physical examination. If the candidate continues to pursue the orthopedic problems, allow the patient's VS to worsen. If a CT scan is ordered, delay it but allow a bedside ultrasound to be performed. Have the candidate convince the vascular surgeon to come in to treat the patient.

2.1. Introduction:

A 68 y/o man presents, via ambulance, complaining of pain in the mid-back and right groin secondary to a fall. The patient is accompanied by his wife.

Vital signs: BP 100/70, P 100, R 22, T 99.0°F.

2.2. Primary Survey:

- General: Obese, white male lying supine, with a hand near his right groin. He is awake but pale, anxious, and in obvious discomfort.
- Airway: Intact.
- Breathing: Normal breath sounds but tachypneic.
- Circulation: Tachycardic.
- Disability: Negative.
- Exposure: No obvious injuries.
- Finger: Normal rectal, hemoccult negative.

2.3. Management:

- Determine that the patient fell because of a syncopal episode.
- Start two large bore IVs with an NS or LR bolus.
- Place on O_2, pulse oximeter, and cardiac monitor.
- Perform frequent VS and mental status checks.
- Perform a bedside ultrasound of the abdomen.
- Order screening laboratory studies and the ECG.

2.4. History: A 68 y/o male presents with a dull ache located in the mid-back region radiating to his right groin. He states this pain started suddenly, 3 days ago but worsened today. Today he was on the first rung of a stepladder when he "slipped" and fell hurting his right groin and back. No chest pain, n/v, weakness, dizziness, or LOC.

- Allergies: None.
- Medications: Furosemide, 40 mg po bid, and metoprolol, 50 mg po bid, aspirin 325 mg po bid.
- PMH: Hypertension, coronary artery disease, cholecystectomy, renal stone 10 years ago.
- Last meal: 1 hour ago.
- Family: Parents died from a heart attack in their sixties.
- Records: Available upon request.
- Immune: Up to date.
- Narcotics: No illicit drug use.
- Doctor: Consultants are available.
- Social history: No alcohol or tobacco use. Lives with his wife, who is an accountant by profession.

2.5. Secondary Survey:

- General: Continues to be anxious, uncomfortable, with VS unchanged.
- Skin: Pale, dry, no bruising.
- HEENT: Normal.
- Neck: Normal.
- Chest: Nontender.
- Lungs: Clear.
- Heart: Normal S1, S2 with the PMI displaced laterally. Grade II/VI systolic ejection murmur heard at the apex without an S3, S4, or rub.
- Abdomen: Obese, with a scar in the right upper quadrant. Bowel sounds are normal and no pain to palpation is noted. An 8 cm tender, pulsatile mass is palpated above the umbilicus.
- Perineum/GU: Normal.
- Rectal: Normal.
- Back: No CVA tenderness.
- Extremity: The right hip is flexed 45 degrees, but good range of motion is noted. Good capillary refill is <2 seconds and all pulses are equal.
- Neuro: No focal deficits.

2.6. Laboratory:

- CBC: WBC 9.8, Hgb 11.2, Hct 32.5, Plt 180,000.
- Chemistry: Na 138, K 4.1, Cl 98, CO_2 20.
- BUN/Cr: 22/1.5.
- Glucose: 170.
- Ca/Mg: Normal.
- LFTs: Normal.
- Amylase/Lipase: Normal.
- PT and PTT: Normal.
- CPK: Normal.
- Troponin: Normal.
- Lactate: Normal.
- D-dimer: Elevated.
- U/A: Trace blood and protein, otherwise no significant findings.

2.7. X-rays:

- Chest x-ray: Cardiomegaly.
- Pelvis x-ray: Normal.
- Ultrasound: 8 cm aortic dilation.

2.8. Special Tests:

- ECG: Left bundle branch block.

2.9. Critical Actions:

- Elicit a history of passing out and falling.
- Identify the presence of a pulsatile mass in the abdomen.
- Start a normal saline bolus.
- Start two large bore IVs.
- Type and crossmatch for 6 to 10 units.
- Obtain early consultation with a vascular surgeon.

2.10. Pearls:

❍ **What is the primary cause of an abdominal aortic aneurysm?**

Atherosclerosis, which weakens the aortic wall. It is present in 96% of these cases. Other causes such as congenital abnormalities, infection, and trauma are relatively uncommon.

❍ **What is the mechanism by which the aneurysm produces pain?**

Pain may be caused by (1) a rapid expansion of the aneurysm, (2) pressure of the aneurysm on surrounding structures such as the femoral nerve, (3) the presence of free blood in the abdomen or retroperitoneum from a leaking or ruptured aneurysm.

CASE 3 (Shock in an Infant)

Examiner

This child is very dehydrated and requires aggressive fluid resuscitation. If this does not happen the patient will have a seizure possible requiring intubation. A septic workup is required even though the seizure is caused by hyponatremia. Make it impossible for a peripheral line to be started so the candidate has to start an intraosseous or central line. Have the candidate describe the procedure in detail.

3.1. Introduction:

An 11 m/o female presents with her mother with a 3-day history of diarrhea, vomiting, and poor feeding. Mom has been giving tap water as that is the only fluid the child will drink and not vomit.

Vital signs: BP 50, Doppler, P 190, R 56, T 100.2°F, Wt 9 kg.

3.2. Primary Survey:

- General: An 11 m/o infant lying quiet, toxic appearing.
- Airway: Intact.
- Breathing: Tachypneic without retractions.
- Circulation: Capillary refill >4 seconds, distal pulses absent.
- Disability: Pupils normal, child moans to painful stimuli.
- Exposure: No gross abnormalities.

3.3. Management:

- Initiate IV rehydration with NS in 20 mL/kg boluses. It will take a total of three boluses to normalize the vital signs and stop the seizures.
- Order appropriate laboratory studies, x-rays, including blood, urine, and stool cultures.
- Access intravenously by intraosseous or central route.
- Place on O_2, cardiac monitor, and pulse oximeter.

3.4. History: An 11 m/o previously healthy, female presents with 3 days of vomiting and diarrhea. Two siblings have also been ill with similar symptoms. Mother has been giving tap water as that is the only thing the child can drink without vomiting.

- Allergies: None.
- Medications: None.
- PMH: Normal spontaneous vaginal delivery, full-term, uncomplicated pregnancy. No significant illnesses or injuries.

- Last meal: 24 hours ago.
- Family: No family history of seizures.
- Records: None.
- Immune: Up to date.
- Doctor: Family doctor is available to answer any questions.
- Social: Child lives with parents and two siblings. Mother is unaware of the dangers of giving tap water. No indications of any social problems.

3.5. Secondary Survey:

- General: If given adequate fluid, the child will become more alert.
- Skin: Doughy, poor turgor, no lesions or petechiae.
- HEENT: Sclera nonicteric, PERRL, eyes sunken, oral mucosa dry, pharynx normal, TMs normal.
- Neck: Supple, no meningeal signs.
- Chest: Nontender to palpation.
- Lungs: Clear, no grunting, no retractions.
- Heart: Tachycardic, no murmur.
- Abdomen: Nontender, no masses, no organomegaly.
- Perineum/GU: Normal.
- Rectal: Hemoccult negative.
- Back: Normal.
- Back: Extremities: Cool extremities with the absence of distal pulses and a capillary refill >4 seconds.
- Neuro: No focal deficits, normal DTRs.

3.6. Laboratory:

- CBC: WBC 14, Hgb 14.1, Hct 43, Plt 225,000.
- Differential: Polys 75, bands 3, lymphs 20, eos 0, mono 2.
- Chemistry: Na 111, K 3.5, Cl 80, CO_2 13.
- BUN/Cr: 56/0.9.
- Glucose: 130.
- Ca/Mg: Normal.
- LFTs: Normal.
- PT/PTT: Normal.
- ABG: pH 7.27, pO_2 98, pCO_2 30, HCO_3 14.
- Cultures: Blood/urine/stool all pending.
- U/A: RBC 0 to 2, WBC 0 to 2, ketones 2+, specific gravity 1.025.

3.7. X-rays:

- CXR: Normal.

3.8. Special Tests:

- CSF: RBC 0, WBC 0, protein/glucose normal, no organisms present, bacterial antigens negative.

3.9. Critical Actions:

- Obtain vascular access via a central line or intraosseous insertion.
- Start a fluid bolus (20 mL/kg) with 0.9 NS or LR.
- Reevaluation of VS following each bolus.
- Lumbar puncture.
- Monitor cardiac responses.
- Obtain appropriate laboratory tests.
- Obtain a history of tap water ingestion.

3.10. Pearls:

❍ **What are the signs of shock in an infant?**

Tachycardia, tachypnea, delayed capillary refill, altered mental status, weak or absent pulses, dry mucous membranes, sunken eyes, and decreased skin turgor. Hypotension is a late sign implying at least 25% loss of intravascular volume.

❍ **What are the indications for rapid correction of hyponatremia?**

Patients with a serum sodium level of less than 110 and an acute alteration in mental status, seizures, or focal findings should have their levels raised about 4 to 6 mEq/dL over a few hours.

CASE 4 (Injured Child)

Examiner

This child has been abused and the mother's story is inconsistent. The mother becomes upset and tries to take the child home. Security must detain the mother and child. A complete body survey is mandatory. The child requires a social service consult, referral to the Department of Children and Family Services, and the police must be contacted.

4.1. Introduction:

A 4 y/o girl is brought to the ED by her mother with a complaint of left elbow pain.

Vital signs: BP 85/65, P 110, R 20, T 103°F, Wt 17 kg.

4.2. Primary Survey:

- General: A 4 y/o WN/WD girl sitting quietly, but not responding to questions. She appears in moderate discomfort.
- Airway: Intact.
- Breathing: Normal.
- Circulation: Normal.
- Disability: Normal.
- Exposure: Old bruises noted.

4.3. Management:

- IV with a 20 mL/kg fluid bolus.
- Consider IV pain medication
- Obtain an elbow x-ray
- Treat the fever with acetaminophen or ibuprofen

4.4. History:

- Allergies: None.
- Medication: None.
- PMH: Born 4 weeks premature with a cleft palate.
- Last meal: 2 hours ago.
- Events: A 4 y/o female presents with elbow swelling and pain. Mom states she fell while at the babysitter's house then later states she fell off of the couch earlier today. This was witnessed with no LOC and the child fell asleep afterward. When she awoke, she could not bend her elbow. The mother states "she hasn't been well a day in her life."
- Family: Noncontributory.
- Records: Old records indicate a sibling died 2 years ago secondary to an unexplained head injury. The patient has had many ED visits for multiple different problems.
- Immune: Up to date.
- Doctor: The mother says she fired her last pediatrician and is looking for another one.
- Social: The mother states she has no job, no money, and is late on her rent payment. The patient was born out of wedlock and she has no family support.

4.5. Secondary Survey:

- General: Patient doesn't speak and sits close to mom.
- Skin: Bruise to left buttocks, approximately 1 to 2 w/o.
- HEENT: The left TM is red and bulging. Remainder of the examination is normal.
- Neck: Normal.

- Chest: Normal.
- Lungs: Normal.
- Heart: Normal.
- Abdomen: Normal.
- Perineum/GU: Normal.
- Rectal: Normal.
- Back: Two small bruises to the right scapular area, 7- to 10-day-old.
- Extremities: The left elbow is swollen and tender, including the distal half of the humerus. Pulse and sensation are normal, but passive flexion and extension at the elbow is limited.
- Neuro: Normal.

4.6. Laboratory:

- CBC: WBC 8, Hgb 14, Hct 48, Plt 300,000.
- Chemistry: Na 140, K 4, Cl 101, CO_2 24.
- BUN/Cr: 12/1.0.
- Glucose: 95.
- Ca/Mg: Normal.
- LFTs: Normal.
- PT/PTT: Normal.
- U/A: Normal.

4.7. X-rays:

- Elbow: There is an oblique fracture through the supracondylar area 2 cm proximal to the epiphysis of the capitellum. The radial head is intact and a posterior fat pad is present.
- Baby gram: Total body radiographic survey reveals multiple old, and healed fractures of the ribs with the skull and other long bones being normal.

4.8. Critical Actions:

- Identify a fractured humerus.
- Obtain a social history to identify risk factors associated with child abuse.
- Obtain a complete radiographic evaluation (total body).
- Admit with consultation of a pediatrician and social worker.
- File a report with the police and Department of Children and Family Services.
- Obtain help from hospital security, when the mother and child attempt to leave.
- Give pain medication.

4.9. Pearls:

❍ **What is the most common cause of death in children suffering child abuse?**

Intracranial injuries. One-sixth of survivors suffer significant neurologic sequelae.

❍ **What is the significance of retinal hemorrhages in children younger than 2 years?**

They are pathognomonic for a subdural hematoma secondary to severe shaken baby syndrome. These children are too small to participate in activities, which could produce significant head trauma.

CASE 5 (Uncooperative Elderly Female)

Examiner

This is a patient with severe digoxin toxicity with stable bradycardia. The toxicity has occurred over a long period of time due to new renal insufficiency and significant dehydration. The patient refuses to answer questions but her family can give all the information needed. As the case continues, the patient's condition will worsen requiring digibind. The family doctor will try to persuade the candidate to admit to a general medical floor.

5.1. Introduction:

A 70 y/o female presents with poor appetite, nausea, vomiting, and blurred vision. The patient's family is in the waiting room.

Vital signs: BP 130/94, P 52 irregular, R 22, T 98.2°F, Wt 80 kg.

5.2. Primary Survey:

- General: Uncooperative, 70 y/o female, alert, slightly tachypneic, and in no distress.
- Airway: Intact.
- Breathing: Bilateral crackles in both bases.
- Circulation: Pulses diminished, capillary refill normal.
- Disability: Pupils equal and reactive, disoriented.
- Finger: Rectal normal.

5.3. Management:

- Start IV, O_2, and place on cardiac monitor.
- Obtain an ECG
- Start IV, O_2, and place on cardiac monitor
- Draw a "rainbow" of blood tubes and hold.
- Give antiemetic of choice

5.4. History:

- Allergies: None.
- Medication: Furosemide, 40 mg qd digoxin, 0.25 mg qd, and an unknown blood pressure pill.
- PMH: Hypertension, acute myocardial infarction 3 years ago with stent placement, cholecystectomy 20 years ago.
- Last meal: 10 hours ago.
- Events: The patient refuses to answer questions. Family states the patient has become more dependent and detached for the past 4 to 6 weeks. Over the past 4 days, the patient has been experiencing nausea, vomiting, blurred vision, loss of appetite, lethargy, increasing confusion, and mild respiratory difficulty.
- Family: Noncontributory.
- Records: None.
- Immune: Up to date.
- Doctor: The family physician is available for admission and consultation.
- Social: Lives alone in her house.

5.5. Secondary Survey:

- General: Patient is resistant to questioning and is becoming more confused.
- Skin: Warm, dry, no rash.
- HEENT: PERRLA, fundi normal.
- Neck: No JVD, no bruits.
- Chest: Normal.
- Lungs: Crackles in both bases.
- Heart: RRR normal S1, S2, S3 present. Grades II to VI systolic murmur present.
- Abdomen: Old, well-healed scar, otherwise normal.
- Pelvic: Normal.
- Rectal: Normal.
- Back: Normal.
- Extremities: Normal and equal pulses.

5.6. Laboratory:

- CBC: WBC 9.6, Hgb 12.1, Hct 38, Plt 220,000.
- Chemistry: Na 140, K 2.3, Cl 110, CO_2 30.
- BUN/Cr: 60/2.1.

- Glucose: 105.
- Ca/Mg: 5.2/1.8.
- LFTs: Normal.
- Amylase/Lipase: Normal.
- PT/PTT: Normal.
- CPK: Normal
- ABG: pH 7.39, pO_2 69, pCO_2 33, HCO_3 28.
- U/A: Normal.
- Troponin: Normal.
- Lactate: Normal.
- BNP: 655 ng/L.
- D-dimer: Normal.
- Digoxin: 10.5 ng/mL (normal = 0.8–2.0 ng/mL).

5.7. X-rays:
- CXR: Mild pulmonary vascular congestion with cardiomegaly.

5.8. Special Test:
- ECG: Sinus bradycardia without ectopy.

5.9. Critical Actions:
- Obtain the history from family.
- Obtain a potassium level.
- Place on monitor.
- Obtain a digoxin level.
- Give Digibind.
- Admit to the ICU.
- Start IV or po KCl.

5.10. Pearls:

❍ **What are the common cardiac rhythm disturbances seen in digoxin toxicity?**

PVCs are the most common arrhythmia seen. Others include sinus bradycardia, AV blocks, PAT with block, junctional tachycardia, ventricular tachycardia, ventricular fibrillation, and atrial fibrillation. Atrial flutter is uncommon.

❍ **What conditions contribute to digoxin toxicity?**

Advanced age, hypoxia, myocardial ischemia, renal impairment, hypothyroidism, hypokalemia, hypomagnesemia, and hypercalcemia.

CASE 6 (Multiple Trauma)

Examiner

The candidate should identify all of the life-threatening injuries in a systematic fashion and treat them. Aggressive fluid resuscitation is required, and O negative or positive blood should be started. Allow the patient to go to the CT scan with a nurse once the patient has been stabilized, intubated, and a chest tube has been inserted.

6.1. Introduction:

A 20 y/o, unresponsive male is brought in by paramedics secondary to an MVA. The patient was unrestrained and was found outside a vehicle. The vehicle was severely damaged as a result of crashing into a tree.

Vital signs: BP 80/40, P 120, R 8, Wt 81 kg.

6.2. Primary Survey:
- General: WN/WD male, unresponsive, in respiratory distress, with a cervical collar, and on a spine board.
- Airway: Airway is patent, but trismus is present.
- Breathing: Agonal, no paradoxical movement of the chest wall.
- Circulation: Pulses diminished in all four extremities.
- Disability: No eye opening or verbal response. Patient responds to pain with decorticate (flexion) posturing.
- Exposure: Multiple bruises to the head, face, chest, and abdomen.
- Finger: Rectal normal, no gross blood, and pelvis stable.

6.3. Management:
- Initiate two large bore IVs with rapid infusion of 2 L of NS or LR.
- Place on monitor and pulse oximeter.
- Preoxygenate with a nonrebreather mask at 15 L/min.
- Perform a rapid sequence intubation by using appropriate medications.
- Check for proper placement of the endotracheal tube.
- Ventilator management. Start with a low respiratory rate of 12 to 16 bpm, to keep the pCO_2 around 35 mm Hg. Assist control with an FiO_2 set at a level to keep the pulse oximeter >95%.
- Place on a continuous CO_2 monitor.
- Start O– or O+ blood.
- Type and cross for 6 to 10 units of PRBCs or call for a massive transfusion protocol (MTP).
- Insert a Foley catheter and an OG tube after appropriate examination.
- Administer tetanus, 0.5 cc IM.
- When the patient has been stabilized, obtain a CT scan. Ensure that a nurse accompanies the patient to the CT scanner.

6.4. History:
- Allergies: Unknown.
- Medications: Unknown.
- PMH: Unknown.
- Last meal: Unknown.
- Events: A 20 y/o unresponsive male arrives via EMS. According to the paramedics, he was the unrestrained driver that hit a tree at 80 mph. He was found outside the car and significant damage was noted.
- Family: Unable to contact family.
- Records: None.
- Immune: Unknown.
- EMS. Paramedics are the source of information but they must leave on another call.
- Narcotics: Unknown.
- Doctor: Unknown.
- Social history: Unknown.

6.5. Secondary Survey:
- General: Patient remains unresponsive, blood pressure increases, if 2 L is given. Temperature is 95°F rectal, if the candidate requests it.
- Skin: Multiple bruises to the head, face, chest, and abdomen.
- HEENT: Large left parietal scalp hematoma. Left pupil is 8 mm with the right at 4 mm, both nonreactive. TMs clear and the nose and oropharynx are normal.
- Neck: Immobilized, trachea midline, no distended veins.
- Chest: No palpable crepitus. No paradoxical movement.
- Lungs: Unequal breath sounds with bagging.
- Heart: Tachycardia without a murmur or rub.
- Abdomen: Decreased bowel sounds, firm, distended, with bruising in the right upper quadrant.
- Pelvis: Stable, no crepitance.

- Rectal: Normal prostate, no gross blood.
- Back: Normal.
- Extremities: No deformities and pulses are weak but equal.
- Neuro: GCS 3. Patient paralyzed for intubation, unable to perform a complete examination.

6.6. Laboratory:
- CBC: WBC 17, Hgb 9.0, Hct 25, Plt 250,000.
- Chemistry: Na 138, K 3.8, Cl 102, CO_2 22.
- BUN/Cr: 16/0.9.
- Glucose: 106.
- Ca/Mg: Normal.
- LFTs: Normal.
- Amylase/Lipase: Normal.
- PT/PTT: Normal.
- Cardiac enzymes: Normal.
- ETOH: 220.
- Toxicology: Negative.
- ABG #1: Postintubation pH 7.32, pO_2 130, pCO_2 35, HCO_3 21, FIO_2 99%.
- U/A: Negative for blood.

6.7. X-rays:
- CXR: 50% right pneumothorax. Normal mediastinum.
- Pelvis: Normal.
- CT head: Large epidural hematoma at the left parietal lobe with a moderate midline shift.
- CT abd/pelvis: Grade III liver laceration with free fluid present in the abdomen.
- CT c-spine: Normal.

6.8. Special Tests:
- ECG: Sinus tachycardia, otherwise normal.
- FAST examination: Fluid in Morison's pouch.

6.9. Management:
- Rapid insertion of a chest tube.
- Consult neurosurgery and a general or trauma surgeon.
- Continue to monitor vital signs.

6.10. Critical Actions:
- Intubate and maintain an appropriate pCO_2 level.
- Administer 2 L fluid bolus with warm NS or LR.
- Identify the pneumothorax and insert and describe proper chest tube placement.
- Consult neurosurgery for drainage of the epidural hematoma.
- Consult general surgery for repair of the liver laceration.
- Ensure that a nurse accompanies the patient to the CT scan.

6.11. Pearls:

❍ **What are the causes of an epidural hematoma, and what is the characteristic CT scan finding?**

The most common cause is a fracture of the temporal bone causing a laceration to the middle meningeal artery. An epidural may also be due to a tear in the dural sinus or bleeding through a fracture from the calvarial diploe. CT scan demonstrates a focal, smooth-margined, biconvex high-density accumulation adjacent to the inner table of the skull.

❍ **Describe the complications associated with insertion of a chest tube.**

Damage to the intercostal nerve, artery, or vein, damage to intrathoracic and/or abdominal organs, incorrect tube position, damage to the internal mammary vessels, infection, hematoma, subcutaneous emphysema, and a persistent pneumothorax.

CASE 7 (Triple)

Patient #1 (Abdominal Pain and Rash in a Child)

Examiner

The first patient presents experiencing abdominal pain for one day. It is not mandatory to obtain the diagnosis of Henoch–Schönlein purpura (HSP). Children with mild symptoms can be safely managed as outpatients, but this patient's pediatrician is out of town so admit for observation. The workup of first patient can be interrupted and the other two patients can be completely treated and dispositioned first.

7.1. Introduction: (**Patient #1**)

A 6 y/o girl presents to the ED with a complaint of abdominal pain. She is carried in by her father and her mother is also present with her.

Vital signs: BP 97/62, P 110, R 22, T 101.8°F, Wt 21 kg.

7.2. Primary Survey:

- General: WN/WD 6 y/o girl appears uncomfortable but in no acute distress.
- Airway: Intact.
- Breathing: Normal.
- Circulation: Normal.
- Disability: Normal.
- Finger: Deferred to secondary survey.

7.3. History:

- Allergies: None.
- Medication: None.
- PMH: No illnesses or surgeries.
- Last meal: Patient ate breakfast 5 hours ago, but vomited. She has not eaten since then.
- Events: *A 6 y/o female presents with abdominal pain that is sharp, generalized, and nonradiating. She has nausea, vomiting, one episode of diarrhea and decreased po intake. No fever, chills, dysuria, hematuria, or urinary frequency noted. She does complain of pain to both knees. No sick contacts, recent travel, or new food/medication exposure.*
- Family: Noncontributory.
- Records: None.
- Immune: Up to date.
- Doctor: The patient's pediatrician has called twice before she ever arrived to the ED. She is available for information but will be unable to admit because of being out of town.
- Social: No risk factors for child abuse. She lives with both natural parents and an 8 y/o brother.

7.4. Management:

- Order appropriate laboratory studies and x-rays.
- Consider calling the pediatrician early in the workup.

Before completing the examination, the nurse asks you to see another patient who is in severe pain.

Patient #2 (Hand Pain)

Examiner

This is a simple case of a hydrofluoric acid (HF) burn to the hand. He can be completely worked up and dispositioned without interruption. If the candidate takes too long, have the third patient arrive, who requires immediate attention. Regardless of the disposition, close follow-up (within 12–24 hours) by a plastic/hand surgeon is required.

7.1. Introduction: (**Patient #2**)

A 45 y/o male presents with a complaint of pain to the digits of his left hand.

Vital signs: BP 122/75, P 112, R 16, T 98.8°F, Wt 102.7 kg

7.2. Primary Survey:

- General: A 45 y/o male is sitting upright on the cart. He is in moderate discomfort, cooperative, but is in no obvious distress.
- Airway: Intact.
- Breathing: Normal.
- Circulation: Normal.
- Disability: Normal.

7.3. History:

- Allergies: None.
- Medication: None.
- PMH: No significant illnesses or injuries. No past surgeries.
- Last meal: 2 hours ago.
- Events : Patient states that while at work his fingers started to burn. He denies trauma but says he works with many different chemicals of unknown composition.
- Family : The employer is available over the phone and states the patient spilled hydrofluoric acid on his workbench approximately 4 hours ago. He reported the spill, but denied cutaneous exposure at that time. The employer also states that the patient was reprimanded earlier for not wearing gloves when working with hazardous material.
- Records: None.
- Immune: Up to date.
- Narcotics: Denies illicit drug use.
- Doctor: Occupational physician is available for consultation or information.
- Social: No alcohol or tobacco use.

7.4. Secondary Survey:

- General: Unchanged.
- Skin: Erythema, swelling, and blistering present on the dorsal and volar aspects of the distal phalanges of the left hand.
- HEENT: Normal.
- Neck: Normal.
- Chest: Normal.
- Lungs: Normal.
- Heart: Normal.
- Abdomen: Normal.
- Perineum/GU: Normal.
- Rectal: Deferred.
- Back: Normal.
- Extremities: Pulses equal, capillary refill <2 seconds, full range of motion with associated pain to all digits of the left hand.
- Neuro: Normal.

7.5. Laboratory:

- None required, but if ordered all will be normal.

7.6. X-rays:

- Left hand: Normal.

7.7. Management:

- Wash the hand with large volumes of water.
- Subcutaneously inject 10% calcium gluconate into the affected areas.

- Give IV or po pain medications.
- Call a plastic/hand surgeon and admit or arrange follow-up (within 12–24 hours).
- Consider giving magnesium sulfate, 2 g IV over 20 minutes.

The nurse informs you that a new patient is in room 3 with a complaint of chest pain.

Patient #3 (65 y/o Male with Chest Pain)

Examiner

This patient is having an acute, inferior, myocardial infarction. The candidate should attempt to transfer the patient to a hospital with a cardiac cath laboratory. The weather will not allow timely transfer so thrombolytic therapy should be instituted after screening for contraindications. In consultation with a cardiologist, heparin, nitroglycerin drip, and aspirin should be started.

7.1. Introduction: (**Patient #3**)

A 65 y/o male presents via EMS with a complaint of chest pain and nausea.

Vital signs: BP 150/70, P 62, R 20, T 98.6°F, Wt 140 kg.

7.2. Primary Survey:
- General: A 65 y/o male is sitting on the cart. He is pale, diaphoretic, and in acute distress.
- Airway: Intact.
- Breathing: Tachypneic and labored. Speaking in full sentences.
- Circulation: Normal.
- Disability : Normal.
- Exposure: Medic alert tag with "Diabetes" on it.
- Finger: Hemoccult negative otherwise, normal.

7.3. Management:
- Initiate two IVs and O_2 at 4 to 6 L. Place on pulse oximeter and cardiac monitor.
- Aspirin 325 mg po.
- Pain relief with sublingual nitroglycerin or morphine sulfate.
- Order appropriate laboratory studies, CXR, and an ECG.

7.4. History:
- Allergies: Sulfa.
- Medication: Glipizide, 10 mg po bid, and Procardia, XL 60 mg po daily.
- PMH: Diabetes and hypertension.
- Last meal: 10 hours ago.
- Events: A 65 y/o male presents with constant chest pain that started 4 hours ago while sitting in a chair. The pain is "pressure-like" radiating to the neck and left arm. He has vomited twice and feels "light-headed."
- Family: Father died of a "heart attack" when he was 50 y/o. His wife is in the waiting room.
- Records: None.
- Immune: Up to date.
- EMTs: No other information to add.
- Narcotics: No illicit drug use.
- Doctor: The patient's family physician is available for consultation and information about the patient.
- Social history: Married, has four children and six grandchildren. He has smoked one pack of cigarette per day for 40 years. Denies alcohol use.

7.5. Secondary Survey:
- General: Patient feels better with O_2 and is breathing easier.
- Skin: Pale, cool, and moist.
- HEENT: Normal.

- Neck: No JVD or bruits.
- Chest: Normal.
- Lungs: Normal.
- Heart: RRR without a murmur or S3, S4.
- Abdomen: Soft, nontender, no pulsatile mass, no organomegaly.
- Perineum/GU: Normal.
- Rectal: Normal tone, hemoccult negative.
- Back: Normal.
- Extremities: No edema, pulses equal.
- Neuro: Normal.

7.6. Laboratory:
- CBC: WBC 12, Hgb 15.0, Hct 42.4, Plt 220,000.
- Differential: Normal.
- Chemistry: Na 134, K 4.1, Cl 101, CO_2 23.
- BUN/Cr: 12/1.0.
- Glucose: 450.
- Ca/Mg: Normal.
- LFTs: Normal.
- Amylase/Lipase: Normal.
- PT/PTT: Normal.
- Cardiac enzymes: Pending.
- ABG: pH 7.40, pO_2 80, pCO_2 40, HCO_3 24 (room air).
- U/A: Normal.
- D-dimer: Elevated.

7.7. X-rays:
- CXR: Normal.

7.8. Special Tests:
- Cardiac monitor: Normal sinus rhythm without ectopy.
- Pulse oximeter: 90% on room air; 97% on 4 to 6 L of O_2.
- ECG: Acute ST-segment elevation in leads II, III, and AVF with reciprocal changes.

7.9. Management:
- Confirm the absence of contraindications for lytic therapy.
- Start thrombolytics.
- Consult cardiology.
- Administer aspirin po.
- Administer heparin and nitroglycerin IV.

Patient #1 (Abdominal Pain and Rash in a Child)

7.5. Secondary Survey:
- General: Unchanged.
- Skin: There is a symmetric rash on the buttocks, posterior thighs, and lower legs. The rash is a maculopapular, erythematous, urticarial, and blanches upon application of pressure. Some areas have turned into palpable, petechial lesions that do not blanch. The size varies from 3 mm to several centimeters in diameter.
- HEENT: Normal.
- Neck: Supple, no meningeal signs. No nodes.
- Chest: Normal.

- Lungs: Normal.
- Heart: Normal.
- Abdomen: Soft with mild tenderness diffusely; Bowel sounds are present, no masses, no rebound or guarding, no organomegaly.
- Perineum/GU: Normal.
- Rectal: Hemoccult positive stool otherwise, normal.
- Back: Normal.
- Extremities: Both knees have small effusions without redness or warmth. The patient has full range of motion of all joints but cries and limps when she tries to walk.
- Neuro: Normal.

7.6. Laboratory:

- CBC: WBC 16, Hgb 14, Hct 42, Plt 400,000.
- Differential: Polys 65, bands 10, lymphs 20, eos 10, mono 3.
- Chemistry: Na 139, K 4.2, Cl 101, CO_2 25.
- BUN/Cr: 10/0.6.
- Glucose: 96.
- Ca/Mg: Normal.
- LFTs: Normal.
- Amylase/Lipase: Normal.
- PT/PTT: Normal.
- Sed rate: 30.
- Blood cultures: Pending.
- U/A: Blood 3+, protein 2+, RBC 50/hpf, WBC 0, specific gravity 1.021.

7.7. X-rays:

- CXR: Normal.
- Abdominal US: Normal.
- CT abdomen/pelvis: Normal.
- X-ray bilateral knees: Normal.

7.8. Management

- IV saline lock.
- Consider corticosteroids in severe cases.
- Treat the pain and nausea.
- Consider a H_2 blocker or PPI.
- Abdominal x-ray series: Normal.

7.9. Critical Actions:

- Complete the history and physical examination.
- Check the platelets.
- Obtain the kidney function tests.
- Obtain the urine for analysis.
- Recognize the multisystem nature of the patient's problem.

7.10. Pearls: (**Patient #1** HSP)

❍ **What is the cause of HSP?**

The cause is unknown but 50% have a history of a recent URI. It is believed that "something" elicits an allergic reaction, which results in deposition of antibody-antigen complexes in the small vessels of the skin, synovium, kidney, and bowel leading to a vasculitis.

❍ **What are the potential complications of HSP?**

Chronic renal failure is the most common and serious complication with gastrointestinal hemorrhage and intussusception occurring less frequently.

Patient #2 (Hand Pain)

7.8. Critical Actions:
- Obtain a history of HF acid exposure.
- Treat with calcium gluconate.
- Call a plastic or hand surgeon and arrange a follow-up in 12 to 24 hours.

7.9. Pearls: (**Patient #2** Hand Pain)

❍ **Can calcium chloride be used for local infiltration?**

No. Calcium chloride causes tissue necrosis when injected within the skin.

❍ **What metabolic abnormalities occur with systemic HF poisoning?**

Metabolic acidosis, severe hypocalcemia (because of the complexing of calcium by fluoride ions), hypomagnesemia, and hyperkalemia.

Patient #3 (65 y/o Male with Chest Pain)

7.10. Critical Actions:
- Initial treatment with O_2, monitor, NTG, or morphine for pain.
- Give aspirin po.
- Start nitroglycerin drip.
- Administer heparin bolus and hourly infusion.
- Talk with a cardiologist.
- Evaluate for absolute contraindications to thrombolytic therapy.
- Start thrombolytic therapy.
- Admit to the CCU until transfer is available.

7.11. Pearls: (**Patient #3** Myocardial Infarction)

❍ **What is the clinical presentation in a patient with a right ventricular (RV) infarction?**

Hypotension, jugular venous distention, clear lungs, Kussmaul's sign, and high-grade AV blocks are seen. RV infarcts are the result of a total occlusion of the right coronary artery and are present in 20% to 40% of patients with an inferior myocardial infarction.

❍ **What are the ECG criteria for thrombolytic therapy?**

One or more of the following: (1) ≥1 mm ST-segment elevation in ≥2 contiguous limb leads, (2) ≥2 mm ST-segment elevation in ≥2 contiguous precordial leads, (3) new left bundle branch block in the context of symptoms consistent with infarction.

CASE 8 (Unresponsive Patient)

Examiner

This patient is in full cardiopulmonary arrest. His wife states that her husband was doing well, ate lunch, and walked upstairs to bed. She discovered him not breathing. The candidate should give appropriate telemetry orders and follow ACLS guidelines when the patient arrives. Once asystole has occurred, the candidate should verify this, terminate the code, and inform the family.

8.1. Introduction:

A telemetry calls from the paramedics: "We have a 60 y/o male, unresponsive for 5 minutes prior to our arrival. He is in cardiopulmonary arrest and we are unable to intubate or start an IV. Our estimated time of arrival is 5 minutes."

8.2. Management:
- Instruct the paramedics to initiate CPR.

- Deliver O_2 at 100% by a bag-valve-mask system.
- Order a rhythm strip sent, interpret this as ventricular fibrillation, and order immediate defibrillation at 120 to 200 J (monophasic or biphasic).

The patient arrives with his wife. Paramedics inform you, they defibrillated at 200 J.

Vital signs: BP 0, P 0, R 0, T 97.0°F, Wt 128.5 kg.

8.3. Primary Survey:
- General: Obese, 60 y/o male, cyanotic, in cardiopulmonary arrest.
- Airway: Clear with absent gag reflex.
- Breathing: No spontaneous respirations.
- Circulation: No pulses, no dependent lividity.
- Disability: Pupils fixed and dilated, GCS 3.
- Exposure: No medic alert tags; atraumatic skin.
- Finger: Rectal hemoccult negative, normal prostate.

8.4. Management:
- Continue CPR at a chest compression rate of >100/min.
- Place the patient on a cardiac monitor and pulse oximeter.
- Recognize V-fib and immediately defibrillate at 200 J.
- Intubate.
- Start two IVs or IO lines.
- Continue CPR and follow the ACLS protocol.

8.5. History:
- Allergies: Sulfa.
- Medication: Lisinopril, 20 mg po qd, propranolol, 40 mg po tid, nitroglycerin, SL prn chest pain.
- PMH: Hypertension, angina, and gout. No surgeries or hospitalizations.
- Family: A younger brother died last year from an acute myocardial infarction.
- Records: None.
- Immune: Up to date.
- Narcotics: No history of illicit drug use.
- Doctor: His family physician is available for consultation.
- Social history: The patient is a local police officer. He is married, has four children and three grandchildren. He smokes two packs of cigarettes per day for 45 years, but he does not consume alcohol.

8.6. Secondary Survey:
- General: No change in the patient's status.
- Skin: Cyanosis present; no bruises, abrasions, or lacerations.
- HEENT: Normocephalic and atraumatic head. ET tube in place. Pupils remained fixed and dilated.
- Chest: Rises and falls equally when bagged.
- Lungs: Breath sounds equal but not spontaneous.
- Heart: No heart sounds. Unable to palpate a PMI.
- Abdomen: Obese, distended, no bowel sounds.
- Perineum/GU: Normal.
- Back: Normal.
- Extremities: No pulses, 3+ pitting edema to the lower legs.
- Neuro: GCS 3, no response to pain, No DTRs.

8.7. Management:
- The rhythm decompensates to asystole.
- Check for proper lead placement and confirm asystole in two contiguous leads.
- Confirm the absence of vital signs and terminate the code.
- Ultrasound: No myocardial motion.
- Inform the family.

8.8. Critical Actions:

- Recognize V-fib in the field and defibrillate.
- Use appropriate ACLS protocol for V-fib.
- Establish an airway.
- Verify asystole and terminate code.
- Talk with family and offer further assistance.

8.9. Pearls:

❍ **What is the mechanism of action of nitroglycerin?**

Nitroglycerin is a smooth muscle dilator resulting in dilatation of large coronary arteries and veins. This results in an increased oxygen delivery to the heart and peripheral pooling of blood, thereby decreasing venous return, ventricular filling pressure, and left ventricular work.

❍ **How does defibrillation of a fibrillating heart work?**

Passing a current through a fibrillating heart depolarizes the cells and allows them to repolarize uniformly, thus restoring organized, coordinated contractions.

CASE 9 (Male with Lower Abdominal Pain)

Examiner

This patient has an acute, testicular torsion requiring immediate intervention. His parents are not present but care should still be given. The urologist tells you he is unavailable for 30 to 45 minutes, so obtain an ultrasound to secure the diagnosis. When results are obtained, immediately call the urologist back. He will try to convince you to allow him to finish rounds in 1 to 2 hours before he sees the patient. Be polite but firm and the urologist will give in and see the patient immediately in the OR. The parents arrive before the patient goes to the OR and sign the consent form.

9.1. Introduction:

A 15 y/o boy presents with an acute abdominal pain. He is accompanied by his high school coach and you are unable to locate his parents.

Vital signs: BP 130/92, P 116, R 30, T 99.6°F, Wt 65.9 kg.

9.2. Primary Survey:

- General: The patient is a WN/WD male, pale, diaphoretic, in severe discomfort.
- Airway: Intact.
- Breathing: Normal.
- Circulation: Normal.
- Disability: Normal.
- Exposure: No medic alert tags.
- Finger: Normal rectal examination.

9.3. History:

- Allergies: None.
- Medications: None.
- PMH: No hospitalizations or surgeries.
- Last meal: 4 hours ago.
- Events: A 15 y/o male presents with right lower abdominal pain that started abruptly, 1 hour ago while running in gym class. The pain is constant, severe, and "hurts all over." He complains of nausea, vomiting, anorexia, and has no diarrhea or constipation. A similar episode occurred 2 days ago but was not as intense and resolved spontaneously.
- Family: Noncontributory.
- Records: None.
- Immune: Up to date.

- Narcotics: No illicit drug use.
- Doctor: None.
- Social: Patient is not sexually active. No alcohol or tobacco use.

9.4. Secondary Survey:

- General: If medicated, patient is more comfortable but still in pain.
- Skin: Normal.
- HEENT: Normal.
- Neck: Supple, no nodes.
- Chest: Normal.
- Lungs: Normal.
- Heart: Normal.
- Abdomen: Unable to fully evaluate because of diffused guarding. Bowel sounds are present, no point tenderness, no organomegaly.
- Perineum/GU: The scrotum appears tense and slightly edematous. The right testicle is very tender and difficult to examine. The epididymis and spermatic cord cannot be localized as the source of pain. The cremasteric reflex is absent, the testicle is elevated, and is in a horizontal position.
- Rectal: Normal.
- Back: No CVA tenderness.
- Extremities: No edema.
- Neuro: Normal.

9.5. Management:

- Immediately consult a urologist (who states he will be in the OR for another 30–45 minutes).
- Obtain a color-flow duplex Doppler ultrasound.
- Keep the patient NPO.
- Obtain appropriate laboratory studies.
- Try to contact his parents.
- Start IV.
- Give pain medication.
- Give an antiemetic.
- Consider manual detorsion.

9.6. Laboratory:

- CBC: WBC 15,000, Hgb 14.5, Hct 44, Plt 250,000.
- Chemistry: Normal.
- BUN/Cr: 13/0.9.
- Glucose: 98.
- Ca/Mg: Normal.
- LFTs: Normal.
- Amylase/Lipase: Normal.
- PT/PTT: Normal.
- U/A: Normal.

9.7. Special Tests:

- Color-flow Doppler US: Normal arterial flow to the left testicle with markedly diminished flow to the right testicle noted.

9.8. Critical Actions:

- Attempt to contact parents, but do not delay care while seeking consent.
- Recognize right testicular tenderness.
- Suspect testicular torsion and consult urology before obtaining a testicular scan.
- Prepare the patient for surgery.
- Attempt manual detorsion.
- Provide pain relief.

9.9. Pearls:

❍ **What are the limits of viability for a torsed testicle?**

A 100% salvage rate is seen with detorsion within 6 hours after an onset of pain. Beyond 12 hours, the rate drops to 20%. After 24 hours, the salvage rate approaches zero.

❍ **What is the procedure for manually detorsing a testicle?**

Elevate the affected testicle toward the inguinal ring and rotate 1½ turns in a medial to lateral manner (similar to opening a book). Relief of pain indicates success however, increasing pain should cause you to stop immediately.

CASE 10 (Male with Syncope)

Examiner

The EMTs are the key to an early diagnosis. If the candidate interviews them, he/she will find out the patient lives in an old house and the entire family (including the family dog) have been sick with "the flu." The patient should be treated with 100% O_2 and arrangement should be made to transfer the patient to a hyperbaric chamber. The family should be instructed to present to the ED for evaluation.

10.1. Introduction:

A 60 y/o male presents, via ambulance, with a complaint of chest pain, dyspnea, and fainting.

Vital signs: BP 160/90, P 110, R 26, T 99.2°F, Wt 63.6 kg.

10.2. Primary Survey:

- General: The patient is a pale, cachectic 60 y/o male, diaphoretic, and hyperventilating.
- Airway: Intact.
- Breathing: Tachypneic; breath sounds distant.
- Circulation: Pulses equal and strong.
- Disability: Pupils equal and reactive, GCS 15.
- Exposure: Medic alert tag stating "Heart disease."
- Finger: Rectal normal, hemoccult negative.

10.3. Management:

- Initiate O_2 100% nonrebreather.
- Place on cardiac monitor and pulse oximeter.
- Order appropriate laboratory studies, ECG, and CXR.
- Start IV.

10.4. History:

- Allergies: None.
- Medication: NTG prn and various inhalers.
- PMH: COPD and angina. No previous surgery.
- Last meal: 4 hours ago.
- Events: A 60 y/o male presents with chest pain and syncope. He states he developed substernal chest pain while walking upstairs from the basement to his bedroom. The pain was "pressure-like" without radiation, but with associated dyspnea, nausea, and diaphoresis. He took one nitroglycerin pill after which he felt faint and passed out. He presently has chest pain, mild dyspnea, nausea, and a severe headache.
- Family: Mother and father died from a "heart attack" in their fifties.
- Records: Available along with an old ECG.
- Immune: Unknown.
- EMTs: EMTs state that everyone in the family has been sick with the flu.
- Narcotics: No illicit drug use.

- Doctor: The patient has a pulmonary specialist, who is available for consultation.
- Social: Smokes 1 pack of cigarettes per day.

10.5. Secondary Survey:
- General: Anxiety has decreased since he was placed on O_2.
- Skin: Pale, diaphoretic.
- HEENT: Normal.
- Neck: Supple without lymphadenopathy.
- Chest: Normal.
- Lungs: Decreased breath sounds bilaterally with few basilar crackles and a prolonged expiratory phase.
- Heart: Tachycardia without an S3, S4, or murmur.
- Abdomen: Normal.
- Perineum/GU: Normal.
- Rectal: Normal.
- Back: Normal.
- Extremities: Normal.
- Neuro: Cranial nerves, motor/sensory examination, coordination, and cerebellar signs are all normal. He is oriented to person and place but thinks it is 1958. He also has lapses in short-term memory.

10.6. Laboratory:
- CBC: WBC 12, Hgb 14.4, Hct 45.4, Plt 260,000.
- Chemistry: Na 138, K 4.2, Cl 101, CO_2 20.
- BUN/Cr: 18/1.4.
- Glucose: 110.
- Ca/Mg: Normal.
- LFTs: Normal.
- Amylase/Lipase: Normal.
- PT/PTT: Normal.
- Cardiac enzymes: CPK 200, LDH 230, SGOT 26, CKMB 1%.
- ABG: pH 7.39, $pO_2$70, pCO_2 30, HCO_3 21, saturation 95%.
- CO Hgb: 35%.
- U/A: Normal.
- D-dimer: Normal.

10.7. X-rays:
- CXR: Changes consistent with COPD, no acute infiltrate.

10.8. Special Tests:
- ECG: Sinus tachycardia without ectopy. No changes as compared to old ECGs.
- Cardiac monitor: Sinus tachycardia.
- Pulse oximeter: 96% on room air.

10.9. Management:
- Once the CO results are known, call the family and have them come to the ED for evaluation.
- Arrange for transfer to a hyperbaric chamber.
- Continue treating with 100% O_2 and consider administering nebulized albuterol.

10.10. Critical Actions:
- Assess ABCs. Place on O_2, IV, and cardiac monitor.
- Interview the EMTs to determine why the whole family has the flu.
- Obtain an ECG, ABG, and CO Hgb level.
- Recognize CO poisoning.
- Treat with 100% O_2.
- Contact family members and arrange for evaluation and testing.
- Transfer the patient to a hyperbaric chamber.

10.11. Pearls:

❍ **What are the indications for hyperbaric oxygen therapy in CO poisoning?**

All patients with coma or loss of consciousness, neurologic findings, ischemic chest pain (ECG changes or arrhythmias), CO Hgb level greater than 30%, and mental status changes that do not resolve after 3 hours of 100% oxygen therapy. Also consider its use for pregnant women, patients with a history of coronary artery disease, and a CO Hgb level greater than 25% to 30%.

❍ **What is the effect of 100% oxygen therapy in the treatment of CO poisoning?**

The half-life of CO is decreased to 40 to 80 minutes from about 6 hours on room air. Hyperbaric oxygen therapy decreases the elimination half-life to ≤20 minutes.

CASE 11 (Female with a Headache)

Examiner

This is a case of meningitis in a young female with focal neurologic deficits. You must order a temperature early and obtain a CT scan of the head before an LP because she has neuro deficits. The physician should start antibiotics before allowing the patient to go to the radiology department for her scan. You may use any of the appropriate approved antibiotic regimes as long as it covers the potential organisms involved. Consult a neurologist or internist and admit the patient to the ICU.

11.1. Introduction:

The paramedics present with a 21 y/o female with a complaint of headache and weakness.

Vital signs: BP 128/70, P 108, R 16, Wt 59 kg.

11.2. Primary Survey:

- General: This is a WN/WD 21 y/o female, appearing lethargic. However, she is arousable and is able to follow commands.
- Airway: Intact.
- Breathing: Normal.
- Circulation: Rapid full pulses. Normal capillary refill.
- Disability: Pupils equal and reactive, GCS 15.
- Exposure: Normal.
- Finger: Normal.

11.3. History:

- Allergies: None.
- Medications: None.
- PMH: No significant illnesses or surgeries. Last menstrual period, 3 weeks ago.
- Last meal: 6 hours ago.
- Events: A 21 y/o female college student presents with a headache. Several days before admission, she was suffering from a severe sore throat. This resolved but last night she started having a headache with a fever that did not subside with acetaminophen. The pain is severe, "throbbing'" located throughout the head and radiating to the neck. No recent trauma. She is nauseated, photophobic, and lightheaded.
- Family: Noncontributory.
- Records: None.
- Immune: Up to date.
- Narcotics: No illicit drug use.
- Social history: No alcohol or tobacco use. She lives with her parents and attends college.

11.4. Secondary Survey:

- Temperature: 103.7°F.
- General: Unchanged.
- Skin: Warm, dry intact, no petechiae.

- HEENT: She does not look past the midline when asked to look right. The right pupil is 2 mm larger than the left and discs are flat. Oropharynx is red without exudates.
- Neck: Rigid, no adenopathy. Positive Kernig's and Brudzinski's signs.
- Chest: Normal.
- Lungs: Clear to auscultation.
- Heart: Tachycardic, normal S1, S2, no S3, S4 or murmur.
- Abdomen: Normal.
- Perineum/GU: Normal.
- Rectal: Normal.
- Back: Normal.
- Extremities: Normal.
- Neuro: Cranial nerves—Right homonymous hemianopsia with a right facial droop, right upper extremity weakness, and decreased sharp/dull discrimination to that extremity. DTRs are normal.
  No Babinski reflex. Unable to fully cooperate for an adequate cerebellar examination. She is oriented only to person and birthday, no dysarthria.

11.5. Laboratory:
- CBC: WBC 16.8, Hgb 12.7, Hct 36.4, Plt 250,000.
- Differential: Polys 80, bands 46%, lymphs 15, eos 1, mono 4.
- Chemistry: Na 142, K 3.7, Cl 101, CO_2 24.
- BUN/Cr: 12/0.7.
- Glucose: 194.
- Ca/Mg: Normal.
- Liver function: SGOT 21, SGPT 24, Alk Phos 60, GGTP 10, Bili 0.8.
- Amylase/Lipase: Normal.
- PT/PTT: Normal.
- ABG: pH 7.42, pCO_2 32, pO_2 97, HCO_3 23.
- U/A: Normal.

11.6. X-rays:
- CXR: Normal.
- CT head: Normal.

11.7. Special Tests:
- ECG: Normal.
- CSF results: Opening pressure 500, protein 480, glu 8, WBC 17,000, Segs 93%, lymphs 3%, mono 4%, RBCs 660. Gram stain positive for gram-positive cocci with many PMNs.

11.8. Management:
- Start IV.
- Place on cardiac monitor and pulse oximeter.
- Administer antibiotics before the CT scan.
- Perform an LP.
- Admit to the ICU on isolation.
- Consult a neurologist or internist.
- Give Decadron 8 to 10 mg IV.

11.9. Critical Actions:
- Examine the neck.
- Determine the temperature.
- Perform a thorough neurologic examination.
- Perform a CT scan before an LP.
- Perform an LP.
- Administer antibiotics (given before allowing patient to go for the CT scan). Vancomycin + ceftriaxone or cefotaxime.

- Admit to the ICU.
- Consult a neurologist or internist.

11.10. Pearls:

❍ **What are the common bacterial pathogens that cause meningitis in this age group?**

Streptococcus pneumoniae is the most common followed by Neisseria meningitidis then Haemophilus influenzae serotypes b, a, e, f.

❍ **Which patients are at risk for meningitis?**

It most often occurs in the very young or the very old age. Other individuals at risk include immunocompromised patients (HIV-infected or splenectomized patients), immunosuppressed patients, alcoholics, patients with recent neurosurgical procedures, and patients with underlying infections such as pneumonia, sinusitis, mastoiditis, or otitis media.

CASE 12 (Burn)

Examiner

Immediate rapid sequence intubation is required and should be performed using in-line c-spine stabilization. The candidate should administer fluids per the Parkland formula and may use the Lund and Browder chart or rule of nines to calculate the percent of body involvement. This patient requires transfer to a burn unit.

12.1. Introduction:

A 45 y/o male presents with burns, soot, and blistering to the face and neck.

Vital signs: BP 100/60, P 120, R 24, T 98.2°F, Wt 80 kg.

12.2. Primary Survey:

- General: Patient is sitting upright, anxious, alert, tachypneic, and is in obvious discomfort.
- Airway: Redness and swelling to the oropharynx with soot present in the nose and mouth.
- Breathing: Tachypnea with a cough present.
- Circulation: Capillary refill is delayed, all pulses are equal.
- Disability: He is alert and oriented to person, place, and time, GCS 15.
- Exposure: Second-degree burns are present on the face, neck, chest, and both upper extremities.
- Finger: Rectal normal.

12.3. Management:

- Perform immediate rapid sequence intubation.
- Protect c-spine.
- Place on cardiac monitor and pulse oximeter. Start two large bore IVs.
- Use the Parkland formula to calculate fluid requirements.
- Administer tetanus prophylaxis.
- Administer pain medication and an H_2 blocker.
- Order appropriate laboratory studies and x-rays.

12.4. History:

- Allergies: None.
- Medications: None.
- PMH: No previous illnesses or injuries.
- Last meal: 1 hour ago.
- Events: A 45 y/o male is brought in by his wife who states that he was burning a pile of wood 10 minutes ago. A flash occurred and the gas can exploded while in his hands. He was thrown 10 ft but did not lose consciousness. He complains of pain to his face and neck but has no respiratory distress.

- Family: Noncontributory.
- Records: None.
- Immune: 15 years ago.
- EMTs: They have no new information to add.
- Narcotics: No history of illicit drug use.
- Doctor: None.
- Social: Married, has two children. No alcohol or tobacco use.

12.5. Secondary Survey:

- General: Patient paralyzed, sedated, and intubated.
- Skin: The total surface involved is approximately 20%, all of which are second degree (deep partial thickness) in nature. The areas include the volar aspect of each arm (hands are spared), the anterior neck, the entire face, and chest.
- HEENT: The entire face is burned. PERRLA, EOM-I, fundi normal, conjunctiva injected.
- Neck: Redness and swelling present.
- Chest: No burns present. The chest rises and falls without difficulty.
- Lungs: Coarse breath sounds bilateral.
- Heart: Tachycardia presents with a regular rate and rhythm, normal S1 and S2, without a murmur.
- Abdomen: Normal.
- Back: Normal.
- Extremities: Normal.
- Neuro: Patient intubated, paralyzed, and sedated. Before intubation no focal deficits were noted.

12.6. Laboratory:

- CBC: WBC 17, Hgb 13.2, Hct 44, Plt 240,000.
- Chemistry: Na 135, K 4.5, Cl 108, CO_2 24.
- BUN/Cr: 6/1.0.
- Glucose: 150.
- Ca/Mg: Normal.
- LFTs: Normal.
- Amylase/Lipase: Normal.
- PT/PTT: Normal.
- Cardiac enzymes: Normal.
- ABG: pH 7.42, pO_2 75, pCO_2 28, HCO_3 22 (preintubation).
- CO Hgb: 1%.
- U/A: No myoglobin or blood.

12.7. X-rays:

- CXR: Diffused infiltrates bilateral. Normal heart size and mediastinum. ETT in place.
- CT c-spine: Normal.
- CT head: Normal.

12.8. Special Tests:

- ECG: Sinus tachycardia without ectopy.

12.9. Management:

- Cleanse all wounds.
- Dress the burns with sterile gauze or sheets.
- Examine the cornea for burns.
- Do not apply antibiotic ointment to the burns or start parenteral antibiotics.
- You may debride blisters to prevent further damage to burned tissue.
- IV fluid hydration with LR or NS.

12.10. Critical Actions:

- Perform a rapid sequence intubation.
- Correctly calculate the fluid requirements.

- Administer tetanus prophylaxis.
- Evaluate c-spine.
- Consult with and transfer to a burn unit.
- Relieve patient's pain.
- Apply dry sterile dressings to burns.

12.11. Pearls:

❍ **What conditions mandate transfer to a burn unit?**

(1) Major partial-thickness burns of >25% in the 10 years to 50 years age group
(2) Major partial-thickness burns of >20% in children younger than 10 years or in adults older than 50 years.
(3) Any full-thickness burn greater than 10% of total body surface area.
(4) Any burn involving the hands, face, feet, perineum, joints, circumferential in nature, associated inhalation injury, or complicated by fractures or trauma.
(5) Electrical burns and burns in patients, who are at risk because of underlying conditions, should also be considered for transfer.

❍ **What is the role of prophylactic parenteral antibiotics?**

They are not to be started in the ED.

CASE 13 (Triple)

Patient #1 (Neck Stiffness)

Examiner

This patient has tetanus, is stable but the candidate should perform a complete body search for injuries. An immunization history is important. If the candidate focuses completely on a c-spine injury, have the patient complain of trismus, increasing pain, and dysphagia. Make the candidate work to get the patient into the ICU by having the consulting internist be resistant to this idea.

13.1. Introduction: (**Patient #1**)

A 68 y/o male presents with a complaint of stiffness to the neck for 4 hours.

Vital signs: BP 140/82, P 110, R 30, T 98.9°F, Wt 80 kg.

13.2. Primary Survey:

- General: Poorly nourished male presents in moderate discomfort. He moves his head, neck, and upper torso as a unit. He is in no respiratory distress.
- Airway : Normal
- Breathing: Normal.
- Circulation: Normal.
- Disability: GCS 15, PERRLA.
- Exposure: No medic alert tags. If the candidate asks for skin lesions, contusions, or lacerations, make them specifically ask about the left lower leg.
- Finger: May be deferred to secondary survey.

13.3. Management:

- Initiate c-spine immobilization.
- You may order appropriate diagnostic studies now or after the history and secondary survey.
- Start IV and place on a pulse oximeter and monitor.

13.4. History:

- Allergies: None.
- Medications: Hydrochlorothiazide 25 mg daily.
- PMH: Hypertension. Hernia repair in 1980.
- Last meal: 24 hours ago.
- Events: A 68 y/o male awoke from sleep with pain, stiffness, and a muscle spasm in his neck, jaw, and shoulders. He is unable to fully open his mouth and he complains of odynophagia and dysphagia, if asked. No fever, chills, nausea vomiting, or abdominal pain. No recent trauma or known insect bites. He thinks he may have fallen in the about 4 days ago while on a drinking binge. As a result, he hit his left lower leg but he did not lose consciousness.
- Family: Noncontributory, no family members or friends are present for information.
- Records: None.
- Immune: "Many years" since his last Td immunization.
- EMTs: N/A.
- Narcotics: No illicit drug use.
- Doctor: None.
- Social: Drinks one case of beer a day and smokes two packs of cigarettes per day.

13.5. Secondary Survey:

- General: Poorly nourished, poorly kept male, who is alert but uncomfortable. He is not in respiratory distress.
- Skin: Well hydrated, 5 cm full-thickness laceration to the left lower leg at the calf. The wound edges are necrotic and red streaks are present. It is very painful to the touch.
- HEENT: Cataract in the left eye, otherwise, normal examination.
- Jaw: The patient is unable to open his mouth more than 3 cm. No palpable tenderness, TMJ crepitation, or deformity noted. There is tightness noted to the masseter and temporalis muscles.
- Neck: Paraspinal and midline tenderness is present. Negative Brudzinski's and Kernig's. Greatly diminished range of motion.
- Chest: Normal.
- Lungs: Normal.
- Heart: Normal.
- Abdomen: Normal.
- Perineum/GU: Normal.
- Rectal: Normal.
- Back: Normal.
- Extremities: Large laceration to the left lower leg at the calf. Pulses are present and equal, no edema or crepitance. Inspection of the wound reveals an embedded sliver of wood.
- Neuro: A/O X 3, GCS 15. Cranial nerves intact. Motor and sensory examination is normal and symmetric. DTRs are brisk without clonus. Negative Trousseau's and Chvostek's signs. Toes downgoing. Normal cerebellar examination.

13.6. Management:

- Don't suture the wound.
- Administer tetanus immune globulin (TIG), 500 to 5,000 units IM.
- Administer 0.5 mL of tetanus toxoid IM.
- Treat the pain and spasm.
- Continue c-spine care until x-rays are back.
- Obtain blood and wound cultures and start antibiotics. You may use metronidazole, tetracycline, erythromycin, penicillin, or a cephalosporin.
- Administer thiamine and folic acid IV or po.
- Consider magnesium sulfate because of his poor nutrition and chronic alcohol abuse.

The nurse informs you that another patient is in room 2. He is upset and wants to sign out against medical advice.

Patient #2 (Sore Throat)

Examiner

This patient has an uncomplicated sore throat but is very upset because of his discomfort and his perceived long wait. It is important that the candidate calms the patient and helps ease his discomfort. This patient may be discharged but a follow-up should be arranged.

13.1. Introduction: (**Patient #2**)

A 22 y/o male presents with a complaint of a sore throat.

Vital signs: BP 120/60, P 110, R 18, T 102.3°F, Wt 82.5 kg.

13.2. Primary Survey:

- General: WN/WD male appearing upset about waiting to be seen.
- Airway: Intact.
- Breathing: Normal.
- Circulation: Normal.
- Disability: GCS 15, PERRLA.
- Exposure: Patient refuses to disrobe.
- Finger: Deferred at this time.

13.3. Management:

- The patient is stable, laboratory studies and treatment may be deferred until completion of the history and secondary survey.

13.4. History:

- Allergies: None.
- Medications: None.
- PMH: No illnesses or injuries. No past surgeries.
- Last meal: 2 hours ago.
- Events: A 22 y/o male presents with a sore throat. This has been hurting for the past 2 days. Pain is worse today and a fever started. He is also complaining of nausea headache, dysphagia, and neck pain. No recent sick contacts.
- Family: Noncontributory.
- Records: None.
- Immune: Up to date.
- EMTs: Not applicable.
- Narcotics: No illicit drug use.
- Doctor: None.
- Social: No alcohol or tobacco use.

13.5. Secondary Survey:

- General: The patient appears uncomfortable but more relaxed, if the candidate's interaction is appropriate.
- Skin: No rash or petechiae.
- HEENT: The oropharynx is injected with enlarged palatine tonsils and exudates present. The uvula is midline with no asymmetric enlargement of the tonsils or swelling of the pharynx. PERRLA, EOM-I, TMs normal. No swelling or fluctuant.
- Neck: No meningeal signs, many anterior cervical lymph nodes.
- Chest: Normal.
- Lungs: Clear.
- Heart: Tachycardia, regular rhythm, no murmur.
- Abdomen: No organomegaly.
- Perineum/GU: Appropriate to defer

- Rectal: Appropriate to defer.
- Back: Normal.
- Neuro: Intact.

13.6. Laboratory:
- CBC: WBC 17,000, Hgb 15, Hct 45, Plt 250,000.
- Chemistry: Normal.
- BUN/Cr: Normal.
- Glucose: Normal.
- LFTs: Normal.
- Monospot: Negative.
- Rapid Strep: Positive.

13.7. X-rays:
- CXR: Normal.
- Lateral neck: Normal.
- CT neck: Normal if ordered.

13.8. Management:
- Establish good relations and convince the patient to stay.
- Treat the patient's fever with acetaminophen or ibuprofen.
- Treat with penicillin, IM, or po.
- Arrange follow-up with a primary care doctor by phone or instruct to return to the ED in 1 to 2 days for recheck.

The charge nurse informs you that a "bad" trauma is in room 3.

Patient #3 (Multiple Trauma)

Examiner

This patient is unable to communicate and has sustained a bladder rupture, tibial fracture, c-spine injury, and a pelvic fracture. The patient appears pale, with shallow and sonorous respirations. He also smells of alcohol. RSI while maintaining c-spine precaution is required. If rapid fluid resuscitation is not performed, have a nurse continually announce a BP of 80/P. Insertion of a Foley catheter before a urethrogram is a dangerous act. Have the candidate describe how to perform a urethrogram.

13.1. Introduction: (**Patient #3**)

The EMTs present with a 50 y/o male who was struck by a car and thrown 20 ft.

Vital signs: BP 88/45, P 118, R 22, Wt 80 kg.

13.2. Primary Survey:
- General: The patient appears pale, with shallow and sonorous respirations, smelling of alcohol.
- Airway: Pooling of secretions and diminished gag reflex.
- Breathing: Shallow sonorous respirations, lungs clear to auscultation.
- Circulation: Pale skin, rapid and thready pulse, and delayed capillary refill.
- Disability: GCS 8. Pupils equal and reactive. Responds to pain by incomprehensible sounds.
- Exposure: No medic alert tags, bruising, and swelling to the left leg.
- Finger: High-riding prostate, no blood per rectum. Blood at the meatus. No scrotal swelling or hematoma. Pelvis stable.

13.3. Management:
- Recognize the airway problem and perform a jaw-thrust or chin-lift maneuver to relieve the obstruction. Perform rapid sequence intubation with head injury and c-spine precautions.

- Evaluate for proper placement of the ETT.
- Recognize shock and treat with two large bore IVs, infusing 2 L of LR or NS.
- Order appropriate laboratory studies, and x-rays.
- Place the patient on a cardiac monitor and pulse oximeter.
- Insert an OG tube.
- DO NOT insert a Foley catheter.
- Check vital signs frequently.

13.4. History:
- Allergies: Unknown.
- Medications: Unknown.
- PMH: Unknown.
- Last meal: Unknown.
- EMTs: The patient was hit by a car and thrown a long distance. No witnesses are available. No identification was found on the patient.

13.5. Secondary Survey:
- Vital signs: BP 120/80, P 100, R 18 (bagged), T 99.0°F.
- General: Patient is intubated, respirations per bag-valve-mask without difficulty.
- Skin: Bruising to the left knee.
- HEENT: There is soft tissue swelling and an abrasion to the forehead but no palpable fracture. Eyes open to painful stimuli, PERRLA, EOM-I. Fundi normal.
- Neck: Immobilized with a c-collar. There is no palpable defect.
- Chest: No obvious injury, no crepitus.
- Lungs: Clear to auscultation.
- Heart: Tachycardia without murmur.
- Abdomen: Distended and firm to palpation. Bowel sounds are absent.
- Perineum/GU: Blood at meatus, perineal hematoma present.
- Pelvis: Pain and crepitus on compression of the symphysis pubis.
- Back: Normal.
- Extremities: Bruising and swelling of the left knee, with ligaments intact and a tense effusion are present. All pulses are present and equal. No other deformities noted.
- Neuro: No focal findings, DTRs are equal, GCS 8 prior to intubation.

13.6. Laboratory:
- CBC: WBC 14, Hgb 15.2, Hct 45.5, Plt 295.
- Chemistry: Na 140, K 4.2, Cl 101, CO_2 23.
- BUN/Cr: 14/1.0.
- Glucose: 125.
- Ca/Mg: Normal.
- LFTs: Normal.
- ABG: pH 7.39, pO_2 65, pCO_2 13, HCO_3 22 (room air).
- ETOH: 350.
- U/A: Gross blood.

13.7. X-rays:
- CXR: Normal.
- C-spine: C6 to C7 unilateral facet dislocation.
- Pelvis: Fractured symphysis pubis and left pubic rami.
- Left knee: Nondisplaced tibial plateau fracture.
- Retrograde urethrogram: Urethra intact. Extraperitoneal bladder rupture with extravasation of dye present.
- Cystogram: Extravasation of dye.
- CT head: Normal.

- CT c-spine: Normal.
- CT chest Normal.
- CT abdomen/pelvis: Grade II liver laceration.

13.8. Special Tests:
- ECG: Sinus tachycardia.
- FAST examination: Fluid present in the rectovesical pouch.

13.9. Critical Actions:
- Consult neurosurgery for the c-spine fracture.
- Maintain c-spine precautions.
- Consult urology for bladder repair.
- Splint the right leg and consult orthopedics.
- Consult a trauma or general surgeon.
- Recognize hypotension and treat with fluids.
- Intubate early.
- Do not insert a Foley catheter until urethrogram is completed and it shows an intact urethra.

Patient #1 (Neck Stiffness)

The nurse has irrigated the patient's leg wound and asks which suture you would like.

13.10. Laboratory:
- CBC: WBC 11, Hgb 15, Hct 45, Plt 300,000.
- Chemistry: Normal.
- BUN/Cr: Normal.
- Glucose: 110.
- Ca/Mg: Normal.
- LFTs: Normal.
- Amylase/Lipase: Normal.
- PT/PTT: Normal.
- Blood cultures: Pending.
- Gram's stain: Gram-positive club-shaped rods.
- U/A: Normal.

13.11. X-rays:
- C-spine: Normal.
- CT c-spine: Normal.
- CXR: Normal.
- L. Tib/fib: Normal, foreign body present.

13.12. Special Tests:
- ECG: Sinus tachycardia, no other abnormality noted.
- Pulse oximeter: 100% on room air.
- Cardiac monitor: Sinus tachycardia.

13.13. Critical Actions:
- Obtain a history of the fall with a leg laceration.
- Obtain immunization history.
- Don't suture the wound.
- Administer tetanus toxoid and tetanus immune globulin.
- Treat the spasm and pain.
- Admit to the ICU.
- Consult a surgeon to explore, debride, and remove the foreign body.

13.14. Pearls: (**Patient #1 Tetanus**)

❍ **What is the differential diagnosis of tetanus?**

Strychnine poisoning, dystonic reaction, hypocalcemia tetany, peritonsillar abscess, parotitis, meningitis, subarachnoid hemorrhage, rabies, temporomandibular joint disease.

❍ **What is the role of TIG in the treatment of tetanus?**

TIG neutralizes circulating tetanospasmin in the wound, but not the toxin that is already present in the nervous tissue. The administration of TIG decreases mortality.

Patient #2 (Sore Throat)

13.15. Critical Actions:

- Establish good rapport with the patient and convince him to stay.
- Diagnose streptococcal pharyngitis.
- Treat with the appropriate antibiotics.
- Arrange follow-up.
- Treat the fever.

13.16. Pearls: (**Patient #2**)

❍ **What are the objectives in treating streptococcal pharyngitis?**

Prevent rheumatic fever, peritonsillar abscess and cellulitis, suppurative cervical lymphadenitis, and retropharyngeal abscess. Treatment also hastens clinical recovery.

❍ **What is the antibiotic of choice for the treatment of Group A β-hemolytic Streptococcal pharyngitis?**

A single dose of penicillin, 1.2 million units IM, or oral penicillin, 500 mg po bid, tid or qid for 10 days, effectively eradicates the infection and prevents rheumatic fever. Alternatives to penicillin include erythromycin, clindamycin, and azithromycin.

13.17. Pearls: (Patient #3)

❍ **In evaluating genitourinary trauma, what is the proper sequence of studies to evaluate the kidneys, bladder, and urethra?**

If blood is present at the urethral meatus, perform a retrograde urethrogram first. If a bladder injury is suspected, a cystogram is performed, after a urethrogram, to avoid residual contrast from obscuring the urethra.

❍ **What are the contraindications to insertion of a Foley catheter?**

Blood at the urethral meatus, "floating" or "high-riding" prostate, perineal hematoma, and a midline pelvic fracture or dislocation. A urethrogram should be performed first when any of these findings are present.

CASE 14 (52 y/o Male Who Feels Funny)

Examiner

This patient has unstable V-tach requiring cardioversion. The candidate may try adenosine first, but this will not work. If the candidate does not identify V-tach and does not treat appropriately, the patient will decompensate. Consult cardiology and admit to the ICU.

14.1. Introduction:

A 52 y/o male presents, via a private automobile, with a complaint of not "feeling well."

Vital signs: BP 80/P, P 120, R 24, T 98.3°F, Wt 84.5 kg.

14.2. Primary Survey:

- General: WN/WD male appears anxious, uncomfortable, in mild respiratory distress.
- Airway: Intact.
- Breathing: Tachypneic but not labored.
- Circulation: Pulses are equal and thready.
- Disability: Normal.
- Exposure: No medic alert tags.
- Finger: Normal rectal. Heme negative.

14.3. Management:

- Start IV and O_2. Place on pulse oximeter and cardiac monitor.
- Order appropriate laboratory studies, x-rays, and an ECG.
- Give sedation and perform synchronized cardioversion at 100 J biphasic and 200 J monophasic. You may use adenosine first.
- Give an amiodarone, lidocaine, or procainamide loading dose followed by an appropriate infusion.
- Give aspirin 325 mg po.

14.4. History:

- Allergies: None.
- Medications: None.
- PMH: None.
- Last meal: 2 hours ago.
- Events: A 52 y/o previously healthy male presents, stating he does not "feel well." He was sitting at his desk at work when he started feeling "funny." He denies chest pain or pressure, but does have nausea and is diaphoretic. He has no history of similar complaints and the event started 1 hour before arrival to the ED. He drove himself to the ED.
- Family: No family history of heart disease.
- Records: None.
- Immune: Up to date.
- Narcotics: Denies use of illicit drugs.
- Doctor: No family physician.
- Social: Denies alcohol use but smokes one pack of cigarettes per day and has done so for 32 years. He is married, has two children.

14.5. Secondary Survey:

- Vital signs: BP 120/80, P 80, R 16.
- General: After treatment he feels and looks better.
- Skin: Initially, it was pale, cool, and moist but after treatment it is warm and dry with good color.
- HEENT: Normal.
- Neck: Normal.
- Chest: Normal.
- Lungs: Normal.
- Heart: RRR with a normal S1, S2 no S3 or S4, and no murmur; Normal PMI.
- Abdomen: Normal.
- Perineum/GU: Normal.
- Rectal: Normal.
- Extremities: Normal.
- Neuro: Normal.

14.6. Laboratory:

- CBC: WBC 9, Hgb 14, Hct 45, Plt 250,000.
- Chemistry: Na 135, K 4.0, Cl 102, CO_2 24.
- BUN/Cr: 10/1.0.
- Glucose: 102.
- Ca/Mg: Normal.

- LFTs: Normal.
- Amylase/Lipase: Normal.
- PT/PTT: Normal.
- Cardiac enzymes: Troponin 0.11
- ABG: pH 7.45, pO_2 95, pCO_2 30, HCO_3 24, saturation 100%.
- U/A: Normal.
- D-dimer: Elevated.

14.7. X-rays:

- CXR: Normal.

14.8. Special Tests:

- ECG: Ventricular tachycardia at a rate of 140. The posttreatment ECG reveals normal sinus rhythm.

14.9. Critical Actions:

- Recognize V-tach on the ECG.
- Cardiovert.
- Admit to the ICU.
- Obtain a cardiology consult.

14.10. Pearls:

❍ **What ECG findings are suggestive of ventricular tachycardia?**

Wide-QRS complex, rate greater than 100, regular rhythm, extreme right axis deviation, and concordance in the precordial leads.

❍ **What are the causes of ventricular tachycardia?**

The most common causes are ischemic heart disease and acute myocardial infarction. Other less common causes include hypertrophic cardiomyopathy, mitral valve prolapse, toxicity from drugs (digoxin, quinidine, procainamide, sympathomimetics), and electrolyte abnormalities.

CASE 15 (Unconscious Male)

Examiner

This is a case of organophosphate poisoning. The patient requires immediate intubation with c-spine immobilization, IV rehydration, nasogastric suctioning, and Foley catheterization. A coma protocol should be instituted but the patient will not respond. During the initial stabilization, one of the treating EMTs complains of nausea. Candidate should recognize a potential toxic exposure and take protective measures, such as bag patient's clothing, wear protective mask and gloves, decontaminate the patient's skin by washing with soap and water, and decontaminate the GI tract with activated charcoal.

15.1. Introduction:

A 17 y/o male in an acute respiratory distress arrives by a basic EMT ambulance. No treatment in the field has been given and his brother is on the way by a private auto. The EMTs complain of nausea.

Vitals signs: BP 80/40, P 48, R 45, T 100.5°F, Wt 88 kg.

15.2. Primary Survey:

- General: A WN/WD 17 y/o male presents unconscious with vomitus on clothing.
- Airway: Excessive oral secretions are present and the gag reflex is absent.
- Breathing: Rapid shallow respirations are present.
- Circulation: Capillary refill is delayed, peripheral pulses are weak.
- Disability: Eyes do not open to painful stimuli, verbal response is absent, and decerebrate posturing is present. Pupils are pinpoint.
- Exposure: No medic alert tags; no lesions, abrasions, burns, or lacerations.
- Finger: Rectal normal. Patient is incontinent of urine and stool.

15.3. Management:

- Give naloxone 2 mg IV.
- Check the glucose or give 1 amp of D50.
- Intubate with c-spine immobilization.
- Start IV with aggressive fluid resuscitation.
- Insert an NG tube and Foley catheter.
- Place on cardiac monitor and pulse oximeter.
- Decontaminate the patient.
- Have the EMTs decontaminated and begin treating them.
- Give activated charcoal to decontaminate the GI tract.

The nurse tells you the patient's brother has arrived and is in the waiting room.

15.4. History:

- Allergies: None.
- Medications: None.
- PMH: No significant past illnesses or injuries. No past surgeries.
- Last meal: Unknown.
- Events: According to his patient's brother, he started a new job with an exterminating company. He was previously healthy and had no complaints before leaving for work today.
- Family: Noncontributory.
- Records: None.
- Immune: Unknown.
- EMTs: They were called to the scene by a bystander, which noticed the patient unconscious in an unmarked private van. The EMTs noted no signs of trauma, no unusual smells, no drug paraphernalia, no alcohol bottles or cans, and no pill bottles.
- Narcotics: No history of drug or alcohol abuse according to the brother.
- Doctor: No family physician.
- Social: No tobacco or alcohol use. He lives with his brother and is a freshman in college.

15.5. Secondary Survey:

- Skin: Normal color but diaphoretic.
- HEENT: Pupils are pinpoint, profuse tearing is present, oropharynx is full of secretions.
- Neck: Normal.
- Chest: Normal.
- Lungs: Shallow respirations, expiratory wheezes are present with few bibasilar crackles.
- Heart: Bradycardia with normal heart tones and no murmur present.
- Abdomen: Bowel sounds are hyperactive.
- Perineum/GU: Normal.
- Rectal: Normal sphincter tone. Hemoccult negative. Brown colored, liquid stool.
- Back: Normal.
- Extremities: Muscle fasciculations are diffusely present.
- Neuro: Minimal flexion response to pain. DTRs are hyperactive and symmetric and toes are downgoing.

15.6. Laboratory:

- CBC: WBC 15, Hgb 13.5, Hct 39.5, Plt 300,000.
- Chemistry: Na 138, K 3.0, Cl 108, CO_2 14.
- BUN/Cr: 18/1.1.
- Glucose: 120.
- Ca/Mg: Normal.
- LFTs: Normal.
- Amylase/Lipase: Normal.
- PT/PTT: Normal.
- Cardiac enzymes: Normal.

- ABG: pH 7.12, pO_2 145, pCO_2 52 (on arrival).
- ABG: pH 7.34, pO_2 90, pCO_2 30 (after intubation).
- Lactate: 5.0 mEq/L.
- Serum osm: 298 mOsm/kg.
- U/A: Protein 3+, glucose 2+, specific gravity 1.020.

15.7. X-rays:
- CXR: Mild pulmonary vascular congestion.
- CT head: Normal.
- CT c-spine: Normal.

15.8. Special Tests:
- ECG: Sinus bradycardia.
- Serum cholinesterase and RBC cholinesterase: Pending.

15.9. Management:
- Contact the patient's employer to determine which insecticide was used (organophosphate called parathion).
- Contact Poison Control.
- Order atropine, 0.05 mg/kg/dose IV q 5 to15 minutes and 2-PAM (pralidoxime) 25 to 50 mg/kg/dose IV.
- Consult an internist and admit to the ICU.

15.10. Critical Actions:
- Intubate with c-spine immobilization.
- Start IV rehydration.
- Recognize the toxidrome and decontaminate.
- Initiate coma protocol (naloxone and glucose).
- Consult Poison Control.
- Contact the employer to determine which insecticide was used.

15.11. Pearls:

❍ **What is the most frequent cause of treatment failure in organophosphate poisoning?**

Inadequate atropinization. Large doses of atropine, 20 to 40 mg/d, may be required.

❍ **What is the difference between organophosphate and carbamate poisoning?**

Carbamates are less toxic and have a shorter duration of action. Signs and symptoms usually disappear within 8 hours after exposure. Carbamates are more rapidly absorbed through the skin than organophosphates, but CNS effects are less, because of poor penetration of the blood-brain barrier.

CASE 16 (Febrile Infant)

Examiner

This patient has experienced a simple febrile seizure secondary to the Tdap, rotavirus, HIB, and poliovirius shots. The candidate may either admit the patient or discharge with follow-up in 24 hours. The family will ask detailed questions regarding febrile seizures which the candidate must be able to answer.

16.1. Introduction:

A 4 m/o male infant, who is actively seizing presents in the arms of his mother.

Vital signs: BP 70, P 140, R 32, Wt 5 kg.

16.2. Primary Survey:
- Airway: Patent, no pooling of secretions, gag reflex intact.
- Breathing: Stridorous and irregular respirations.

- Circulation: Decreased capillary refill, normal pulses.
- Disability: Pupils equal and reactive. Spontaneous eye opening, localizes to pain, grunting verbal response.
- Exposure: No rash, petechiae, or signs of trauma.
- Finger: Normal.

16.3. Management:

- Stabilize the airway and start O_2.
- Place the patient on a cardiac monitor and pulse oximeter.
- Obtain a bedside blood glucose.
- Obtain a rectal temperature.
- After determining the patient to be febrile (103.5°F), administer acetaminophen 15 mg/kg po or pr, or ibuprofen, 10 mg/kg po.
- Start IV with a 20 mL/kg bolus of normal saline.
- Obtain appropriate laboratory studies and x-rays.
- Give an appropriate benzodiazepine IV or pr, if the seizure persists.
- If a head CT scan is ordered, give antibiotics before the patient leaves the department.

16.4. History:

- Allergies: None.
- Medications: None.
- PMH: No significant illnesses, normal spontaneous vaginal delivery at 41 weeks of gestation. Birth weight 7 lb, 8 oz. No past surgeries.
- Last meal: Drank 2 oz of formula 3 hours ago.
- Events: A 4 m/o male presents with seizures. Earlier today he seemed irritable, warm to the touch, and refused his bottle. He was sitting on his mother's lap when he stiffened, rolled his eyes back, and began having clonic–tonic movements of all the extremities for approximately 2 minutes. In addition, the patient received a multiple immunization injections yesterday.
- Family: Negative.
- Records: None.
- Doctor: Dr. Pediatrician.
- Social history: Patient lives with natural parents and one sibling. No risk factors for abuse.

16.5. Secondary Survey:

- General: WN/WD, unresponsive, no respiratory distress.
- Skin: Warm, moist, no rash.
- HEENT: Head normocephalic/atraumatic, fontanels open and flat PERRL, TMs normal, nose, and throat are clear.
- Neck: Supple, no nodes, no meningeal signs.
- Chest: Normal.
- Lungs: Tachypnea, no wheezing.
- Heart: Tachycardic rate, regular rhythm, no murmur.
- Abdomen: Soft, BS present, no mass, no organomegaly.
- Perineum/GU: Normal.
- Rectal: Normal sphincter tone, heme negative.
- Back: Normal.
- Extremities: Normal.
- Neuro: Postictal. Cranial nerves intact as best as can be determined. DTRs normal.

16.6. Laboratory:

- CBC: WBC 14, Hgb 11.5, Hct 35.6, Plt 350,000.
- Differential: Normal.
- Chemistry: Na 140, K 3.8, Cl 101, CO_2 24.
- BUN/Cr: 17/0.7.
- Glucose: 102.

- Ca/Mg: 9.0/2.0.
- LFTs: Normal.
- Blood cultures: Pending.
- U/A: Normal.
- Urine culture: Pending.

16.7. X-rays:
- CXR: Normal.
- CT head: Normal.

16.8. Special Tests:
- CSF: Appearance, clear.
- Cell count: WBC 2, RBC 0.
- Glucose: 65.
- Protein: 30.
- Gram stain: No organisms.
- CIE/Latex: Negative.
- Culture: Pending.

16.9. Critical Actions:
- Protect the airway.
- Stat serum glucose.
- Obtain a rectal temperature.
- Lower the temperature with antipyretics.
- Administer antibiotics before obtaining the head CT scan and before admission.
- Instruct follow-up with a pediatrician in 24 hours, if candidate does not admit.

16.10. Pearls:

○ **What are the usual characteristics of a simple febrile seizure?**

(1) Temperature greater than 100°F with a rapid rise.
(2) Age between 3 months and 5 years.
(3) Generalized tonic–clonic, nonfocal.
(4) Short postictal period.
(5) Seizure lasts less than 15 minutes.

○ **What are the risk factors for recurrent febrile seizures?**

(1) First-degree relative with epilepsy.
(2) First-degree relative with febrile seizures.
(3) Complex first febrile seizure.
(4) Age younger than 12 months at the time of the initial febrile seizure.
(5) Increased infectious exposure because of day care attendance.

○ **What is the incidence of developing epilepsy in the future?**

Febrile seizures do not cause epilepsy but there is a 1% chance of developing this by the age of 7 years. The incidence of epilepsy in children without a history of febrile seizures is 0.4%.

CASE 17 (Female with Pelvic Pain)

Examiner

This patient has a ruptured ectopic pregnancy. If IV fluids are started, the patient will respond by "feeling better," and her BP will increase to 100/P. You may have the candidate perform a culdocentesis by making the ultrasound difficult to interpret. Immediately upon finishing the culdocentesis, the ultrasound technician arrives and confirms the presence of an adnexal mass and free fluid in the pelvis.

17.1. Introduction:

A 28 y/o female presents with a complaint of lower abdominal and pelvic pain.

Vital signs: BP 100/70, P 108, R 22, T 98.9°F.

17.2. Primary Survey:

- General: WN/WD female sitting up, appears uncomfortable and pale but is in no immediate distress.
- Airway: Normal.
- Breathing: Tachypnea but no distress.
- Circulation: Strong, rapid, and equal pulses. Normal capillary refill.
- Disability: Normal.
- Exposure: No medic alert tags.

17.3. Management:

- Because the patient is stable, the candidate may not initiate treatment until a full history is completed.

17.4. History:

- Allergies: None.
- Medications: Sulfa.
- PMH: Ectopic pregnancy, 5 years ago, treated with methotrexate. No past surgeries.
- Last meal: 6 hours ago.
- Events: A 28 y/o pregnant women presents with abdominal pain that started 1 week ago and has progressively gotten worse. She describes the pain as diffuse, sharp, constant, and nonradiating. She has experienced nausea but no vomiting, diarrhea, fever or chills. The patient denies vaginal discharge but complains of dysuria without hematuria. No history of similar complaints. Her last menstrual period was approximately 7 weeks ago and she had some vaginal bleeding 3 days ago.
- Family: Noncontributory.
- Records: None.
- Immunizations: Up to date.
- Narcotics: No illicit drug use.
- Doctor: Patient has a gynecologist.
- Social history: The patient is married, has no children, and works as a lawyer for a personal injury firm. She denies alcohol and tobacco use.

During the history, the patient becomes dizzy, nauseated, and complains of increasing abdominal pain. If asked, the new vital signs are BP 80/P, P 120, R 22.

17.5. Management:

- Administer l L bolus of LR or 0.9 NS.
- Place the patient on a pulse oximeter and cardiac monitor.
- Start O_2.
- Consult OB/GYN.
- Obtain appropriate laboratory studies.
- Order a stat pelvic ultrasound.
- Type and cross for 2 to 4 units of packed RBCs.

17.6. Laboratory:

- CBC: WBC 13.2, Hgb 7.1, Hct 21.2, Plt 220,000
- Differential: Normal.
- Chemistry: Na 141, K 4.1, Cl 110, CO_2 24.
- BUN/Cr: 14/0.7.
- Glucose: 105.
- LFTs: Normal.
- Amylase/Lipase: Normal.
- B-HCG: 2,200.
- Type and Rh: B+.

- U/A: Normal.
- Urine pregnancy test: Positive.

17.7. Special Tests:
- Ultrasound: No intrauterine pregnancy, free fluid in the cul-de-sac.

17.8. Secondary Survey:
- General: After a fluid bolus, the nausea and dizziness is gone but the abdominal pain is worse.
- Skin: Pale, cool, dry.
- HEENT: Normal.
- Neck: Normal.
- Chest: Normal.
- Lungs: Normal.
- Heart: Tachycardia without a murmur.
- Abdomen: Mild distention, bowel sounds are diminished, pain to palpation in the suprapubic region. Rebound and guarding present.
- Pelvic: The uterus is 6 to 7 weeks in size with tenderness to palpation of both adnexa. No adnexal mass palpable. The cervical os is closed and no blood is present in the vaginal vault. Positive Hagar and Chadwick's sign.
- Rectal: Normal.
- Extremities: No edema.
- Neuro: Normal.

17.9. Management:
- After the ultrasound is completed, the gynecologist will take the patient to the OR.

17.10. Critical Actions:
- Obtain a menstrual history.
- Start IV rehydration.
- Order a pelvic ultrasound.
- Consult OB/GYN.
- Type and cross for 2 to 4 units of packed RBCs.

17.11. Pearls:

❍ **What is the classic triad of symptoms in ectopic pregnancy?**

Abdominal pain, amenorrhea, and vaginal bleeding. This is seen 15% of ectopic pregnancies.

❍ **What is the most common sign?**

Tenderness on pelvic examination is present in 85% to 97% of cases.

❍ **When can a gestational sac be detected in the uterus by transvaginal ultrasound?**

Five to six weeks of gestation corresponding to a quantitative β-HCG >1,500 mIU/mL.

CASE 18 (Red Painful Rash)

Examiner

The candidate should recognize this as the life-threatening condition called toxic epidermal necrolysis (TEN). Appropriate burn care (including the Parkland formula) should be used along with transfer to a burn center. The candidate should understand the difference between erythema multiforme minor, major, Stevens–Johnson syndrome, and TEN.

18.1. Introduction:

A 26 y/o female arrives by ambulance with a complaint of worsening rash over the past 5 days.

Vital signs: BP 110/60, P 112, R 22, T 100.6°F, Wt 74 kg.

18.2. Primary Survey:
- General: WN/WD female, awake, and oriented but lethargic. She is in no distress but appears uncomfortable.
- Airway: Intact.
- Breathing: Normal.
- Circulation: Capillary refill delayed, rapid pulse rate.
- Disability: Normal.
- Exposure: No medic alert tags. Large areas of denuded skin and blisters are present.
- Finger: Normal.

18.3. Management:
- Recognize the life-threatening dermatoses.
- Start two large bore IVs.
- Use the Parkland burn formula to calculate fluid needs.
- Place the patient on a cardiac monitor and pulse oximeter.
- Order appropriate diagnostic tests.
- Use standard burn treatment.
- Consult a burn specialist and arrange for transfer to a burn unit.

18.4. History:
- Allergies: None.
- Medications: An unknown, large, white pill given to her by a friend.
- PMH: Two pregnancies, both normal spontaneous vaginal deliveries. No other significant illnesses or injuries. No past surgeries.
- Last meal: 3 hours ago.
- Events: A 26 y/o female presents with a rash. She complained of dysuria 5 days ago so a friend gave her an unknown "bladder" antibiotic. After taking two doses of the unknown antibiotic, she noted large, red, painful lesions on her chest, legs, and arms. Within 24 hours, blisters formed and denuded skin developed. She also complained of anorexia, fever, joint aches, and malaise. She stopped taking the medication and disposed of them after the rash appeared.
- Family: Contact her friend and find out whether the medication she gave the patient was a sulfonamide.
- Records: None.
- Immune: Up to date.
- EMTs: In the ED break room.
- Narcotics: Denies illicit drug use.
- Doctor: None.
- Social history: Married, has two children. No alcohol or tobacco use.

18.5. Secondary Survey:
- General: No change since arrival to the ED.
- Skin: Blistering with denuded areas present, positive Nikolsky's sign. Sixty percent of the body surface is involved. Multiple red, target-like lesions, some with central clearing and others with a central grey bulla.
- HEENT: Small oral erosions, and bilateral injected sclera.
- Neck: Normal.
- Chest: Lesions present.
- Lungs: Tachypnea but no respiratory distress. Lungs clear to auscultation.
- Heart: Tachycardia without a murmur.
- Abdomen: Lesions present otherwise, normal.
- Pelvic: No rash, no vaginal discharge, normal bimanual examination.
- Rectal: No lesions, normal tone, hemoccult negative.
- Back: Lesions present.
- Extremities: Lesions that include the dorsum of the hands. The feet are spared.
- Neuro: Normal.

18.6. Laboratory:

- CBC: WBC 19, Hgb 12, Hct 36, Plt 275,000.
- Differential: Poly 45, bands 25, lymphs 25, eos 2, mono 1.
- Chemistry: Na 140, K 4.5, Cl 98, CO_2 14.
- BUN/Cr: 20/2.0.
- Glucose: 90.
- Ca/Mg: Normal.
- LFTs: Elevated.
- Amylase/Lipase: Normal.
- PT/PTT: Normal.
- ABG: pH 7.30, $pO_2$95, pCO_2 36, HCO_3 15.
- B-HCG: Negative.
- Blood cultures: Pending.
- U/A: Specific gravity 1.025, WBC 100, RBC 10, bacteria large amount, protein 3+ ketones 3+.
- Urine culture: Pending.

18.7. Critical Actions:

- Obtain the diagnosis and cause of toxic epidermal necrolysis.
- Use the Parkland formula to determine fluid requirements.
- Use burn techniques in handling the patient.
- Admit to a burn unit.
- Consult a burn specialist.

18.8. Pearls:

❍ **What is the etiology of toxic epidermal necrolysis and Stevens–Johnson syndrome?**

SJS/TEN is precipitated by drugs such as sulfonamides, barbiturates, phenytoin, phenylbutazone, or penicillin. Rare causes include a graft-versus-host reaction (after a bone marrow transplant) or administration of blood products.

❍ **What differentiates staphylococcal scalded skin syndrome (SSSS) from SJS/TEN?**

SSSS contracted by children younger than 5 years and it is because of a *Staph* toxin that spares the mucous membranes. Cleavage occurs within the epidermis, and has a mortality rate of less than 5%. SJS/TEN occurring primarily in adults is usually because of medications and often involves the mucous membranes. Cleavage occurs at the dermal–epidermal junction. The latter condition has a mortality rate of 5% to 50%.

❍ **What differentiates SJS from TEN?**

SJS and TEN are a disease continuum distinguished by severity, based upon the percentage of body surface involved with skin detachment. SJS is the less severe form, with skin detachment of <10% and two or more mucous membrane sites involved. TEN involves detachment of >30% of the body surface area along with mucous membrane involvement. SJS was once considered a severe form of erythema multiforme (major) but is now considered a different entity with different, distinct causes.

CASE 19 (Vomiting and Chest Pain)

Examiner

This is a case of Boerhaave's syndrome due to multiple episodes of forceful vomiting. The patient appears very uncomfortable and toxic. He will require immediate antibiotics and fluid resuscitation. It is appropriate to do a "cardiac" workup, which will be negative.

19.1. Introduction:

A 62 y/o male presents with a complaint of severe chest pain. He is accompanied by his wife.

Vital signs: BP 92/50, P 122, R 26, T 102.5°F, 110 kg.

19.2. Primary Survey:
- General: This is a WN/WD diaphoretic, anxious male in moderate distress.
- Airway: Patent, gag reflex intact.
- Breathing: Breath sounds are diminished on the left side, he is tachypneic, neck veins are flat, and the trachea is midline.
- Circulation: Skin is pale, capillary refill is delayed, and patient is tachycardic.
- Disability: GCS 15, PERRLA.
- Exposure: No medic alert tags.
- Finger: Rectal normal.

19.3. Management:
- Start two large bore IVs of LR or 0.9 NS.
- Administer multiple 250 cc fluid boluses until the pressure increases.
- Place on cardiac monitor and pulse oximeter.
- Order appropriate laboratory studies, x-rays, and an ECG.
- Insert an NG tube and a Foley catheter.

19.4. History:
- Allergies: None.
- Medications: None.
- PMH: Fractured right femur with rod placement 10 years ago.
- Last meal: 10 hours ago.
- Events: A 62 y/o male presents with chest pain. According to his wife, he felt "sick to his stomach" over the past 2 days. After eating breakfast this morning, he began vomiting. He drank some Pepto-Bismol and began complaining of severe left sided chest pain. Two hours ago, he became feverish, short of breath, and the chest pain worsened. He was previously healthy with no recent trauma noted.
- Family: Wife present to answer questions, family history noncontributory.
- Records: None.
- Immune: Up to date.
- Narcotics: Wife denies drug use.
- Doctor: No family physician.
- Social history: Drinks one beer per week, no tobacco use.

19.5. Secondary Survey:
- General: Patient is intubated in mild respiratory discomfort but he responds to commands.
- Skin: Warm, dry mucous membranes, no rash or petechiae.
- HEENT: Normal.
- Neck: Slight crepitance to palpation.
- Chest: Atraumatic, no palpable crepitance.
- Lungs: Diminished breath sounds on the left. Hamman's "crunch" present.
- Heart: Rapid rate, regular rhythm, no murmur.
- Abdomen: Mild epigastric tenderness present. Bowel sounds are normal, no masses, no organomegaly, no rebound, or guarding.
- Rectal: Normal, hemoccult negative.
- Back: Normal.
- Extremities: Normal.
- Neuro: No focal deficits, normal DTRs, patient obeys commands.

19.6. Laboratory:
- CBC: WBC 22, Hgb 13.5, Hct 42, Plt 150,000.
- Differential: Polys 80, bands 5%, lymphs 10, eos 1, mono 3.
- Chemistry: Na 135, K 4.0, Cl 101, CO_2 18.
- BUN/Cr: 12/1.2.

- Glucose: 110.
- Ca/Mg: Normal.
- LFTs: Normal.
- Amylase/Lipase: Normal.
- PT/PTT: Normal.
- Cardiac enzymes: Pending.
- ABG: pH 7.29, $pO_2$85, pCO_2 42, HCO_3 16 (before intubation, on room air).
- Blood cultures: Pending.
- U/A: Normal.
- D-dimer: Elevated.

19.7. X-rays:
- CXR: Large left pleural effusion with a radiopaque substance present. A 30% pneumothorax present on the left side.
- Lateral neck: Air is present in the retropharyngeal space.
- Esophagram: Extravasation of the water-soluble agent is seen in the left pleural space.
- CT chest: Not available.

19.8. Special Tests:
- ECG: Sinus tachycardia with nonspecific ST- and T-wave changes in the anterior leads.

19.9. Critical Actions:
- Initiate a cardiac workup.
- Identify the esophageal rupture and obtain an esophagram.
- Start IV fluid resuscitation.
- Administer broad spectrum antibiotic coverage (include anaerobic coverage).
- Consult a thoracic or general surgeon immediately.
- Insert a chest tube.

19.10. Pearls:

❍ **What is the most common area of rupture in the esophagus?**

Left side of the distal portion, which is a physiologically weakened area.

❍ **What is the role of esophagoscopy?**

This is performed if a perforation is suspected but cannot be confirmed by contrast studies, if there is upper gastrointestinal bleeding associated with a partial-thickness laceration, or if the patient is unconscious and a contrast study cannot be performed.

❍ **Why is early surgical repair important?**

If surgical repair is done in less than 24 hours, the mortality rate is 5%. However, if repair is delayed, the mortality reaches 75%.

CASE 20 (Child with Fever and Poor Appetite)

Examiner

The candidate should recognize this disease, know the diagnostic criteria, and start the appropriate therapy. The patient requires admission, but the parents are resistant until the potential complications are explained by the candidate.

20.1. Introduction:

A 3 y/o boy is brought in by his parents with a complaint of rash and fever.

Vital signs: BP 98/60, P 122, R 26, T 103.6°F, Wt 15 kg.

20.2. Primary Survey:
- General: WN/WD male, sitting with parents, appears uncomfortable, but in no distress.
- Airway: Intact.
- Breathing: Tachypnea, lungs clear.
- Circulation: Normal capillary refill, pulses strong and regular.
- Disability: Intact.
- Exposure: Child undressed except for underwear, no bruising, abrasions, or lacerations. Diffuse rash present.
- Finger: Intact.

20.3. Management:
- Patient is stable, proceed to the history and secondary survey.
- Laboratory and x-rays may be ordered now (not mandatory).

20.4. History:
- Allergies: None.
- Medications: Acetaminophen every 4 hours for past 2 days.
- PMH: No significant illnesses or injuries. No surgeries.
- Last meal: 2 hours ago.
- Events: A 3 y/o male brought in by mother. She states that he has had a fever and poor appetite for the past 6 days. Today, he broke out in a rash and his eyes started to drain. He has had no vomiting, diarrhea, cough, or abdominal pain.
- Family: Noncontributory.
- Records: None.
- Immune: Up to date.
- Doctor: The patient's pediatrician is available.
- Social history: The patient lives with parents and three brothers, all of which have been well. No smoking within the household, no pets, or recent carpet cleaning.

20.5. Secondary Survey:
- General: Nontoxic but ill appearing child.
- Skin: The rash is a raised, painful, deep red (scarlatiniform), plaque-like eruption present on the trunk, extremities (palms and soles), and perineum. No petechia or purpura
- HEENT: Normocephalic/atraumatic, PERRLA, EOM-I, fundi normal, conjunctiva injected. Throat is red, mucous membranes are moist, strawberry tongue present.
- Neck: Three large (2 cm) anterior cervical nodes present. No meningeal signs.
- Lungs: Normal.
- Heart: Tachycardia with a regular rhythm, no murmur or rub.
- Abdomen: Normal.
- Perineum/GU: Desquamation of the perineum present.
- Rectal: Deferred.
- Back: Rash as described above.
- Extremities: Rash as described above with involvement of the palms of the hands and soles of the feet.
- Neuro: Normal.

20.6. Laboratory:
- CBC: WBC 20, Hgb 12, Hct 35, Plt 550,000.
- Differential: Polys 80, bands 15%, lymphs 5, eos 1, mono 0.
- Chemistry: Na 140, K 4.5, Cl 98, CO_2 26.
- BUN/Cr: 10/1.0.
- Glucose: 95.
- Ca/Mg: Normal.
- LFTs: Normal.
- Amylase/Lipase: Normal.
- PT/PTT: Normal.

- Cardiac enzymes: Pending.
- Sed rate: 52.
- CRP: Elevated.
- Blood cultures: Pending.
- U/A: Normal.

20.7. X-rays:
- CXR: Normal.

20.8. Special Tests:
- ECG: Sinus tachycardia.
- Echocardiogram: Normal.

20.9. Critical Actions:
- Start IV gamma globulin infusion at 2 g/kg over 8 to 12 hours. (May refer to a reference).
- Administer aspirin, 80 to 100 mg/kg/d divided q 6 hours.
- Obtain CBC, Plt, and blood culture.
- Determine LFTs.
- Order an ECG.
- Admit.

20.10. Pearls:

❍ **Why should infusion of gamma globulin be started immediately?**

Early infusion of gamma globulin decreases the incidence of coronary artery aneurysms and promotes resolution of established aneurysms.

❍ **What are the diagnostic criteria for Kawasaki syndrome?**

Fever for at least 5 days along with the presence of four out of the following five conditions:

(1) Bilateral conjunctivitis
(2) Polymorphous rash
(3) Cervical adenopathy
(4) Extremity changes (erythema of palms and soles, edema of hands and feet, skin desquamation).
(5) Oral mucosa involvement

❍ **What is the purpose of aspirin therapy?**

Aspirin may reduce the tendency toward thrombosis and associated coronary artery aneurysms.

CASE 21 (Hand Numbness)

Examiner

This is a difficult case and obtaining an exact diagnosis is not required. The candidate should acquire an in depth history and physical examination, and should be able to develop a detailed differential diagnosis.

21.1. Introduction:

A 52 y/o female is brought in by wheelchair with a complaint of weakness and numbness in the arms and legs.

Vital signs: BP 138/60, P 60, R 21, T 99.6°F.

21.2. Primary Survey:
- General: WN/WD female, looks younger than the stated age, is in no apparent distress.
- Airway: Intact.
- Breathing: Tachypnea, lungs clear.
- Circulation: Normal.
- Disability: GCS 15, PERRLA.

- Exposure: No medic alert tags, no rash, bruising, or abrasions.
- Finger: Rectal deferred to secondary survey.

21.3. Management:

- No acute treatment is required at this time, may proceed to the history and secondary survey.
- Consider starting an IV of LR or 0.9 NS now.
- Consider placing on a pulse oximeter and cardiac monitor.

21.4. History:

- Allergies: None.
- Medications: None.
- PMH: No past illnesses or injuries. No past surgeries.
- Last meal: 3 hours ago.
- Events: A 52 y/o female states she was feeling well until about 2 days ago. She felt numbness to both hands which progressed to her arms, followed by both feet and legs. She awoke today unable to get out of bed and walk. She denies no recent illnesses, fever, chills, night sweats, blurred or double vision, cough or difficulty swallowing. In addition, she has not traveled recently and has no known tick exposure.
- Family: Noncontributory.
- Records: None.
- Immune: Last tetanus shot 15 years ago.
- Narcotics: Denies illicit drug use.
- Doctor: No family physician.
- Social history: No alcohol or tobacco use. Lives with husband and two adolescent children all of which have been well.

21.5. Secondary Survey:

- General: Pleasant, 52 y/o female in no acute distress.
- Skin: No rash, no ticks.
- HEENT: Normal.
- Neck: Normal, no meningeal signs.
- Chest: Breast examination normal, no mass.
- Lungs: Clear and equal breath sounds.
- Heart: Normal.
- Abdomen: Bladder is distended and painful to palpation. Otherwise, the examination is normal.
- Pelvic: Normal.
- Rectal: Poor tone, stool in vault, heme negative.
- Back: Normal.
- Extremities: Normal.
- Neuro: Alert and oriented times 3. CN II to XII intact. Patellar and Achilles reflexes absent bilaterally with bicep and tricep reflexes 1/4 and symmetric. The patient has diminished hand grip strength and she is unable to dorsiflex and plantarflex against resistance. All proximal muscle groups are strong and equal. She is unable to distinguish sharp versus dull discrimination to the lower extremities. Toes are downgoing and finger-to-nose test is normal. Unable to assess gait because of her inability to walk.

21.6. Laboratory:

- CBC: WBC 8, Hgb 12, Hct 35.2, Plt 250,000.
- Differential: Polys 58, bands 3%, lymphs 35, eos 1, mono 3.
- Chemistry: Na 140, K 3.5, Cl 99, CO_2 24.
- BUN/Cr: 10/1.0.
- Glucose: 106.
- Ca/Mg: Normal.
- LFTs: Normal.
- Amylase/Lipase: Normal.
- PT/PTT: Normal.
- Cardiac enzymes: Pending.

- ABG: Normal.
- Sedimentation rate: Normal.
- Blood cultures: Pending.
- U/A: Normal.
- ESR: Normal.
- CRP: Normal.

21.7. X-rays:
- CXR: Normal.
- CT head: Normal.

21.8. Special Tests:
- Pulse oximeter: 99%.
- ECG: Normal.
- Lumbar puncture: Color clear, WBC 1, RBC 2, protein 65, glucose 52, Gram stain negative.
- Pulm function tests: Pending.

21.9. Critical Actions:
- Complete a neurologic examination.
- Complete a detailed history, including questioning for tick exposure.
- Perform a lumbar puncture.
- Consult neurology.
- Admit.
- Obtain a CT of the head.

21.10. Pearls:

❍ **Discuss the pathophysiology of myasthenia gravis.**

Myasthenia gravis is the most common disorder of the neuromuscular junction. It is an autoimmune disorder directed against the acetylcholine receptors. It reduces the number of available receptors thereby impairing neuromuscular transmission.

❍ **Describe tick paralysis and its treatment.**

A reversible, rapidly progressive ascending paralysis beginning at the extremities and trunk and moving up to involve the bulbar musculature. Treatment involves finding the tick, removing it, and providing supportive care with resolution of symptoms noted in 24 to 48 hours.

CASE 22 (Male with Leg Pain)

Examiner

This is a sick patient who requires surgical intervention but needs stabilization first. He has a significant infection that has put him in DKA. He needs fluids, antibiotics, and correction of metabolic abnormalities.

22.1. Introduction:

A 51 y/o male presents with left lower leg swelling.

Vital signs: BP 130/80, P 130, R 28, T 102.4°F, Wt 122.6 kg.

22.2. Primary Survey:
- General: Obese male who appears toxic. He is hyperalert and sweating.
- Airway: Intact.
- Breathing: Tachypneic, bilateral breath sounds present.
- Circulation: Capillary refill is diminished.
- Disability: Normal.
- Exposure: No gross findings.
- Finger: Deferred to secondary survey.

22.3. Management:

- Start IV of NS or LR with a bolus of 1 to 2 L.
- Place the patient on a cardiac monitor and pulse oximeter.
- Obtain quick glucose.
- Order appropriate laboratory studies and x-rays.
- Call family members.

22.4. History:

- Allergies: None.
- Medications: Insulin, 45 units NPH and 21 units regular in the AM. Lisinopril 20 mg daily. Xanax, 0.5 mg prn, Lipitor 20 mg qd.
- PMH: IDDM, HTN, and hyperlipidemia.
- Last meal: 24 hours ago.
- Events: *A 51 y/o male states he noticed swelling and increasing pain to his left leg over the past 3 days. He also complained of fever, chills, anorexia, night sweats, and polyuria. He denies nausea, vomiting, or diarrhea. The patient "scratched" his leg 5 days ago while he was working in his garden.*
- Family: Family history of stroke, HTN, and heart disease.
- Records: Medical records department is unable to find his records.
- Immune: Up to date.
- Narcotics: No illicit drug use.
- Doctor: His doctor is out of town.
- Social history: Married, has three children. He does not drink or smoke.

22.5. Secondary Survey:

- General: Patient appears uncomfortable and continues to be diaphoretic and anxious.
- Skin: Pale, moist, no rash.
- HEENT: Normal.
- Neck: Normal.
- Chest: Normal.
- Lungs: Tachypneic, clear to auscultation bilateral.
- Heart: Tachycardia, no murmur, or extra sounds.
- Abdomen: Soft, decreased bowel sounds; mild-to-moderate tenderness in the suprapubic region.
- Perineum/GU: Circumcised penis, nontender testicles.
- Rectal: Normal rectal, normal prostate, heme negative stool.
- Back: Normal.
- Extremities: Left lower leg is large, swollen, with purulent drainage from an open wound. Crepitance is felt.
- Neuro: Normal.

22.6. Laboratory:

- CBC: WBC 25, Hgb 16, Hct 53, Plt 225,000.
- Differential: Polys 35, bands 27%, lymphs 25, eos 4, mono 1.
- Chemistry: Na 148, K 4.8, Cl 108, CO_2 10.
- Anion gap: 30.
- BUN/Cr: 36/1.7.
- Glucose: 730.
- Ca/Mg: 11/1.4.
- LFTs: Normal.
- Amylase/Lipase: Normal.
- PT/PTT/INR: 17/41/1.2.
- Cardiac enzymes: Normal.
- CRP/ESR: Elevated.
- VBG: pH 7.16, pO_2 47, pCO_2 45, HCO_3 13.
- ABG: pH 7.15, pO_2 93, pCO_2 29, HCO_3 12.
- Lactate: 2.7

- Blood cultures: Pending.
- Serum ketone: Moderate.
- U/A: Glucose 4+, ketone 3+, protein 250, nitrite negative, leukocyte negative, RBC 1, WBC 6.

22.7. X-rays:
- CXR: Normal.
- Left leg: Gas present in the tissue. No foreign body, no fracture.
- CT left leg: Gas diffusely present.

22.8. Special Tests:
- ECG: Sinus tachycardia, otherwise normal.

22.9. Critical Actions:
- Start IV fluid rehydration.
- Perform a quick glucose test.
- Determine ABG or VBG.
- Administer insulin with or without a bolus.
- Order an ECG.
- Obtain an x-ray and/or CT to identify free air in the left leg.
- Start appropriate antibiotics (anaerobic) in the ED.
- Obtain intensive care consult.
- Stat surgery consult.

22.10. Pearls:

❍ **What is the initial treatment for DKA?**

IV fluids. Glucose-induced diuresis produces deficits averaging 5 L. Replace fluids with 0.9% normal saline at 1 L/h for the first 2 to 3 hours.

❍ **What are the precipitating factors leading to DKA?**

Noncompliance with medications, infection, myocardial infarction, CVA, trauma, pregnancy, pancreatitis, or emotional stress.

CASE 23 (Triple)

Patient #1 (Altered Level of Consciousness)

Examiner

This patient is in need of a quick diagnosis, glucose check (fingerstick glucose >700), and fluid resuscitation. After a 500 cc bolus of NS, the patient will stabilize. The abdominal pain will persist and IV pain medication is appropriate once the diagnosis is made.

23.1. Introduction: (**Patient #1**)

A 70 y/o female presents, via ambulance, from a nursing home, with a complaint of altered level of consciousness.

Vital signs: BP 80/40, P 130, R 30, T 100.2°F, Wt 89.6 kg.

23.2. Primary Survey:
- General: Chronically ill-appearing female with rapid respirations and tachycardic, moans to painful stimuli.
- Airway: Intact.
- Breathing: Fine bibasilar crackles.
- Circulation: Poor turgor, delayed capillary refill.
- Disability: PERRL, incomprehensible sounds, eyes open to pain.
- Exposure: No medic alert tags.

23.3. Management:

- Perform a quick bedside glucose test.
- Start IV bolus of NS (500 cc). If given, the patient becomes more alert.
- Place on cardiac monitor, pulse oximeter, and O_2.
- Order appropriate laboratory studies and x-rays.

23.4. History:

- Allergies: None.
- Medications: Lasix, 40 mg po daily. Glyburide, 2.5 mg po daily. Colace, daily. Zantac, 150 mg po bid. Lisinopril 20 mg po daily.
- PMH: Dementia, NIDDM, HTN, chronic gastritis.
- Last meal: 3 hours ago.
- Events: Information from EMTs and nursing home records.
- Family: Unknown.
- Records: None.
- Immune: Up to date.
- EMTs: *According to the EMTs, the staff at the nursing home noticed a decreased appetite, altered level of consciousness, and increasing lethargy.*
- Doctor: Private physician available for admission and information.
- Social history: Unknown.

23.5. Secondary Survey:

- General: If a fluid bolus is given the patient appears more awake.
- Skin: Dry mucosa, poor turgor, no rash.
- HEENT: Bilateral cataracts, cracked dry lips.
- Neck: Normal.
- Chest: Normal.
- Lungs: Bilateral fine crackles.
- Heart: Tachycardia, 3/6 systolic ejection murmur.
- Abdomen: Firm, bowel sounds present, tenderness over the epigastric region. No organomegaly, negative Cullen's, negative Grey–Turner's.
- Perineum/GU: Normal.
- Rectal: Heme negative.
- Back: Normal.
- Extremities: Normal.
- Neuro: Patient responds with incomprehensible sounds and localizes to painful stimuli. DTRs normal, no focal deficits. Toes downgoing.

The nurse interrupts stating another patient is in room 2 and appears very uncomfortable. Patient #1 is stable enough for the candidate to completely evaluate patients #2 and #3.

Patient #2 (Child with a Limp)

Examiner

This is a straight forward case of a child with septic arthritis. Allow the candidate to complete the case before patient #3 arrives.

23.1. Introduction: (**Patient #2**)

A 4 y/o male presents with a limp. He is accompanied by his parents.

Vital signs: BP 100/50, P 120, R 20, T 101.2°F, Wt 19.7 kg.

23.2. Primary Survey:
- General: WN/WD 4 y/o male, uncomfortable, but nontoxic appearing.
- Airway: Intact.
- Breathing: Normal.
- Circulation: Normal.
- Disability: Normal.
- Exposure: Swelling to the left knee.
- Finger: Deferred.

23.3. Management:
- Start IV.
- Administer bolus of 400 cc NS (20 mL/kg).
- Order appropriate laboratory studies and x-rays.

23.4. History:
- Allergies: None.
- Medications: None.
- PMH: No significant illnesses or injuries. No past surgeries.
- Last meal: 2 hours ago.
- Events: *The mother states that her child fell in the driveway 4 days ago sustaining an abrasion to the left knee. Yesterday his knee began to swell and today he started to vomit. He is previously healthy and active. No complaints of a rash, abdominal pain, diarrhea, cough, or sore throat.*
- Family: Noncontributory.
- Records: None.
- Immune: Up to date.
- Doctor: Family doctor is available.
- Social history: The patient lives with both natural parents and three older siblings. No indication of physical abuse.

23.5. Secondary Survey:
- General: Alert and happy with no signs of distress.
- Skin: Warm, dry, no rash, or petechiae. Moist mucous membranes.
- HEENT: Normal.
- Neck: Normal.
- Chest: Normal.
- Lungs: Normal.
- Heart: Normal.
- Abdomen: Normal.
- Perineum/GU: Normal.
- Rectal: Deferred.
- Back: Normal.
- Extremities: Warm, swollen, and red left knee. Decreased range of motion, cries when you attempt to examine it. Pulses are present distal to the knee. No other joints are involved.
- Neuro: Normal.

23.6. Laboratory:
- CBC: WBC 19, Hgb 15, Hct 46, Plt 450,000.
- Differential: Poly 80, bands 25, lymphs 15, eos 1, mono 3.
- Chemistry: Na 140, K 4.5, Cl 109, CO_2 22.
- BUN/Cr: 10/1.0.
- Glucose: 80.
- Ca/Mg: Normal.
- LFTs: Normal.

- Amylase/Lipase: Normal.
- PT/PTT: Normal.
- ESR: 88.
- Blood cultures: Pending.
- U/A: Normal.
- Lactate: 1.7
- CRP: 20.4

23.7. X-rays:
- CXR: Normal.
- Left knee: No air, no fracture, or periosteal reaction. Significant soft tissue swelling is present.

23.8. Special Tests:
- Joint fluid: WBC 75,000, Glc 30, Poly 80%, turbid, Gram stain pending.

23.9. Critical Actions:
- Start IV line.
- Order appropriate laboratory studies.
- Admit.
- Start antibiotics in the ED.
- Arthrocentesis.

Patient #3 (55 y/o Female Overdose)

Examiner

This patient has taken an intentional overdose of a β-blocker. The information should be hidden from the candidate until late in the case when her sister brings in the empty bottle and reveals that she has been depressed lately. The patient will be unable to provide any information until treated with glucagon.

23.1. Introduction: (**Patient #3**)

A 55 y/o female is brought by the family who states she is tired and keeps vomiting.

Vital signs: BP 80/P, P 50, R 20, T 98.8°F, Wt 82 kg.

23.2. Primary Survey:
- General: WN/WD female who looks younger than the stated age presents confused, disoriented, and lethargic.
- Airway: Intact.
- Breathing: Normal.
- Circulation: Delayed capillary refill, pulse regular but slow.
- Disability: PERRLA, opens eyes spontaneously, obeys verbal commands, disoriented.
- Exposure: Medic alert tags indicated she has hypertension.
- Finger: Heme negative stools.

23.3. Management:
- Start IV fluids with a 250 cc bolus of NS. May repeat.
- Place on O_2, pulse oximeter, and cardiac monitor.
- Order appropriate laboratory studies, x-rays, and an ECG.
- Interview the family members and have family bring all pill bottles.
- Candidate may administer atropine and dopamine when the pressure doesn't respond to fluids (this will also not work).
- Perform stat bedside glucose check.
- Administer Narcan.

23.4. History:
- Allergies: Unknown.
- Medications: Unknown.
- PMH: HTN, no previous suicide attempts.
- Last meal: Unknown.
- Events: *According to her younger sister, she has been feeling depressed for the past year since her husband died. The family thought she was doing better because she seemed more "content" recently. She currently sold her house and moved in with her sister. She is otherwise in very good health and has no major complaints.*
- Family: Family present for questioning.
- Records: None.
- Immune: Unknown.
- Narcotics: No history of illicit drug use according to the family.
- Doctor: Family doctor is available, if needed.
- Social history: No tobacco use, employed as a lawyer in an accounting firm.

23.5. Secondary Survey:
- General: Confused, but responds to commands.
- Skin: Normal.
- HEENT: Normal.
- Neck: Normal.
- Chest: Normal.
- Lungs: Normal.
- Heart: Bradycardia without a murmur or extra sounds.
- Abdomen: Normal.
- Perineum/GU: Normal.
- Rectal: Heme negative.
- Back: Normal.
- Extremities: Normal.
- Neuro: Normal.

Examiner

The older sister of the patient brings back an empty bottle of propranolol which was refilled 3 days ago. There are 60 pills missing. No other medications were noted but a suicide note was found. The candidate should immediately be treated with glucagon, 3 to 10 mg IV every, 15 to 20 minutes until improvement is seen. If glucagon is given, the patient will get better and become more responsive.

23.6. Laboratory:
- CBC: WBC 11, Hgb 12.2, Hct 39, Plt 255,000.
- Chemistry: Na 144, K 4.4, Cl 115, CO_2 23.
- BUN/Cr: 12/1.0.
- Glucose: 105.
- Ca/Mg: Normal.
- LFTs: Normal.
- Amylase/Lipase: Normal.
- PT/PTT: Normal.
- Cardiac enzymes: Normal.
- ABG: pH 7.43, pO_2 98, pCO_2 40, HCO_3 21 (room air).
- Blood cultures: Pending.
- Salicylate: Negative.
- Acetaminophen: Negative.
- Anion gap: 6.

- Osmolality: 290.
- Osmo gap: 10.
- ETOH: Negative.
- U/A: Normal.
- Urine drug screen: Negative.

23.7. X-rays:
- CXR: Normal.
- CT head: Normal.

23.8. Special Tests:
- ECG: Sinus bradycardia without ectopy or heart block.
- Pulse oximeter: 100% on room air.
- Cardiac monitor: Sinus bradycardia.

23.9. Critical Actions:
- Start IV fluids, O_2, and cardiac monitor.
- Obtain a history of depression and overdose with propranolol.
- Treat the low BP and altered level of consciousness with fluids and appropriate medications (glucose, Narcan, atropine, and possibly dopamine).
- Administer glucagon after determining a β-blocker is involved.
- Check salicylate, acetaminophen, urine drug screen, serum ETOH.
- Admit to the ICU.
- Place the patient on suicide precautions.
- Obtain a psychiatric consult.

Patient #1 (Altered Level of Consciousness)

23.6. Laboratory:
- CBC: WBC 18, Hgb 15.5, Hct 54, Plt 400,000.
- Differential: Polys 60, bands 27%, lymphs 11, eos 2, mono 0.
- Chemistry: Na 150, K 5.6, Cl 120, CO_2 22.
- BUN/Cr: 48/2.7.
- Glucose: 1,205.
- Ca/Mg: 11.0/1.5.
- Phosphorus: 2.2.
- LFTs: Normal.
- Amylase/Lipase: 360/2,102.
- PT/PTT: Normal.
- Cardiac enzymes: Normal.
- ABG: pH 7.35, pO_2 85, pCO_2 46, HCO_3 22.
- Serum ketones: Negative.
- Blood cultures: Pending.
- U/A: Protein 300, glucose 3+, ketone negative, WBC 0, RBC 0.
- Lactate: 2.9.

23.7. X-rays:
- CXR: Normal.
- Abdominal series: Sentinel loop with calcifications in the area of the pancreas. No free air.
- CT abdomen/pelvis: No pseudocyst, pancreatic inflammation, no other abnormalities.

23.8. Special Tests:
- Cardiac monitor: Sinus tachycardia.
- Pulse oximeter: 94% on room air.

23.9. Critical Actions:

- Start IV, O_2, and place on monitor.
- Administer fluid bolus.
- Check bedside glucose.
- Order appropriate laboratory studies.
- Relieve patient's pain.

23.10. Pearls: (**Patient #1** HHS)

❍ **What predisposing factors precipitate hyperosmolar, hyperglycemic state (HHS)?**

Chronic renal insufficiency, pneumonia, gram-negative sepsis, myocardial infarction, pancreatitis, GI bleeding, and medication (thiazide diuretics, phenytoin, propranolol, cimetidine, and corticosteroids).

❍ **What are the indications for insulin in HHS?**

Severe acidosis, hyperkalemia, or renal failure.

23.11. Pearls: (**Patient #2** Septic Arthritis)

❍ **What are the bacterial etiologies of septic arthritis in children and adolescents?**

Staphylococcus aureus and Group B *streptococcus* are the most common pathogens in the first 2 months of life. From 3 months to 3 years, *Haemophilus influenzae* type B and *S. aureus* are the most common. *H. influenzae* has decreased since advent of the HIB vaccine. After the age of 3 years, *S. aureus* predominates until adolescence, when *Neisseria gonorrhea* becomes a frequent cause.

❍ **How does septic arthritis occur?**

Seeding of a joint with bacteria occurs either by hematogenous spread, direct inoculation, or spread from an adjacent site of infection. Hematogenous dissemination is secondary to the spread of colonized invasive organisms that breach mucosal defenses, resulting in bacteremia.

23.12. Pearls: (**Patient #3** β-Blocker Overdose)

❍ **Why is glucagon useful in the treatment of β-blocker overdose?**

IV glucagon enhances myocardial contractility, heart rate, and AV conduction by stimulating the production of intracellular cyclic AMP.

❍ **What are the potential ECG abnormalities seen in a β-blocker overdose?**

Sinus bradycardia, first-degree block, widening of the QRS complex, peaked T-waves, and ST changes.

❍ **What clinical presentation may be seen with β-blocker poisoning?**

Bradyarrhythmias, hypotension, conduction abnormalities, CHF (more likely in those with heart disease), bronchospasm (especially in those with a history of bronchospasm), seizures, altered mental status, and hypoglycemia.

CASE 24 (Uncooperative 70 y/o Male)

Examiner

This patient has alcoholic ketoacidosis with lice and will refuse to cooperate and will be combative. His neighbor gives an accurate history. He will require sedation and IV rehydration will normalize his vital signs and mental status.

24.1. Introduction:

A 70 y/o male is brought by ambulance screaming obscenities.

Vitals signs: BP 140/75, P 114, R 34, T 99.6°F, Wt 98 kg.

24.2. Primary Survey:
- General: Unkept, unshaven, obese male holding his abdomen, and smelling of alcohol with lice covering his body.
- Airway: Intact.
- Breathing: Tachypneic.
- Circulation: Rapid thready pulse.
- Disability: Normal.
- Exposure: No medic alert tags.
- Finger: Trace positive blood in stool.

24.3. Management:
- Start IV of NS with a 500 cc bolus.
- Perform bedside glucose check (35 mg/dL).
- Place on cardiac monitor, pulse oximeter, and O_2.
- Sedate to calm the patient.
- Order appropriate laboratory studies, CXR, head CT scan, and ECG.
- Administer thiamine, 100 mg IM or IV.

24.4. History:
- Allergies: None.
- Medications: None.
- PMH: His neighbor is unsure of his past medical problems. She does not remember whether he had his gallbladder or appendix removed.
- Last meal: 2 days ago.
- Events: *According to a neighbor, the patient drinks alcohol. However, he told her last night that he stopped drinking because of abdominal pain. The neighbor checked on him this morning and he was still complaining of abdominal pain and felt nauseated with one to two episodes of vomiting. She forced the patient to come to the ED.*
- Family: Unknown.
- Records: None.
- Immune: Unknown.
- EMTs: They are present to comment on his appearance.
- Narcotics: No illicit drug use.
- Doctor: None.
- Social history: Retired lawyer. Divorced four times. Smokes two packs of cigarettes per day and drinks about one-fifth of bourbon daily.

24.5. Secondary Survey:
- General: As above. If given a fluid bolus and glucose, he will be more awake and alert.
- Skin: Multiple old well-healed scars and bruises of varying age. Pruritic rash, located in genital region.
- HEENT: Left frontal ecchymosis, beefy red tongue, dental caries, PERRLA, EOM-I. Fundi normal.
- Neck: Normal.
- Chest: Tenderness to palpation along left ribs, old ecchymosis present.
- Lungs: Tachypnea, diffused rhonchi.
- Heart: Tachycardia. No murmur, rub, or gallop.
- Abdomen: Tenderness to the epigastric region without guarding.
- Perineum/GU: Atrophic testicles.
- Rectal: Trace guaiac positive stools, normal prostate.
- Back: Normal.
- Extremities: No clubbing, wasted musculature present, no edema.
- Neuro: Resting tremor is present, otherwise normal.

24.6. Laboratory:
- CBC: WBC 4.4, Hgb 12.3, Hct 34.7, Plt 145,000.
- Differential: Polys 77, bands 2%, lymphs 18, eos 2, mono 5.
- Chemistry: Na 146, K 5.2, Cl 108, CO_2 23.

- BUN/Cr: 30/1.1.
- Glucose: 35.
- Ca/Mg: 8.4/1.6.
- Phosphorus: 2.8.
- LFTs: Normal.
- Amylase/Lipase: 350/200.
- PT/PTT: 13/38.
- Cardiac enzymes: Normal.
- ABG: pH 7.15, pO_2 94, pCO_2 27, HCO_3 10.
- Blood cultures: Pending.
- Anion gap: 13.
- Osmolality: 370.
- Serum acetone: Moderate.
- ETOH: 20.
- U/A: Normal.
- Lactate: 0.7

24.7. X-rays:
- CXR: No pneumothorax or infiltrate.
- CT head: Diffuse cortical atrophy.

24.8. Special Tests:
- ECG: Sinus tachycardia.
- Wood's lamp: Fluoresce nits.
- Microscopic: *Pthirus pubis.*

24.9. Critical Actions:
- Start IV with fluid bolus.
- Perform bedside glucose test with correction of low sugar.
- Order appropriate laboratory studies, x-rays, and ECG.
- Obtain an ABG or VBG.
- Add thiamine, vitamins, and magnesium to IV.
- Order head CT scan.
- Sedate accordingly.
- Admit to a monitored bed.
- Contact isolation.

24.10. Pearls:

❍ **Why would a patient with alcoholic ketoacidosis be negative for ketone bodies?**

There are three types of ketone bodies; acetone and the two acids, β-hydroxybutyrate (β-HB) and acetoacetate (Ac–Ac). The nitroprusside reaction, commonly used to detect ketones, may give a false negative because only Ac–Ac and acetone cause a positive reaction and β-HB is the dominant ketone in AKA.

❍ **What is the classic historical presentation for a patient with AKA?**

The patient is a chronic alcoholic with poor caloric intake, vomiting, anorexia, abdominal pain, and a recent termination of binge drinking. Patients often present 24 to 48 hours after last alcohol use.

CASE 25 (Altered Mental Status)

Examiner

This is a case of hyperthermia (heat stroke) with rhabdomyolysis, requiring rapid immediate cooling. If cooling is performed, the patient will respond by becoming more responsive and the neurologic findings will disappear. Only state the temperature when asked a second time by the candidate. Have the candidate describe their cooling technique of choice, in detail.

25.1. Introduction:

A 70 y/o female arrives, via ambulance, with an acute altered level of consciousness.

Vital signs: BP 90/P, P 120, R 36, Wt 80 kg.

25.2. Primary Survey:

- General: Obtunded female, speaking incomprehensible words.
- Airway: Intact.
- Breathing: Lungs clear, tachypneic.
- Circulation: Rapid thready pulse, delayed capillary refill.
- Disability: PERRL. Opens eyes to verbal command, localizes pain, incomprehensible words.
- Exposure: No medic alert tags.
- Finger: Negative.

25.3. Management:

- Determine rectal temperature (106.5°F) with continuous rectal temperature probe or temperature sensing Foley catheter.
- Start IV of NS and give a 500 mL bolus.
- Place on cardiac monitor, pulse oximeter, and O_2.
- Insert Foley catheter—rose colored urine.
- Order appropriate laboratory studies.
- Begin rapid cooling.
- Administer Narcan and check the glucose.

25.4. History:

- Allergies: Unknown.
- Medications: Unknown.
- PMH: Unknown.
- Last meal: Unknown.
- Events: *A neighbor called the EMTs because the patient has not left her apartment for 4 days and does not answer the door or phone. The neighbor does not know anything else about the history of the patient.*
- Family: Unknown.
- Records: None.
- Immune: Unknown.
- EMTs: They noted the apartment was hot, the windows were closed, and the patient was lying on the bed asleep. No pill bottles or alcohol were present in the house.
- Narcotics: Unknown.
- Doctor: The internist on call is available.
- Social history: Unknown.

25.5. Secondary Survey:

- General: Patient is more awake and gives some history, if appropriate cooling measures and fluids are given.
- Skin: Hot, dry, pale.
- HEENT: Dry, parched mouth. Otherwise, normal.
- Neck: Normal.
- Chest: Normal.
- Lungs: Tachypneic.
- Heart: Tachycardia without murmur.
- Abdomen: Normal.
- Perineum/GU: Normal.
- Rectal: Hemoccult negative.
- Back: Normal.
- Extremities: Normal.
- Neuro: Cranial nerves intact. DTRs hyperactive and equal. Toes upgoing bilateral. Unable to assess cerebellar function.

25.6. Laboratory:

- CBC: WBC 22, Hgb 14, Hct 41, Plt 92,000.
- Chemistry: Na 148, K 4.5, Cl 120, CO_2 24.
- BUN/Cr: 40/1.7.
- Glucose: 80.
- Ca/Mg: Normal.
- LFTs: AST 300, ALT 222, 45, GGT 80, Alk Phosp 110.
- Amylase/Lipase: Normal.
- PT/PTT: 13/25.
- Cardiac enzymes: CPK 31,510, CKMB 2%, Troponin 0.11
- ABG: pH 7.40, pO_2 92, pCO_2 40, HCO_3 23.
- Blood cultures: Pending.
- U/A: 0 WBC, 0 RBC.
- Urine dip: Positive for blood and protein.
- Urine myoglobin: Positive.

25.7. X-rays:

- CXR: Normal.
- CT head: Normal.

25.8. Special Tests:

- ECG: Sinus tachycardia without abnormalities.
- Pulse oximeter: 93% on room air.
- Cardiac monitor: Sinus tachycardia without ectopy.

25.9. Critical Actions:

- Recognize hyperthermia and begin rapid cooling.
- Recognize rhabdomyolysis and initiate treatment with volume resuscitation.
- Place on O_2 and monitor cardiac responses.
- Insert Foley catheter.
- Order CBC, chemistry profile, LFTs, coagulation studies, U/A, urine myoglobin, and ECG.
- Admit to the ICU.

25.10. Pearls:

❍ **What is the etiology and treatment for myoglobinuria?**

The cause is rhabdomyolysis, and the treatment is IV hydration, osmotic diuretics, and alkalinization of the urine.

❍ **Which medications can cause hyperthermia?**

Neuroleptic agents, anticholinergics, salicylate toxicity, PCP, amphetamine, cocaine, and lithium.

CASE 26 (Malnourished Homeless Male)

Examiner

This patient presents with an altered level of consciousness because of hypothermia. The candidate should use a rectal probe because standard thermometers monitor only down to a temperature of 95° F. Implementing a coma protocol is required. If the candidate aggressively warms the patient, he will become more responsive. If not, he will go into VF and will remain in VF until he is warmed.

26.1. Introduction:

A 45 y/o, homeless male presents, via ambulance, unconscious.

Vital signs: BP 90/P, P 50, R 10, Wt 74.6 kg.

26.2. Primary Survey:
- General: Give the temperature as 95°F unless the candidate asks for a rectal probe. The probe will read 80°F. The patient is a poorly nourished male, who is unresponsive to painful stimuli with a poor respiratory effort.
- Airway: Intact.
- Breathing: Decreased respiratory rate.
- Circulation: Capillary refill 4 seconds.
- Disability: Pupils dilated and nonreactive.
- Exposure: No medic alert tags, no gross abnormalities. A bottle of whiskey is in his pocket.
- Finger: Hemoccult negative.

26.3. Management:
- Intubate with c-spine precaution.
- Start two large bore IVs. Infuse 250 mL bolus of warm saline and continue warm saline.
- Apply an external warming device.
- Insert an NG tube and a Foley catheter. Remove all clothing.
- Place on cardiac monitor and pulse oximeter.
- Order appropriate laboratory studies, x-rays, and an ECG.
- Administer naloxone IV, and check the glucose.
- Active core rewarming.

26.4. History:
- Allergies: Unknown.
- Medications: Unknown.
- PMH: Unknown.
- Last meal: Unknown.
- Family: None.
- Records: None.
- Immune: Unknown.
- EMTs: The patient was found behind a building unconscious, wet, cold without signs of trauma.
- Narcotics: Unknown.
- Doctor: Unknown.
- Social history: Unavailable.

26.5. Secondary Survey:
- General: No change from the primary survey.
- Skin: Cold, moist, clammy, poor turgor, old healed scars.
- HEENT: Normocephalic and atraumatic head. Pupils dilated, nonreactive; Fundi normal.
- Neck: Supple, no JVD, no nodes.
- Chest: Atraumatic. No palpable crepitance.
- Lungs: Clear.
- Heart: Bradycardic without a murmur.
- Abdomen: Soft, bowel sounds decreased. No mass, no organomegaly.
- Perineum/GU: Normal.
- Rectal: Normal.
- Back: Normal.
- Extremities: Diminished pulses, abrasions to the left forearm.
- Neuro: No eye opening, incomprehensible sounds, and flexion withdraw reaction to pain. Toes equivocal. DTRs +1/+4 and symmetric.

26.6. Laboratory:
- CBC: WBC 7.5, Hgb 18, Hct 59, Plt 35,000.
- Differential: Polys 70, bands 3%, lymphs 20, eos 1, mono 3.
- Chemistry: Na 140, K 4.5, Cl 106, CO_2 24.
- BUN/Cr: 28/1.6.

- Glucose: 130.
- Ca/Mg: Normal.
- LFTs: Normal.
- Amylase/Lipase: 300/650.
- PT/PTT: 17/45.
- Cardiac enzymes: Normal.
- ETOH: 355.
- ABG: pH 7.16, pO_2 90, pCO_2 50, HCO_3 24.
- Blood cultures: Pending.
- Urine drug: Negative.
- U/A: Negative.

26.7. X-rays:
- CXR: Normal.
- Pelvis: Normal.
- CT head/c-spine: Normal.
- Left forearm: Normal.

26.8. Special Tests:
- Cardiac monitor: Sinus bradycardia.
- Pulse oximeter: 86% on room air initially.
- ECG: Sinus bradycardia with Osborne J-waves.

26.9. Critical Actions:
- Intubate with c-spine precautions.
- Obtain an accurate core temperature.
- Perform active rewarming.
- Insert an NG tube and a Foley catheter.
- Place on cardiac monitor.
- Administer tetanus, 0.5 cc IM.
- Obtain CT scan of the head.
- Admit to the ICU.

26.10. Pearls:

❍ **What constitutes active rewarming?**

Techniques that warm the core of the body directly. Such techniques include heated IV fluids, peritoneal lavage, gastrointestinal and bladder irrigation, heated inhalation, thoracostomy tube irrigation, and extracorporeal rewarming.

❍ **What are the indications for active rewarming?**

When the temperature is below 90°F, cardiovascular instability, neurologic, or endocrinologic insufficiency.

CASE 27 (Child with a Sore Throat)

Examiner

This is a 4 y/o male that presents, via EMS, with epiglottitis on arrival. The candidate should avoid any painful tests or procedures. The crash cart should be available while calls are made to anesthesia, and ENT.

Once initial stabilization is achieved, the emergency physician should be asked to see a patient with an ankle injury that is demanding immediate attention. The candidate should ask the nurse to obtain x-rays but they should not leave the patient's bedside. If they do, the patient requires immediate crash intubation and results in the patient's death. The role of ED physician should be close observation without active intervention until the appropriate consultants are immediately available.

27.1. Introduction:

A 4 y/o child presents, via EMS, with a sore throat, drooling, and difficulty in breathing.

Vital signs: BP N/A, P 120, R 30, T N/A, Wt 19 kg.

Nurse should be instructed to take P and RR, avoid BP and T.

27.2. Primary Survey:

- General: Toxic appearing child is sitting propped up on his hands with his head forward and his tongue out.
- Airway: Avoid examination of airway. If airway is examined the child immediately goes into respiratory distress, intubation is impossible, and the child dies.
- Breathing: Child is moving air. Stridor. Lungs clear and equal.
- Circulation: Distal pulse intact, rate of 120.
- Disability: Alert, moving all extremities.
- Exposure: Avoid.
- Finger: Avoid.

27.3. Management:

- Ensure that a pediatric crash cart is located at bedside.
- Place an immediate call to anesthesiology.
- Call ENT.
- Allow the mother to remain with child.

27.4. History:

- Allergies: None.
- Medications: None.
- PMH: None.
- Last meal: 8 hours ago.
- Events: Child has had a cough, sore throat, and fever today, which has quickly worsened.
- Family: None.
- Records: None.
- Immune: Child is Hispanic and his family is visiting the United States. The child has not received the Haemophilus B vaccine.
- EMTs: No treatment given.
- Narcotics: None.
- Doctor: Pages to Dr. Pediatrician, Dr. Anesthesiologist, and Dr. ENT.
- Social history: None.

27.5. Secondary Survey:

- General: Toxic 4 y/o in moderate respiratory distress. Distress increases, if any active intervention occurs.
- Skin: Warm and dry.
- HEENT: Drooling.
- Neck: Avoid.
- Chest: Tachypnea.
- Lungs: Clear.
- Heart: Regular and tachycardic.
- Abdomen: Avoid.
- Rectal: Avoid.
- Back: No gross abnormality.
- Extremities: No gross abnormality.
- Neuro: Toxic. Moving all extremities.

27.6. Laboratory:

- Avoid laboratory draws.
- Pulse oximeter 96%.

27.7. X-rays:
- CXR: Avoid.
- Soft tissue neck: Avoid.

27.8. Critical Actions:
- Ensure that intubation equipment is readily available, including needle cricothyrotomy.
- Page anesthesiology and ENT quickly.
- Prepare OR for patient.
- Avoid unnecessary interventions (blood draws, monitors, and radiographs).
- Allow patient to remain with parent.
- Avoid leaving patient's bedside.

27.9. Pearls:

❍ **What is the most common cause of epiglottitis in children and in adults?**

Children: *Haemophilus influenzae* type B. Adults: *Staph aureus*, Group A Streptococcus *Haemophilus influenzae* type B.

❍ **If *Haemophilus influenzae* is isolated, what should be done for family members and close contacts?**

Close contacts and family members younger than 4 years, should be treated with rifampin.

CASE 28 (Bite Wound)

Examiner

The patient is intoxicated. With some difficulty, the physician learns the patient was bitten in the buttocks when he sat on a snake while at a campfire. He has had increasing pain and swelling of the buttock and feels light-headed since the event occurred 1 hour ago. The patient has a high envenomation bite and eventually requires antivenom.

28.1. Introduction:

A 24 y/o male, very intoxicated, complaining of pain.

Vital signs: BP 80/60, P 128, R 20, T 99°F, Wt 89.5 kg.

28.2. Primary Survey:
- General: Intoxicated, very wild, poor historian, complaining of severe pain.
- Airway: Intact.
- Breathing: Regular.
- Circulation: Tachycardic.
- Disability: None.
- Exposure: Buttocks swelling and two clear puncture wounds.
- Finger: Normal rectal tone, hemoccult negative.

28.3. Management:
- IV, O_2, and place on monitor.
- Orders laboratory studies.
- Fluid challenge.

28.4. History:
- Allergies: None.
- Medications: None.
- PMH: Previous rattlesnake bite.
- Last meal: Had several beers in the last few hours.
- Events: A 24 y/o male presents intoxicated, combative after sitting on a snake. This occurred 1 hour ago. He has felt increasing pain, nausea, weakness, and feels like passing out.
- Family: None.
- Records: None.
- Immune: None.

- EMTs: None.
- Doctor: Consult private MD for the ICU admission.
- Social history: A history of excessive alcohol use.

28.5. Secondary Survey:

- VS: Minimal response to fluid challenge.
- General: Vomiting, complaining of pain.
- Skin: Two fang marks on buttock, extensive soft tissue swelling, and edema.
- HEENT: Numbness and tingling to mouth and tongue.
- Neck: Normal.
- Chest: Normal.
- Lungs: Normal.
- Heart: Tachycardia.
- Abdomen: Mild nonfocal tenderness.
- Rectal: Normal.
- Back: Normal.
- Extremities: Normal.
- Neuro: Decreased motor strength, muscle fasciculations, somnolent.

28.6. Laboratory:

- CBC: WBC 12, Hgb 11, Hct 33, Plt 200.
- Chemistry: Na 135, K 4.8, Cl 110, CO_2 24.
- BUN/Cr: 18/1.2.
- Glucose: 130.
- Ca/Mg: Normal.
- LFTs: Normal.
- Amylase/Lipase: Normal.
- PT/PTT: 16/30.
- U/A: +3 Glucose, protein, and blood.
- ETOH: 146.
- Type and cross: Pending.
- Drug screen: Negative.

28.7. X-rays:

- CXR: Normal.

28.8. Critical Actions:

- Determine Tetanus status.
- Relieve pain with narcotics or Tylenol.
- Crotalidae Polyvalent Immune FAB (CroFab)
  - 4 to 6 vials until initial control of envenomation syndrome.
  - Dilute in 250 mL 0.9% NaCl infused over 60 minutes.
  - Infused slowly over first 60 minutes at 25 to 50 mL/h with careful observation for allergic reaction.
- Avoid NSAIDs and ASA, which may increase bleeding.
- Admit to the ICU.

28.9. Pearls:

❍ **What percentage of rattle snake bites are dry bites?**

25%.

❍ **What signs and symptoms suggest the need for antivenom?**

Systemic symptoms such as tachycardia, hypo/hypertension, muscle fasciculations, and change in mental status.

❍ **How much antivenom is typically required?**

Up to 30 vials may be required for severe envenomation (most effective, if given within 6 hours).

CASE 29 (Blunt Trauma)

Examiner

This is a 24 y/o female that was an unrestrained driver of a car that hit a parked car. She was found passed out, behind the wheel with extensive damage to the front end of her car. The patient has a C5 fracture, left pneumothorax, and is pregnant with the uterus placing pressure on the vena cava until she is rolled. The patient also has a bladder rupture, an abruption, a pelvic fracture, and a dislocated open fracture of the left ankle. The reason for the accident was severe hypoglycemia and opiate-induced somnolence. The examiner should be careful not to give anything away. The candidate must remember to roll the patient 30 degrees to the left or the vital signs will continue to drop. The fetus also is in distress until the patient is rolled. In addition, the patient only responds to pain until both dextrose and naloxone are given.

The physician must consult several specialists, including the trauma surgeon, urologist, obstetrician, and orthopedic surgeon. However, all of the specialists are unavailable until all the patient's problems are diagnosed and treated appropriately.

29.1. Introduction

A 24 y/o female crashes her car into another parked car. Backboard, but no c-collar.

Vital signs: BP 90/60, P 128, R 30, T 97.6°F, Wt 88 kg.

29.2. Primary Survey:

- General: Unresponsive female.
- Airway: No gag.
- Breathing: Tachypnea. No breath sounds on the left.
- Circulation: Capillary refill 4 seconds.
- Disability: Does not respond to painful stimuli. Pupils reactive.
- Exposure: No medic alert tags. Trachea deviated to the right. Left ankle is deformed. Patient is obviously pregnant but this information is only provided if the candidate asks or examines the abdomen.
- Finger: Rectal tone intact, no blood. Blood in vaginal vault, os closed.

29.3. Management:

- Apply a cervical collar.
- Intubate by using in-line immobilization.
- Insert left chest tube. Obtain 200 cc of blood.
- Start large bore IVs, 1 to 2 L wide open. Place on O_2 and monitor.
- Insert an NG tube but do not insert a Foley catheter because of blood.
- Draw a type and Rh and other trauma labs.
- Administer Narcan, and check the glucose.
- C-spine, CXR, and pelvis x-rays.
- Relocate ankle, apply a splint, and order x-rays.
- Administer antibiotics for open fracture.
- Roll the patient on the left side by placing a blanket roll under the right side of the backboard.
- Give Tetanus immunization.

29.4. History:

- Allergies: Unknown.
- Medications: Unknown.
- PMH: Unknown.
- Last meal: Unknown.
- Events: Hit a parked car. Found passed out behind the wheel of the car. No seatbelt. Extensive damage to the front end of the vehicle.
- Family: Unknown.
- Records: Unknown.
- Immune: Unknown.
- EMTs: Extensive vehicle damage.

- Narcotics: Search reveals empty bottle of hydrocodone 10/325 mg (40 tabs).
- Doctor: Dr. Abacus on pill bottle. If called, answering service says the dentist is not in until tomorrow morning.
- Social history: Unknown.

29.5. Secondary Survey:
- General: Nonresponsive unless given Narcan and dextrose.
- Skin: Multiple tattoos.
- HEENT: Normal.
- Neck: Palpable step off at C5.
- Chest: Palpable crepitance on the left side.
- Lungs: Breath sounds equal with tube placement.
- Heart: Tachycardic.
- Abdomen: BS+. Soft. Pelvic mass present. If specifically asked, palpably enlarged uterus, 6 months.
- Perineum/GU: Blood in vaginal vault and around urethra.
- Rectal: Guaiac negative.
- Back: Normal.
- Extremities: Dislocated left ankle, open fracture, pulseless until relocated.
- Neuro: Minimal response to painful stimuli while moving all extremities. The patient wakes up and fights tube if given naloxone and glucose.

29.6. Laboratory:
- CBC: WBC 18, Hgb 11, Hct 33, Plt 400.
- Chemistry: Na 135, K 4.0, Cl 110, CO_2 24.
- BUN/Cr: 18/1.2.
- Glucose: 20; 150 if given glucose.
- LFTs: Normal.
- Amylase/Lipase: Normal.
- PT/PTT: Normal.
- ABG: pH 7.4, pO_2 95, pCO_2 24, HCO_3 20.
- U/A: Large blood.
- Urine pregnancy test: Positive.
- Drug screen: Opiates.

29.7. X-rays:
- CXR: Good placement ETT. No pneumothorax after chest tube. Left pulmonary contusion.
- C-spine: Step off at C5–6.
- Pelvis: Left pubic rami fracture. Fetus present.
- CT abdomen/pelvis: No liver or spleen injury. Free fluid and fetus in pelvis.
- Urethrogram: Bladder extravasation.
- Left ankle x-ray: Trimalleolar fracture.

29.8. Special Tests:
- US Pelvis: Partial placental abruption. Free fluid in pelvis. FHTs 136.
- Fetal monitor: Shows distress until mother put in left lateral position.
- ECG: Tachycardia.

29.9. Critical Actions:
- Place a cervical collar on the patient.
- Intubate by using in-line immobilization.
- Insert left chest tube.
- Use large bore IVs, 1 to 2 L wide open.
- Order a type and Rh.
- Administer naloxone, and check glucose.
- Relocate ankle, apply splint, and order x-rays.

- Administer antibiotics for open fracture.
- Roll patient on left side.
- Obtain fetal evaluation, that is, ultrasound and fetal monitor.
- Consult trauma, ortho, OB/GYN, and urology.
- Diagnosis: C-spine fracture, pneumothorax, bladder rupture, pelvic fracture, and fracture/dislocation to ankle.

29.10. Pearls:

❍ **What percentage of patients with bladder rupture have hematuria?**

94%.

❍ **What are common risk factors for bladder rupture?**

Full bladder at the time of the trauma and prior pelvic or bladder surgery.

CASE 30 (28 y/o with Dyspnea)

Examiner

A patient with a history of asthma is brought in by paramedics. The paramedics indicate that shortly before arrival the patient became significantly worse. All attempts at medical therapy fail, such as subcutaneous and IV epinephrine, Solu-Medrol, magnesium, and inhalers. Intubation does not help. The patient is very tight and breath sounds cannot be distinguished. The only x-ray technician in the hospital is in the ICU at a code.

The patient has a pneumothorax that can only be diagnosed by performing a needle thoracostomy. The physician must needle both sides to find the pneumothorax. Following needle thoracostomies it is critical that chest tubes are placed in both sides. Have the candidate describe the steps in performing a needle thoracostomy.

30.1. Introduction:

A 28 y/o female with a history of asthma arrives, via paramedics, in acute respiratory distress.

Vital signs: BP 160/80, P 130, R 34, T 98.6°F, Wt 91.5 kg.

30.2. Primary Survey:

- General: Acute distress, unable to speak.
- Airway: No gag.
- Breathing: No breath sounds.
- Circulation: Capillary refill 3 seconds.

30.3. Management:

- Start IV, O_2, and place on monitor.
- Intubate. Consider sedating with Ketamine 5 mg/kg.
- Administer β-agonists.
- Administer epinephrine.
- Administer Solu-Medrol 1 to 2 mg/kg IV.
- Consider magnesium 2 to 4 g IV over 20 minutes.
- Order laboratory studies and an ABG.
- CXR ordered but is not available.
- Needle both sides of the chest (rush of air).
- Place a chest tube bilaterally.

30.4. History:

- Allergies: None.
- Medications: Albuterol inhaler, prednisone, and Ciprofloxacin.
- PMH: N/A.

- Last meal: N/A.
- Events: Family says patient ran out of inhalers and steroids 2 days ago and today she became much worse. No past admits, intubations, or other significant complications from her asthma.
- Family: None.
- Records: None.
- Immune: N/A.
- EMT: Administered two breathing treatments when she suddenly worsened.
- Narcotics: None.
- Doctor: Available for admission.
- Social history: None.

30.5. Secondary Survey:
- General: Acute distress.
- Skin: Warm.
- HEENT: Normal.
- Neck: Retractions.
- Chest: Retractions and tachypnea.
- Lungs: No breath sounds until chest tube placement and then diffuse wheezes.
- Heart: Tachycardia.
- Abdomen: Normal.
- Pelvic: Deferred.
- Rectal: Deferred.
- Back: Normal.
- Extremities: Normal.
- Neuro: Unconscious, GCS 3 after sedation and paralysis.

30.6. Laboratory:
- CBC: WBC 15, Hgb 12, Hct 36.
- Chemistry: Normal.
- BUN/Cr: Normal.
- Glucose: Normal.
- ABG: pH 7.3, pO_2 60, pCO_2 40, HCO_3 22 (before intubation).
- U/A: + Bacteria and WBCs.

30.7. X-rays:
- CXR: Bilateral chest tubes, ETT in place.

30.8. Critical Actions:
- Intubate.
- Administer β-agonists.
- Administer epinephrine.
- Administer Solu-Medrol.
- Ventilator settings of low tidal volume and prolonged expiratory time.
- Needle L and R chest.
- Place bilateral chest tubes.
- Describe the technique for performing a needle thoracostomy.

30.9. Pearls:

❍ **What risk factors increase the mortality from asthma?**

Greater than three ED visits/year or greater than two hospitalizations/year, nocturnal symptoms, previous ICU admissions, previous mechanical ventilation, steroid dependence, and frequent steroid use.

❍ **The decision to intubation should be determined by the pO_2 and pCO_2 levels on an ABG?**

False. The decision to intubate should be made clinically. Indications include cardio/respiratory arrest, severe hypoxia, exhaustion, or deterioration of mental status.

CASE 31 (Triple)

Patient #1 (Abdominal Pain and Dehydration in an Infant)

Examiner

This patient has Intussusception. Just prior to the physician's evaluation, the child sustained a miraculous recovery. The mother is in the process of bundling up the child to take him home when the physician walks into the room. The mother says that she is tired of waiting and wants to take the patient home. Only with reluctance is the physician able to persuade the mother to stay for a complete history and physical examination. At this time, red-tinged stool becomes apparent which mother attributed to beets. The child suddenly starts to cry and grabs at his stomach. Tests are ordered, including a barium enema.

The case is interrupted by Cases 2 and 3. Eventually the patient comes back from x-ray with a diagnosis of intussusception and is admitted for observation following the procedure.

31.1. Introduction: (**Patient #1**)

An 8 m/o infant is brought by his mother with intermittent crying, impossible to console, and multiple episodes of vomiting.

Vital signs: BP N/A, P 130, R 28, T 100.2°F, Wt 30 kg.

31.2. Primary Survey:

- General: Fussy child, crying in mother's arms. Listless.
- Airway: Intact.
- Breathing: Normal.
- Circulation: Normal.
- Disability: None.
- Exposure: Normal.
- Finger: Hemoccult positive stool with current jelly stool.

31.3. Management:

- CBC, CMP, PT/PTT/INR, UA, Lipase, LFTs, Lactate.
- NS fluid bolus at 20 cc/kg.
- Abdominal x-rays and CXR.
- Barium or air contrast enema.
- Consult surgery before enema.

31.4. History:

- Allergies: None.
- Medications: Amoxicillin for otitis.
- PMH: Recent diagnosis of otitis in right ear 4 days ago.
- Last meal: Milk, 8 hours ago.
- Events: An 8 m/o child presents with intermittent intense crying. When the pain starts the child flexes his legs, cries, and vomits. These episodes last 10 to 20 minutes and spontaneously resolve. Mom has now noted fever and a red-colored, jelly-like stool in his diaper.
- Family: None.
- Records: Normal birth.
- Immune: Up to date.
- EMTs: Via private vehicle.
- Narcotics: None.
- Doctor: Dr. Meconium.
- Social history: Lives at home with parents.

31.5. Secondary Survey:
- General: Lethargic, irritable, and listless.
- Skin: Decreased turgor.
- HEENT: Mucous membranes dry.
- Neck: Supple.
- Chest: Normal.
- Lungs: Clear.
- Heart: Regular.
- Abdomen: Distended and swollen, oblong mass RLQ.
- Perineum/GU: Normal.
- Rectal: Hemoccult positive, currant jelly stool.
- Back: Normal.
- Extremities: Normal.
- Neuro: Listless.

At this point the nurse asks you to see a patient that is having a stroke.

Patient #2 (40 y/o with Slurred Speech)

Examiner

This patient has thrombotic thrombocytopenic purpura. The physical examination is consistent with a CVA; however, the CT scan comes back negative and the patient's symptoms resolve while in the scanner. Her primary care doctor thinks she is having a TIA and wants to send her home for an outpatient workup. This should be resisted by the candidate. The diagnosis is verified by checking the platelet count, which is very low. The candidate may actually be given a second chance at the diagnosis as the private physician may ask if any of the laboratory studies are abnormal.

31.1. Introduction: (**Patient #2 50 y/o with Slurred Speech**)

A 40 y/o female presents with slurred speech and tingling to the right side of the face, arm, and hand.

Vital signs: BP 126/90, P 96, R 20, T 98.6°F, Wt 102 kg.

31.2. Primary Survey:
- General: Normal.
- Airway: Normal.
- Breathing: Normal.
- Circulation: Normal.
- Disability: Slurred speech.
- Exposure: Bruising and diffuse petechiae on extremities.
- Finger: Normal.

31.3. Management:
- IV, pulse oximeter, and monitor.
- CT head.
- Order laboratory studies and ECG.

31.4. History:
- Allergies: None.
- Medications: Doans pills.
- PMH: Bladder infections.
- Last meal: 4 hours ago.
- Events: Patient has had two episodes of slurred speech and tingling in the right arm, hand, and face. The first episode occurred yesterday, lasting 1 hour and spontaneously resolved. The next episode occurred 1 hour prior to arrival and is improving.

- Family: DM and cancer.
- Records: None.
- Immune: Up to date.
- EMTs: None.
- Narcotics: None.
- Doctor: Dr. Manage Care.
- Social history: Nonsmoker, nondrinker.

31.5. Secondary Survey:

- General: Alert, no distress.
- Skin: Petechiae on extremities.
- HEENT: Normal.
- Neck: Normal.
- Chest: Normal.
- Lungs: Normal.
- Heart: Normal.
- Abdomen: Normal.
- Perineum/GU: Normal.
- Rectal: Normal.
- Back: Normal.
- Extremities: Bruising and diffuse petechiae on extremities.
- Neuro: Slurred speech, decreased sensation right arm compared to left, otherwise normal examination.

At this point, the nurse asks you to see a third patient that is experiencing severe eye pain.

Patient #3 (Eye Pain)

Examiner

This non-English speaking patient has severe eye pain due to acute angle closure glaucoma. The pain began shortly after attending a movie with her daughter and grandchild.

The diagnosis may be obtained by using the English speaking daughter and from the clinical examination, but you must get a medically trained interpreter at some time during the case. Give extra points if the candidate comments on the potential complications from giving timolol to an asthmatic, and acetazolamide to a sulfa-allergic patient.

31.1. Introduction: (**Patient #3 Eye Pain**)

A 52 y/o Hispanic female in severe distress complaining of left eye pain, nausea, and vomiting.

Vital signs: BP 160/90, P 105, R 22, T 98.6°F, Wt 123 kg.

31.2. Primary Survey:

- General: Severe distress.
- Airway: Normal.
- Breathing: Normal.
- Circulation: Normal.
- Disability: None.
- Exposure: Normal.
- Finger: Normal.

31.3. Management:

- None at this time.

31.4. History:

- Allergies: Sulfa causes severe anaphylaxis.
- Medications: None.

- PMH: Asthma.
- Last meal: None.
- Events: Severe eye pain began shortly after attending a movie with her daughter and grandchild. The pain is constant and nonradiating with associated nausea and vomiting.
- Family: None.
- Records: None.
- Immune: Up to date.
- EMTs: None.
- Narcotics: None.
- Doctor: None.
- Social history: Nonsmoker, nondrinker.

31.5. Secondary Survey:
- General: Ill appearing due to pain.
- Skin: Normal.
- HEENT: Diffused injection with watery discharge. Vision is markedly blurred in the left eye. Cornea is hazy. Pupils are mid-dilated with little reaction to light. Anterior chamber is shallow. Intraocular pressure is 80 mm Hg (<20 mm Hg is normal). Visual acuity 20/100 OS, 20/30 OD.
- Neck: Normal.
- Chest: Normal.
- Lungs: Rare wheeze.
- Heart: Normal.
- Abdomen: Normal.
- Perineum/GU: Normal.
- Rectal: Normal.
- Back: Normal.
- Extremities: Normal.
- Neuro: Normal.

31.6. Laboratory:
- Not indicated.

31.7. X-rays:
- CXR: Not indicated.

31.8. Special Tests:
- ECG: Not indicated.

31.9. Critical Actions:
- Consult ophthalmology.
- Visual acuity.
- Evaluate intraocular pressure.
- Avoid β-blockers such as timolol in an asthmatic.
- Pilocarpine hydrochloride 1%, one drop every 30 minutes until the pupil constricts, followed by one drop every 6 hours.
- Acetazolamide po or IV.
- Mannitol IV.

Patient #1 (Abdominal Pain and Dehydration in an Infant)

31.6. Laboratory:
- CBC: WBC 18,000, Hgb 14, Hct 42, Plt 385.
- Differential: Pending.
- Chemistry: Na 132, K 4.2, Cl 98, CO_2 10.

- BUN/Cr: 30/1.0.
- Glucose: 130.
- Ca/Mg: Pending.
- LFTs: Pending.
- Amylase/Lipase: Pending.
- Lactate: Pending.
- PT/PTT/INR: Pending.
- Blood cultures: Pending.
- U/A: Spec G 1.036, 2 + ketones. Otherwise normal.

31.7. X-rays:
- CXR: Normal.
- Abdominal x-ray: Decreased bowel gas and fecal material in right colon. Small bowel distention and multiple air-fluid levels.
- Ultrasound: Target and pseudokidney sign present.
- Barium enema: Diagnostic and therapeutic for intussusception.

31.8. Special Tests:
- ECG: None.

31.9. Critical Actions:
- Start IV fluid bolus of 20 cc/kg of NS.
- Obtain a surgical consult.
- Order a barium enema.
- Admit for observation.
- Start antibiotics for potential perforation, that is, ampicillin, 100 to 200 mg/kg, or clindamycin, 30 to 40 mg/kg, or gentamicin, 5.0 to 7.5 mg/kg.

Patient #2

31.6. Laboratory:
- CBC: WBC 13, Hgb 8.5, Hct 30, Plt 13.
- Differential: Segs 55%, lymphs 38%, mono 5%, eos 1%.
- Chemistry: Na 140, K 3.8, Cl 105, CO_2 28.
- BUN/Cr: 15/1.0.
- Glucose: 120.
- Ca/Mg: Pending.
- LFTs: Pending.
- Amylase/Lipase: Pending.
- PT/PTT/INR: 12/28/1.0.
- Cardiac enzymes: Not indicated.
- ABG: Not indicated.
- Blood cultures: Not indicated.
- U/A: Normal.

31.7. X-rays:
- CXR: Normal.

31.8. Special Tests:
- ECG: NSR.
- CT head: Normal.
- MRI head: Normal.

31.9. Critical Actions:
- Do not allow the patient to go home.
- Note the petechiae on physical examination.

- Obtain a CBC.
- Steroids.
- Plasmapheresis coupled with FFP infusion.
- Admit to the ICU.
- Consult hematology.

31.10. Pearls: (**Patients# 1–3**)

❍ **What are the common complications of intussusception?**

Perforation, peritonitis, shock, sepsis, and reintussusception.

❍ **When do you expect to see currant jelly stools?**

Within 12 to 24 hours, mucus or blood may be found per rectum.

❍ **What is the classic pentad of TTP?**

(1) Fever, (2) microangiopathic hemolytic anemia, (3) thrombocytopenia, (4) renal impairment, and (5) CNS impairment. Only 40% of patients present with all five components.

❍ **What is the differential of an acutely painful red eye?**

Keratitis, iritis, ulcer, erosion, foreign body, conjunctivitis, glaucoma, and trauma.

CASE 32 (Female in Respiratory Distress)

Examiner

This patient has pneumonia which has made her chronic hypothyroid state significantly worse. In the last few days, she has had a fever, chills, and a productive cough. She now presents in acute distress but does not require intubation. The daughter can give the history and if candidate treats appropriately, she gets better at the time of admission.

32.1. Introduction:

A 62 y/o female in mild respiratory distress.

Vital signs: BP 90/60, P 60, R 14, T 96°F, Wt 97.4 kg.

32.2. Primary Survey:

- General: Obese female in moderate respiratory distress.
- Airway: Gag reflex present.
- Breathing: Crackles at left base, rare rhonchi. Coughs during examination.
- Circulation: Capillary refill >2 seconds.
- Disability: None.
- Exposure: No gross abnormality.
- Finger: Deferred.

32.3. Management:

- Start IV, O_2, and place on monitor and pulse oximeter.
- Order CXR.
- Order CBC, CMP, thyroid studies, cardiac enzymes, and U/A.
- Obtain blood, urine, and sputum cultures.

32.4. History:

- Allergies: None.
- Medications: None.
- PMH: Appendicitis with appendectomy.
- Last meal: Light breakfast earlier today.

- Events: A 62 y/o female has had 2 days of fever, chills, weakness, and a productive cough. For the last several weeks, she has noticed increasing episodes of constipation, fatigue, muscle cramps, and a sensation of always being cold. She has also been gaining weight and has been "slowing down" lately.
- Family: Noncontributory.
- Records: N/A.
- Immune: Normal.
- EMTs: No further information.
- Narcotics: None.
- Doctor: Dr. Fermi.
- Social history: Drinks alcohol socially.

32.5. Secondary Survey:
- General: Mild lethargy.
- Skin: Dry, yellow skin, course hair, diffuse, nonpitting edema.
- HEENT: Large tongue, puffy eyes and face, loss of lateral part of eyebrows.
- Neck: Normal.
- Chest: No retractions.
- Lungs: Crackles in the left base.
- Heart: Regular and slow.
- Abdomen: Slight abdominal distention, bowel sounds low pitched.
- Perineum/GU: Normal.
- Rectal: Normal.
- Back: Normal.
- Extremities: Puffy hands and legs.
- Neuro: Slow DTRs, ataxia, and paresthesias.

32.6. Laboratory:
- CBC: WBC 16, Hgb 11, Hct 39, Plt 350.
- Differential: Bands 33%.
- Chemistry: Na 121, K 5.2, Cl 102, CO_2 25.
- BUN/Cr: 18/1.4.
- Glucose: 60.
- Ca/Mg: Normal.
- LFTs: Mild elevation SGOT, LDH.
- Amylase/Lipase: Pending.
- PT/PTT: Pending.
- Cardiac enzymes: Pending.
- CHF peptid (BNP): Pending
- ABG: pH 7.36, pO_2 77, pCO_2 26, HCO_3 24.
- Blood cultures: Pending.
- U/A: Normal.
- T4, TSH: Pending.

32.7. X-rays:
- CXR: Cardiomegaly, LLL pneumonia.
- Abdominal series: Mild ileus.

32.8. Special Tests:
- ECG: Bradycardia, low voltage, prolonged PR interval and inverted T-waves.

32.9. Critical Actions:
- Administer hydrocortisone, 300 mg IV.
- Administer glucose.

- Administer L-thyroxine, 500 to 800 μg slow IV.
- Admit to the ICU.
- Obtain appropriate cultures
- Start antibiotics for pneumonia.

32.10. Pearls:

❍ **What treatment has been shown to decrease mortality in patients with pneumonia?**

Early antibiotic therapy.

❍ **What laboratory abnormalities available in the ED are expected in severe hypothyroidism?**

Anemia, elevated cholesterol, LDH, AST, CPK, and hyponatremia.

CASE 33 (Female with Weight Loss and Dyspnea)

Examiner

This patient is in thyroid storm and presents in moderate CHF with atrial fibrillation.

A thorough history and physical examination reveals that the patient is suffering from severe hyperthyroidism. The patient's CHF is relieved by standard therapy and she does not require intubation.

33.1. Introduction:

A 52 y/o female presents SOB, sitting up, and in respiratory distress.

Vital signs: BP 140/70, P 130, R 28, T 103°F, Wt 60 kg.

33.2. Primary Survey:

- General: Obvious respiratory distress, diaphoretic, cool, and clammy.
- Airway: Gag reflex present.
- Breathing: Diffused crackles at bases, respiratory retractions.
- Circulation: Capillary refill 3 seconds.
- Disability: Able to make very brief gasping statements "I," "can't," "breath."
- Exposure: No gross abnormalities.
- Finger: Deferred.

33.3. Management:

- Start IV, O_2, pulse oximeter, and place on monitor.
- Order CBC, CMP, thyroid studies, U/A, CXR, and ECG.
- CXR and ECG.
- ECG.
- Administer Lasix.
- Administer nitroglycerin IV.
- Place patient on BiPAP.

33.4. History:

- Allergies: None.
- Medications: None.
- PMH: N/A.
- Last meal: N/A.
- Event: *This evening the daughter found her mother in respiratory distress. She states her mom has had intermittent episodes of palpitations and dyspnea. For the last week, she has been having diarrhea, nausea, and vomiting with crampy abdominal pain. She has also noticed that her mother is more nervous than usual, has lost a lot of weight, and has been complaining of being "hot" all the time.*
- Family: None.

- Records: None.
- Immune: None.
- EMTs: None.
- Narcotics: None.
- Doctor: Dr. Purkinje is available to admit the patient.
- Social history: Rarely consumes alcohol and is a nonsmoker.

33.5. Secondary Survey:
- General: Middle-aged female in moderate respiratory distress.
- Skin: Warm and moist, hair is fine and silky, if asked.
- HEENT: Exophthalmos, inflamed conjunctiva.
- Neck: Enlarged thyroid with bruit over the gland.
- Chest: Nontender.
- Lungs: Diffused crackles.
- Heart: Tachycardic and irregular.
- Abdomen: Soft, BS +, No focal tenderness.
- Perineum/GU: Normal.
- Rectal: Hemoccult negative.
- Back: Normal.
- Extremities: Normal.
- Neuro: Brisk DTRs, symmetrical decreased muscle strength, slight tremor.

33.6. Laboratory:
- CBC: WBC 15, Hgb 12, Hct 36, Plt 400.
- Differential: Pending.
- Chemistry: Na 140, K 4.4, Cl 102, CO_2 29.
- BUN/Cr: 11/1.2.
- Glucose: 180.
- Ca/Mg: Normal.
- LFTs: Normal.
- Amylase/Lipase: Pending.
- PT/PTT: Pending.
- Cardiac enzymes: Normal.
- CHF peptid (BNP): Pending
- ABG: pH 7.38, pO_2 76, pCO_2 30, HCO_3 22.
- Blood cultures: Pending.
- U/A: Normal.
- Thyroid studies: Pending.

33.7. X-rays:
- CXR: Pulmonary vascular congestion.

33.8. Special Tests:
- ECG: Atrial fibrillation.

33.9. Critical Actions:
- Administer Tylenol and cover with cooling blanket.
- Give PTU 900 to 1,200 mg po initially.
- Give Iodine 1 hour after starting antithyroid therapy.
- Administer Lasix.
- Administer nitroglycerin IV
- Avoid propranolol.
- Administer hydrocortisone, 300 mg IV.
- Admit to the ICU.

33.10. Pearls:

❍ **What is the mortality rate of thyroid storm?**

10% to 20%.

❍ **What are the most common causes?**

Infection, trauma, vascular accident, diabetes, and nonthyroidal surgery.

❍ **What are the common diagnostic criteria?**

T >100°F, tachycardia, peripheral manifestations, and CNS, CV, and GI dysfunction.

CASE 34 (5 w/k Male Spitting Up)

Examiner

A 5 w/o Hispanic male presents with a classic history for pyloric stenosis. Symptoms have been progressing over the past 3 to 4 weeks and now the infant has blood-tinged vomit. The parent speaks very little English and you will be unable to obtain any specific details until an interpreter arrives.

34.1. Introduction:

A 5 w/k Hispanic infant presents with mother who speaks very little English.

Vital signs: BP N/A, P 100, R 26, T 100.1°F, Wt 5 kg.

34.2. Primary Survey:

- General: Awake, hungry, mildly lethargic.
- Airway: Intact.
- Breathing: Normal.
- Circulation: Normal.
- Disability: Normal.
- Exposure: Normal.
- Finger: Normal.

34.3. History:

- Allergies: None.
- Medications: None.
- PMH: None.
- Last meal: 2 hours ago.
- Events: A 5 w/o born via normal spontaneous vaginal delivery with an uncomplicated prenatal course presents with 3 days of spitting up. Symptoms have worsened to the point that he vomits "across the room." Vomiting is clear with occasional streaks of blood. He continually appears hungry and finishes his bottle. Ten to 15 minutes after a feed the vomiting occurs. No diarrhea, fever, cough but he is lethargic and appears yellow.
- Family: Normal.
- Records: None.
- Immune: Up to date.
- EMTs: None.
- Narcotics: None.
- Doctor: Dr. Banks.
- Social history: None.

34.4. Secondary Survey:

- General: A 5 w/o infant, lethargic, feeding on a bottle.
- Skin: Jaundiced.
- HEENT: Normal.
- Neck: Normal

- Chest: Normal.
- Lungs: Clear.
- Heart: Normal.
- Abdomen: Palpable mass just below the liver edge on the right side.
- Perineum/GU: Normal.
- Rectal: Hemoccult negative.
- Back: Normal.
- Extremities: Normal.
- Neuro: Normal.

34.5. Laboratory:
- CBC: WBC 16, Hgb 14, Hct 42, Plt 400.
- Differential: Pending.
- Chemistry: Na 136, K 3.2, Cl 96, CO_2 35.
- BUN/Cr: 28/1.2.
- Glucose: 130.
- Ca/Mg: Pending.
- LFTs: Pending.
- Amylase/Lipase: Not indicated.
- PT/PTT: Pending.
- Blood cultures: Pending.
- U/A: Pending.

34.6. X-rays:
- CXR: Normal.

34.7. Special Tests:
- Abdomen films: Gastric dilation.
- Ultrasound: Pyloric stenosis (hypertrophied pyloris 5 mm in diameter).
- Gastrografin or barium upper GI: String sign (elongated pyloric canal).

34.8. Critical Actions:
- Administer 0.9 NS at 20 mL/kg over 20 minutes.
- Insert NG tube at low-intermittent suction.
- Obtain surgery consult.
- US or UGI.

34.9. Pearls:

❍ **What is the cause of pyloric stenosis?**

Hypertrophy and hyperplasia of the circular antral and pyloric musculature resulting in a gastric outlet obstruction.

❍ **Which type of chemical imbalance is expected in pyloric stenosis?**

Hypochloremic metabolic alkalosis due to loss of hydrochloric acid from vomiting.

CASE 35 (7 y/o Lethargic Male)

Examiner

A 7 y/o male presents after drinking an unknown liquid that contained ethylene glycol. The patient is unable to answers questions due to an altered level of consciousness. When pressured, the 9 y/o brother provides details. Send the police or paramedics to find the ethylene glycol containing liquid. Otherwise, the diagnosis is made by finding crystals in the urine. He will require intubation and treatment with a specific antidote.

35.1. Introduction:

A 7 y/o male lying on the cart appears very lethargic.

Vital signs: BP 90/60, P 90, R 20, T 100.5°F, Wt 28 kg.

35.2. Primary Survey:

- General: Slurred speech and very lethargic.
- Airway: + Gag reflex present.
- Breathing: Equal breath sounds.
- Circulation: Capillary refill 3 seconds.
- Disability: Responds to verbal stimuli with confused unclear response.
- Exposure: No gross abnormalities.
- Finger: NG tube, Foley catheter.

35.3. Critical Event:

- Child has a tonic–clonic seizure.

35.4. Management:

- Start IV, O_2, and place on monitor and pulse oximeter.
- Administer diazepam, lorazepam, or midazolam. Seizure stops if given.
- Intubate.
- 20 mL/kg NS bolus.

35.5. History:

- Allergies: Unknown.
- Medications: Unknown.
- PMH: Unknown
- Last meal: 4 hours ago.
- Events: A 7 y/o male presents via EMS, with altered mental status for unknown reason. His 9 y/o brother is also brought by EMS. After frequent questioning he states, they were playing in a barn and the patient drank an unknown fluid 3 hours ago. The patient started vomiting and "felt funny" about 1 hour ago. His brother ran to a local house and called 911. The brother denies drinking the fluid but says it was a greenish color in a plastic container.
- Family: Unknown.
- Records: Unavailable.
- Immune: Unknown.
- EMTs: Police or paramedics sent to site and find ethylene glycol.
- Narcotics: None.
- Doctor: Dr. I. Robi.
- Social history: Parents cannot be located.

35.6. Secondary Survey:

- General: Appears intoxicated with a faint, sweet, aromatic odor detected on the child's breath.
- Skin: Dry.
- HEENT: Vertical and horizontal nystagmus.
- Neck: Supple.
- Chest: Normal.
- Lungs: Normal.
- Heart: Regular rhythm, tachycardic.
- Abdomen: Soft, BS+.
- Perineum/GU: Normal.
- Rectal: Normal.
- Back: Normal.
- Extremities: Normal.
- Neuro: Responds to pain by moving all extremities and making incomprehensible sounds.

35.7. Laboratory:

- CBC: WBC 14.0, Hgb 13.0, Hct 39.0.
- Chemistry: Na 140, K 5.0, Cl 90, CO_2 10.
- BUN/Cr: 9/1.0.
- Glucose: 180.
- Ca: 6.
- O_2 sat: 95%
- ABG: pH 7.05, pO_2 110, pCO_2 20, $HCO_3$12.
- U/A: Protein 3+, blood 2+, calcium oxalate crystal 1+.
- Amylase: 140.
- Lactate: 4.2
- Measured serum osm: 350.
- Calculated serum osm: 303.
  - [2(Na + K) + Glu/18 + BUN/3]
  - [2(140 + 5) + 180/18 + 9/3] = 303
- Tox screen: Pending.
- Anion gap: 40 [Na – (Cl + HCO_3)].

35.8. X-rays:

- CXR: Normal.

35.9. Special Tests:

- ECG: Sinus tachycardia.
- Ethylene glycol: 55 mg/dL.
- Methanol: Negative.
- Isopropyl: Negative.
- Wood's lamp: Fluorescence of urine.

35.10. Critical Actions:

- Intubate.
- Administer IV bicarbonate.
- Treat hypocalcemia with IV calcium chloride or gluconate.
- Treat seizures with a bezodiazepine.
- Give an ethanol IV loading dose of 7.5 mL/kg (10% ethanol in D5W) then 1 to 1.5 mg/kg/h or Fomepizole (Antizol) 15 mg/kg IV loading dose. Then 10 mg/kg q 12 hours times 4 doses.
- Give IV pyridoxine and thiamine.
- Admit to the ICU.

35.11. Pearls:

❍ **Explain the competitive metabolism of ethylene glycol and ethanol.**

EG is metabolized to glycoaldehyde by alcohol dehydrogenase. Alcohol dehydrogenase has a much higher affinity for ethanol than for EG. When both alcohols are present, ethanol is metabolized. Thus, ethanol inhibits the metabolism of EG.

❍ **What is the significance of calcium oxalate crystals in EG ingestion?**

EG results in the accumulation of glycolic acid resulting in decreased bicarbonate levels, acidotic symptoms, renal tubular damage, interstitial edema, and increased mortality. Glycolic acid metabolism results in the production of oxalic acid which precipitates as calcium oxalate crystals.

❍ **What is the lethal dose of EG?**

0.1 mL/kg may produce toxic levels, even a mouthful could be hazardous. Less than 60 mL has resulted in death.

CASE 36 (Female with Shoulder Pain Demanding Narcotics)

Examiner

This is a 37 y/o female that presents with a complaint of acute on chronic right shoulder pain. The patient appears to be drug seeking but a careful examination will reveal severe anemia. The patient is an evasive historian and does not provide this information nor does she reveal the signs and symptoms of her anemia unless specifically asked. She concentrates on her shoulder pain and requests a large dose of Dilaudid. Furthermore, she denies shortness of breath, headaches, black stools, or vomiting blood.

After the pain shot, the patient wants to leave. At this point the laboratory studies return and the diagnosis of severe anemia is made. She does not want to stay in the hospital and, for religious reasons, she refuses a transfusion.

The patient continues to refuse admission until the candidate asks the husband to come in from the waiting room. With his help the patient agrees to stay in the hospital. If the candidate should send the patient home, an AMA form should be completed; however, she returns to the ED immediately, vomiting blood and arrests.

36.1. Introduction:

A 37 y/o female presents with complaint of severe right shoulder pain.

Vital signs: BP 100/80, P 114, R 26, T 99.1°F, Wt 72 kg.

36.2. Primary Survey:

- General: Poorly nourished female appearing much older than her stated age.
- Airway: Intact.
- Breathing: Shallow rapid breaths. Crackles at the right base which clear with coughing.
- Circulation: Capillary refill 4 seconds.
- Disability: None.
- Exposure: Normal.
- Finger: Hemoccult negative.

36.3. History:

- Allergies: Penicillin, tramadol, ibuprofen
- Medications: Oxycontin.
- PMH: Rotator cuff surgery, anemia, and hysterectomy.
- Last meal: 4 hours ago.
- Events: A 37 y/o female presents with severe R shoulder pain for the past 2 days. She had rotator cuff surgery 10 months ago and the pain started after she took her last oxycontin pill. No recent injury, swelling, redness, or numbness to that shoulder. Dilaudid is the only shot that works for her. She has been feeling weak and sleeping a lot lately but denies shortness of breath, headaches, black stools, or hematemesis.
- Family: Husband is in the waiting room.
- Records: Rotator cuff repair 10 months ago.
- Immune: Up to date.
- EMTs: None.
- Narcotics: Ran out of oxycontin 2 days ago.
- Doctor: Dr. Bone and Dr. Medicine.
- Social history: Smokes 1 pack of cigarettes per day.

36.4. Secondary Survey:

- General: Cachectic white female.
- Skin: Pale.
- HEENT: Pale conjunctiva.
- Neck: Supple.
- Chest: Normal.
- Lungs: Crackles at right base, which clears with cough.
- Heart: RRR with no murmur.
- Abdomen: Soft.

- Perineum/GU: Normal.
- Rectal: Hemoccult negative.
- Back: Normal.
- Extremities: Severe pain with all any movement of the right shoulder.
- Neuro: Unable to assess motor strength of R upper extremity due to pain. All other muscles groups are normal.

36.5. Management:
- Give pain medication IM or IV.
- Order laboratory studies.
- CXR.
- R shoulder x-ray.

36.6. Laboratory:
- CBC: WBC 12, Hgb 4.1, Hct 14.6, Plt 590.
- MCV: 57.
- Differential: Pending.
- Chemistry: Na 134, K 4.0, Cl 104, CO_2 24.
- BUN/Cr: 10/1.0.
- Glucose: 120.
- Ca/Mg: Normal.
- LFTs: Normal.
- Amylase/Lipase: Normal.
- PT/PTT: Normal.
- Type and screen: Pending.
- Cardiac enzymes: Normal.
- Saturation: 98% on room air.
- Blood cultures: Not indicated.
- U/A: Normal.

36.7. X-rays:
- CXR: Cardiomegaly.
- R shoulder x-ray: No acute fracture. Surgical pins in place.

36.8. Special Tests:
- ECG: Sinus tachycardia.

36.9. Critical Actions:
- Diagnose anemia
- Convince the patient to be admitted.
- Treat pain.

36.10. Pearls:

❍ **What are the 3 causes of anemia?**

(1) Blood loss, (2) decreased RBC production, (3) increased RBC destruction (hemolysis).

❍ **What is the most common cause of microcytic anemia?**

Iron deficiency.

CASE 37 (Child with a Bug Bite)

Examiner

An 8 y/o child presents with a black widow spider bite. He is not able to provide much of a history other than he was playing in a wood pile. The patient is brought in by the grandmother who was watching the child. According to his grandmother, he came into the house with a complaint of crampy abdominal pains as well as pain in the neck, back, and legs. The candidate may or may not use the antivenom after discussion with poison control.

37.1. Introduction:

An 8 y/o child presents with a complaint of abdominal pain.

Vital signs: BP 150/110, P 110, R 24, T 99.0°F, Wt 32 kg.

37.2. Primary Survey:

- General: Moderate distress.
- Airway: Intact.
- Breathing: Normal.
- Circulation: Normal.
- Disability: None.
- Exposure: If specifically asked, the child has a circular area of pallor surrounded by a ring of erythema located on his upper back.
- Finger: Hemoccult negative.

37.3. Management:

- Candidate may order initial screening laboratory studies at this time.

37.4. History:

- Allergies: None.
- Medications: None.
- PMH: None.
- Last meal: 5 hours ago.
- Events: This 8 y/o male has been playing in the wood pile all day. According to his grandmother, he came into the house with a complaint of crampy abdominal pain. He has had nausea, vomiting, headaches, facial swelling, and muscle pain in the neck, back, and legs. He tells the candidate that a bug stung him on the back.
- Family: None.
- Records: None.
- Immune: Up to date.
- EMTs: None.
- Narcotics: None.
- Doctor: No family doctor, child is visiting grandmother, parents are traveling in Europe.
- Social history: None.

37.5. Secondary Survey:

- General: Child in moderate distress, moving intermittently but unable to find a comfortable position.
- Skin: Circular area of pallor surrounded by a ring of erythema located on the upper back. Two small puncture wounds in center of lesion.
- HEENT: Periorbital swelling.
- Neck: Supple.
- Chest: Normal.
- Lungs: Clear.
- Heart: Tachycardia.
- Abdomen: BS+, tender abdomen with rigid abdominal muscles. Guarding with no rebound.
- Perineum/GU: Child has an erect penis.
- Rectal: Hemoccult negative, nontender.
- Back: Normal. Wound on upper back as described above.
- Extremities: Normal.
- Neuro: Normal.

37.6. Laboratory:

- CBC: WBC 12, Hgb 14, Hct 44, Plt 300.
- Differential: Pending.
- Chemistry: Na 140, K 4.0, Cl 105, CO_2 24.

- BUN/Cr: 10/1.0.
- Glucose: 125.
- Ca/Mg: Normal.
- LFTs: Normal.
- Amylase/Lipase: Normal.
- PT/PTT: Normal.
- Blood cultures: Pending.
- U/A: Normal.

37.7. X-rays:
- CXR: Normal.
- Abdomen: Normal.

37.8. Special Tests:
- ECG: Not indicated.

37.9. Critical Actions:
- Recognize lesion as a black widow spider bite.
- Treat pain.
- Provide muscle relaxation with a benzodiazepine.
- Recognize this as Grade III envenomation.
- Discuss potential use of antivenom with Poison Control.
- If giving antivenom, check skin for antivenom sensitivity before administering this medication. Dose is generally one vial of antivenin regardless of patient's weight. Physician may check with Poison Center for dose or read package insert.

37.10. Pearls:

❍ **What is the role of calcium in the treatment of black widow spider bites?**

There is no scientific evidence that calcium is effective, there are only anecdotal reports of its benefit.

❍ **When is antivenin indicated for a black widow spider bite?**

It is considered for grade II or III envenomation. Indications include severe muscle and abdominal pain, headache, vomiting, diaphoresis, hypertension, and tachycardia.

CASE 38 (Female with Seizures)

Examiner

This 38 y/o female presents via EMS with eclampsia. She is 2 days postpartum after an uncomplicated normal spontaneous vaginal delivery. The Medics have started no treatment and she is actively seizing. The candidate should diagnose and treat eclampsia and possible aspiration pneumonia.

38.1. Introduction:

A 38 y/o female presents seizing.

Vital signs: BP 190/130, P 120, R 24, T 101°F, Wt 96 kg.

38.2. Primary Survey:
- General: Seizing female.
- Airway: Gag absent.
- Breathing: Spontaneous with right-sided crackles.
- Circulation: Capillary refill 3 seconds.
- Disability: Seizing.
- Exposure: No gross deformity.
- Finger: Pending.

38.3. Management:

- IV, O_2, pulse oximeter, monitor.
- Give 4 to 6 g magnesium sulfate IV, over 10 minutes, followed by 1 to 3 g/h.
- Administer lorazepam, midazolam, or diazepam to stop the seizure.
- Intubate to protect airway.
- Order blood work and UA.
- CXR.

38.4. History:

- Allergies: None.
- Medications: Vitamins, Atenolol.
- PMH: G2P2.
- Last meal: 2 hours prior to seizure.
- Events: The husband states she has chronic hypertension and delivered 2 days ago. Since that time she has had headaches and blurry vision. She has not taken her hypotensive medication for the past 5 days. About 10 minutes before arrival she started jerking her arms and legs. This lasted 3 to 4 minutes followed by a postictal period. Upon arrival she started seizing again. She is currently breast-feeding and denies fever, chills, vomiting, or abdominal pain.
- Family: Normal.
- Records: Not available.
- Immune: Up to date.
- EMTs: No further information.
- Narcotics: None.
- Doctor: Dr. Obs.
- Social history: None.

38.5. Secondary Survey:

- General: Seizing, unless benzodiazepine given.
- Skin: Normal.
- HEENT: Normal.
- Neck: Normal.
- Chest: Normal.
- Lungs: Crackles at right side.
- Heart: Regular.
- Abdomen: Soft, BS positive.
- Perineum/GU: Dark discharge per vagina.
- Rectal: Normal.
- Back: Normal.
- Extremities: 3+ edema.
- Neuro: Hyperactive DTRs, and ankle clonus present if not paralyzed for intubation.

38.6. Management:

- Intubate.
- Give 4 to 6 g magnesium sulfate IV, over 10 minutes, followed by 1 to 3 g/h.
- Administer lorazepam, midazolam, or diazepam.
- Consult OB attending.

38.7. Laboratory:

- CBC: WBC 14, Hgb 13, Hct 39, Plt 400.
- Differential: Pending.
- Chemistry: Pending.
- BUN/Cr: Pending.
- Glucose: 140 by glucometer.

- Ca/Mg: Pending.
- LFTs: Pending.
- Amylase/Lipase: Pending.
- PT/PTT: Not indicated.
- Cardiac enzymes: Pending.
- Pulse oximeter: 95%.
- ABG: pH 7.42, pO_2 84, pCO_2 35, HCO_3 40.
- Blood cultures: Pending.
- U/A: Pending.

38.8. X-rays:
- CXR: RUL infiltrate.

38.9. Special Tests:
- ECG: Sinus tachycardia.

38.10. Critical Actions:
- Diagnose eclampsia.
- Administer 2 to 4 g magnesium sulfate as a 20% solution IV over 5 to 10 minutes, followed by 1 to 3 g/h.
- Give a benzodiazepine to stop the seizure.
- Consult OB/Gyn.
- Intubate.
- Recognize possible aspiration pneumonia and start antibiotics.

38.11. Pearls:

❍ **What physical finding is most predictive of impending eclampsia?**

Ankle clonus.

❍ **How do you evaluate a patient for Magnesium toxicity?**

Loss of patellar reflex occurs at 7 to 10 mEq/L and respiratory depression occurs at 12 mEq/L.

CASE 39 (50 y/o Male Overdose)

Examiner

This 50 y/o male presents with a calcium channel blocker overdose with a history of depression. He called EMS after swallowing a full bottle of sustained release diltiazem with a large quantity of alcohol. A suicide note was found at the scene. No other medications were found. There was no evidence of trauma. The physician should treat the patient for a toxic ingestion and altered mental status while protecting the airway before gastric lavage.

39.1. Introduction:

A 50 y/o male is brought to the ED smelling strongly of alcohol, with emesis on clothing, and responding to sternal rub.

Vital signs: BP 90/60, P 46, R 12, T 97°F.

39.2. Primary Survey:
- General: Disheveled male, decreased responsiveness.
- Airway: Patent after chin-lift to clear tongue, decreased gag reflex.
- Breathing: Inspiratory crackles at bases.
- Circulation: Capillary refill 2 seconds, pulses symmetric.
- Disability: PERRL, pupils midrange, strong smells of ethanol, responds slowly to noxious stimuli by withdrawing.

- Exposure: No evidence of trauma, no track marks, no scars.
- Finger: Normal rectal tone, hemoccult negative.

39.3. Management:

- IV, O_2, monitor, and place on pulse oximeter.
- Intubate.
- Establish large bore IV. Obtain stat glucose, electrolytes, renal and liver function tests, PT/PTT, osm, Mg, and Ca. Start bolus with NS 500 mL IV.
- ECG.
- Administer naloxone and check glucose.
- Insert OG tube. Lavage with normal saline until aspirate is clear.
- Administer activated charcoal with sorbitol, 1 g/kg. Consider whole bowel irrigation.
- Administer calcium chloride (works faster than calcium gluconate) 1 to 3 g q 30 minutes times 8 hours.
- Consider glucagon, atropine, isoproterenol, epinephrine, amrinone, dopamine, norepinephrine, pacemaker, or intra-aortic balloon pump as indicated by patient's condition.

39.4. History:

- Allergies: Unknown.
- Medications: Diltiazem, others unknown.
- PMH: Hypertension.
- Last meal: Recent alcohol.
- Events: Upon arrival, the paramedics noted that the patient was lethargic but states he took a full bottle of his blood pressure medication. He vomited once but no pill fragments were seen. Empty vodka bottles, beer cans, an empty pill bottle, and a suicide note were found. No other medications were found. There was no evidence of trauma.
- Family: Unknown.
- Records: None.
- Immune: Unknown.
- EMTs: Less responsive during transport to the ED. Stated wife left him yesterday. A suicide note was found at the scene.
- Narcotics: Unknown.
- Doctor: Name on pill bottle.
- Social history: Married, unknown history of previous drugs or alcohol abuse, smokes cigarettes.

39.5. Secondary Survey:

- General: Intubated, no obvious injuries.
- Skin: Warm, moist, no skin lesions.
- HEENT: Anicteric, oropharynx-normal, TMs-normal.
- Neck: No JVD, supple.
- Chest: Symmetric, no injury.
- Lungs: Inspiratory crackles at bases.
- Heart: Bradycardic, no murmur.
- Abdomen: Normal.
- Perineum/genital: Normal.
- Rectal: Normal tone, hemoccult negative.
- Extremities: Normal.
- Neuro: Paralyzed and sedated. If not intubated, some symmetric movement of extremities to noxious stimuli.

39.6. Laboratory:

- CBC: WBC 11, Hgb 13, Hct 39, Plt 230.
- Chemistry: Na 140, K 4.0, Cl 110, CO_2 22.
- BUN/Cr: 14/1.0.
- Glucose: 140.
- Ca/Mg: 10/2.0.

- LFTs: Normal.
- Amylase/Lipase: Normal.
- PT/PTT: Normal.
- Cardiac enzymes: Normal.
- ABG: pH 7.40, $pO_2$150, pCO_2 30, HCO_3 22 (postintubation).
- U/A: Normal.
- Ethanol: 380.
- Urine drug screen: Pending.
- Salicylate: Negative.
- Acetaminophen: Negative.
- Cardiac enzymes: Pending

39.7. X-rays:
- CXR: Mild failure, borderline increased heart size, ETT in good position.
- KUB: No pills or foreign body.

39.8. Special Tests:
- ECG: Sinus bradycardia with first-degree heart block.

39.9. Critical Actions:
- Intubate to protect the airway.
- Treat hypotension with IV fluids. Consider glucagon, isoproterenol, epinephrine, amrinone, norepinephrine, dopamine, and intra-aortic balloon pump, if refractory.
- Give calcium chloride or gluconate.
- Administer naloxone, and check glucose.
- Gastric lavage with administration of charcoal and cathartic. Consider whole bowel irrigation.
- ICU admission.

39.10. Pearls:

❍ **How do calcium channel blockers exert their therapeutic effect?**

They interfere with calcium entry into the myocardial tissue and the vascular smooth muscle resulting in decreased conduction through the A-V node, decreased S-A node discharge, vasodilation, and decreased cardiac contractility.

❍ **Which calcium channel blocker is associated with hyperglycemia?**

Verapamil may inhibit the release of insulin. Administering calcium can decrease this effect.

CASE 40 (2 y/o Foreign-Body Ingestion)

Examiner

A child is brought in by his parents after swallowing a disc battery 1 hour ago. He will appear normal with no evidence of aspiration or obstruction.

40.1. Introduction:

A 2 y/o child is brought to the ED by his parents who report that he swallowed a disc battery 1 hour ago.

Vital signs: P 100, R 22, T 98.6°F, Wt 13 kg.

40.2. Primary Survey:
- General: Well-developed, well-nourished child in no respiratory distress and is consolable by parents.
- Airway: Patent, normal cry.
- Breathing: Clear, symmetric breath sounds, no use of accessory muscles.
- Circulation: Capillary refill 2 seconds.
- Disability: Alert, responds appropriately to parents.

- Exposure: No evidence of any injury.
- Finger: Deferred.

40.3. Management:
- Order CXR (include view of the neck) and KUB.
- Allow parents to remain with child.
- Keep patient NPO while x-ray is pending.

40.4. History:
- Allergies: None.
- Medications: None.
- PMH: None.
- Last meal: Had bottle enroute to hospital.
- Events: A 2 y/o male is brought in by his parents who report he swallowed a disc battery 1 hour ago. The child is crying but has no drooling and has taken his bottle without difficulty since the ingestion. There is no evidence of aspiration of the battery.
- Family: Noncontributory.
- Records: None.
- Immune: Up to date.
- Narcotics: No other ingestion.
- Doctor: Pediatrician available.
- Social history: Lives with parents.

40.5. Secondary Survey:
- General: Healthy appearing, active child.
- Skin: Normal.
- HEENT: Oropharynx clear, pink, moist, no drooling.
- Neck: No stridor, supple.
- Chest: No use of accessory muscles.
- Lungs: Clear, equal breath sounds.
- Heart: RRR, no murmurs.
- Abdomen: Normal bowel sounds, no tenderness, no distention, no masses, no organomegaly.
- Perineum/GU: Normal.
- Rectal: Deferred.
- Back: Normal.
- Extremities: Normal.
- Neuro: Active, alert, normal examination.

40.6. Laboratory:
- None indicated.

40.7. X-rays:
- CXR: Normal x-ray, no foreign bodies, normal lung fields.
- Abdomen x-ray: Opaque disc detected in the stomach. Object appears intact. Remainder of abdomen is normal.

40.8. Special Tests:
- None indicated.

40.9. Critical Actions:
- Obtain an accurate history of type and time of ingestion as well as history of any vomiting or respiratory distress.
- Avoid inducing vomiting.
- Obtain x-ray to determine the position of the battery and if the battery appears intact.
- Explain follow-up to parents, that is, observe for abdominal pain, distention, vomiting, strain stool to look for battery passage, and repeat x-ray to follow passage through GI tract. Consult with PMD to arrange follow-up x-ray.

40.10. Pearls:

- **Name the materials contained in disc batteries.**

  Disc, or button, batteries may contain salts of metals, including zinc, cadmium, mercury, silver, nickel, and lithium as well as concentrated alkaline media, usually potassium or sodium hydroxide.

- **What are the potential complications of disc battery ingestion?**

  Complications include obstruction, aspiration, heavy metal absorption, and perforation. Lodged batteries may lead to pressure necrosis, liquefaction, necrosis if leakage of contents occurs, or electrical injury through conduction to tissues. Most batteries pass uneventfully in 2 to 3 days.

- **Name possible interventions for a battery lodged in the esophagus.**

  Glucagon, nitrates, or benzodiazepines may be useful in relaxing esophageal tone, allowing the battery to pass into the stomach.

CASE 41 (Cyanide Poisoning)

Examiner

A 32 y/o male laboratory worker is brought to the ED after collapsing while at lunch. Colleagues know of no ingestion or medical conditions. The physician is presented with a comatose patient who is bradycardic and is having agonal respirations. The physician must secure the airway after giving naloxone, and checking the glucose. Obtain appropriate laboratory data/studies in an attempt to discover the etiology of the patient's moribund state.

While working on the patient, a medical student, who worked in a laboratory, recognizes the aroma of bitter almonds associated with cyanide. Patient improves after treatment. The physician then initiates specific treatment for cyanide poisoning and arranges for ICU admission. Further questioning of the patient's colleagues reveals that the he had appeared depressed recently. They report he had access to numerous chemicals, including cyanide.

41.1. Introduction:

Vitals signs: BP 60/p, P 58, R 8, T 98.0°F, Wt 88.3 kg.

41.2. Primary Survey:

- General: Comatose male with no evidence of trauma.
- Airway: Patent.
- Breathing: Agonal respirations, saturation 92% on room air.
- Circulation: Unable to obtain blood pressure, weak carotid pulse, delayed capillary refill.
- Disability: Pupils are equal and reactive, no response to deep pain.
- Exposure: Blisters in oropharynx, no other injury or lesions.
- Finger: Normal rectal tone, hemoccult negative.

41.3. Management:

- O_2, pulse oximeter, and monitor.
- IV 1 L NS bolus.
- Administer naloxone and check glucose.
- Perform RSI and give ventilator settings.
- Order CBC, CMP, ETOH, urine drug screen, UA, salicylate, acetaminophen, lactate, and ABG.
- *A medical student who is working in the adjacent area reports he smells a bitter almond odor, associated with cyanide, emanating from the comatose patient. Management now includes:*
  - Administer sodium nitrite, 300 mg, followed by sodium thiosulfate, 12.5 g, contained in the Lilly Cyanide Antidote Kit.
  - Administer hydroxycobalamin IV

- Lavage patient and administer charcoal.
- Start an inotropic agent for hypotension.
- Admit to the ICU.

41.4. History:

- Allergies: Unknown.
- Medications: Unknown.
- PMH: None.
- Last meal: Last meal 1 hour ago.
- Events: Colleagues report that the patient appeared depressed recently and collapsed at lunch, while sitting in chair. They report he had access to numerous chemicals, including cyanide.
- Family: Unknown.
- Records: None.
- Immune: Unknown.
- EMTs: Confirm above history, no vomiting, no trauma.
- Narcotics: No known drug ingestion.
- Doctor: Unknown.
- Social history: No regular alcohol or cigarette use. Recently overlooked for promotion.

41.5. Secondary Survey:

- General: Comatose male, no cyanosis.
- Skin: Slightly cool, no track marks.
- HEENT: No evidence of trauma. Eyes are clear, retinal vessels appear cherry red. Blistering of oropharynx is evident.
- Neck: No step off, supple, no stridor prior to intubation.
- Chest: No crepitus.
- Lungs: Clear, equal breath sounds bilaterally.
- Heart: RRR, bradycardic, no murmurs.
- Abdomen: Normal bowel sounds, nondistended, no masses.
- Perineum/GU: Normal male.
- Rectal: Normal tone, guaiac negative.
- Back: Normal.
- Extremities: Normal.
- Neuro: Comatose, pupils equal and reactive.

41.6. Laboratory:

- CBC: WBC 10.0, Hgb 14, Hct 40, Plt 232.
- Differential: Normal.
- Chemistry: Na 140, K 4.2, Cl 104, CO_2 8.
- BUN/Cr: 12/1.0.
- Glucose: 86.
- Ca/Mg: Normal.
- LFTs: Normal.
- Amylase/Lipase: Normal.
- PT/PTT: Normal.
- Cardiac enzymes: Normal.
- ABG: pH 7.11, pO_2 90, pCO_2 28, HCO_3 12.
- U/A: Normal.
- Lactate: 5.0.

41.7. X-rays:

- CXR: Clear lung fields, normal heart size.

41.8. Special Tests:

- ECG: Sinus bradycardia.

41.9. Critical Actions:

- Intubate the patient.
- Administer naloxone, and check glucose.
- Administer antidote for cyanide poisoning.
- Lavage and administer charcoal.
- Admit to the ICU with psychiatric evaluation when patient awakens.

41.10. Pearls:

❍ **How does cyanide exert its effect?**

Cyanide combines with the enzyme cytochrome oxidase. Binding with cytochrome oxidase disrupts the final step in mitochondrial oxidative phosphorylation preventing oxygen utilization and aerobic metabolism. The body, therefore, cannot utilize oxygen and anaerobic metabolism ensues.

❍ **What are some sources of cyanide?**

Cyanide is widespread in various industries, including electroplating, fumigation, precious metal refining, photography, and chemical production. It is also found in acetonitrile, a solvent used as an artificial nail remover. Cyanide may also be released when various materials are burned, including silk, wool, synthetic rubber, polyurethane, and nitrocellulose.

CASE 42 (Intoxicated Homeless Male)

Examiner

A patient is brought to the ED appearing severely intoxicated from isopropyl alcohol ingestion. On initial arrival of the paramedics, he complained of abdominal pain but quickly lost consciousness. The physician should stabilize the patient's blood pressure, assess for etiology of altered mental status, and evaluate the abdominal pain. On further questioning the medics report finding an empty bottle of rubbing alcohol and mouthwash at the scene.

42.1. Introduction:

A disheveled, intoxicated male brought in by EMS, unconscious. There is no evidence of trauma.

Vital signs: BP 86/58, P 104, R 14, T 98.0°F, O_2 sat 95%, Wt 74 kg.

42.2. Primary Survey:

- General: Disheveled, intoxicated male, faint odor of acetone.
- Airway: Patent, no gag reflex.
- Breathing: Clear and equal breath sounds.
- Circulation: Symmetric pulses, capillary refill >2 seconds.
- Disability: Withdraws to painful stimuli, pupils equal and reactive.
- Exposure: No evidence of trauma.
- Finger: Normal rectal tone, hemoccult positive stool.

42.3. Management:

- IV, pulse oximeter, monitor.
- Administer naloxone and check glucose.
- Intubate.
- NS bolus.
- Order CBC, CMP, LFTs, PT/PTT/INR, lipase, toxicology screen, ethanol, osmolality, ABG, toxic alcohols, UA, and hold type and screen.
- Insert an NG tube to assess for upper GI bleeding.

42.4. History:

- Allergies: Unknown.
- Medications: Unknown.
- PMH: Unknown.
- Last meal: Unknown, probable recent alcohol ingestion.
- Events: Unknown, probable recent alcohol ingestion. On initial arrival of the paramedics, he complained of abdominal pain. There is no history of trauma. The patient was found wandering in the street.
- Family: None.
- Records: None.
- Immune: Unknown.
- EMTs: Paramedics find, when going through his belongings, an empty bottle of rubbing alcohol.
- Narcotics: Intoxicated, no response to naloxone.
- Doctor: None.
- Social history: Homeless, not known to ED staff.

42.5. Secondary Survey:

- General: Poor hygiene, intoxicated, BP increased with IVF.
- Skin: No track marks, dry, poor turgor.
- HEENT: No evidence of trauma, anicteric, oropharynx dry, poor dentition, normal nose, ears.
- Neck: No deformity, moving head freely on arrival, no meningismus, no nodes, no stridor, no JVD.
- Chest: No deformity or crepitus, gynecomastia.
- Lungs: Clear and equal breath sounds.
- Heart: RRR, no murmurs, rubs, or gallops.
- Abdomen: Normal bowel sounds, tenderness to deep palpation in left upper quadrant, no peritoneal signs, no masses or organomegaly, nondistended
- Perineum/genital: Normal male.
- Rectal: As above.
- Back: No deformity.
- Extremities: No deformity, tobacco stains on fingers.
- Neuro: PERRL, rouses to noxious stimuli, face symmetric, moves all extremities, DTRs symmetric, toes downgoing bilaterally.

42.6. Laboratory:

- CBC: WBC 10, Hgb 10, Hct 30, Plt 53,000.
- Differential: Pending.
- Chemistry: Na 140, K 3.8, Cl 105, CO_2 22.
- BUN/Cr: 10/1.0.
- Glucose: 60.
- Ca/Mg: 10/1.1.
- LFTs: LDH 290, AST 80, ALT 55, GGT 75, Alk Phos 40, Bili 1.3.
- Amylase/Lipase: 120/15.
- PT/PTT: 13/33.
- ABG: pH 7.4, $pO_2$90, pCO_2 40, HCO_3 22.
- Osmolality: 360, osmol gap = 74.
- ETOH: 5 mg/dL.
- U/A: + ketones, – glucose.
- Isopropanol: Pending.
- Methanol: Pending.
- Ethylene glycol: Pending.

- Lactate: Pending.
- Toxicology: Negative.

42.7. X-rays:
- CXR: No acute infiltrate.

42.8. Special Tests:
- ECG: Normal sinus rhythm, no abnormalities.
- NG aspirate: No blood or coffee ground material.

42.9. Critical Actions:
- Intubate.
- Administer naloxone, and check glucose.
- Assess for cause of hypotension/altered mental status/abdominal pain. Eliminate possibility of acute GI bleed.
- Provide supportive care for isopropanol ingestion. Consider hemodialysis, if patient has persistent hypotension or coma, or if isopropanol level is greater than 400 mg/dL.
- Admit to the ICU.

42.10. Pearls:

❍ **What are the findings that are associated with isopropanol intoxication?**

CNS depression, prolonged intoxication, abdominal pain, hemorrhagic gastritis, hypotension, odor of acetone or rubbing alcohol, mild or no acidosis, ketonuria, ketonemia, elevated osmol gap, normal to low glucose.

❍ **What is the major pathway for isopropanol metabolism?**

It is metabolized by alcohol dehydrogenase to acetone in the liver.

CASE 43 (Triple)

Patient #1 (Female with a Headache)

Examiner

This patient presents with a 3-day history of a severe headache due to a subarachnoid hemorrhage. This patient is stable but the candidate should perform a complete examination, order a CT scan, and perform an LP once the CT scan comes back as negative. Since the patient remains stable throughout the case, critical actions involve diagnosing a SAH by LP and instituting appropriate supportive therapy. The patient may be sent to CT while the other patients are evaluated.

43.1. Introduction:

A 45 y/o female presents with a complaint of headache.

Vital signs: BP 198/120, P 88, R 18, T 100.1°F.

43.2. Primary Survey:
- General: WN/WD female in moderate discomfort, sitting still with sun glasses on. She is in no respiratory distress.
- Airway: Intact.
- Breathing: Intact.
- Circulation: Intact.
- Disability: GCS 15, PERRLA.
- Exposure: No medic alert tags.
- Finger: Deferred to secondary examination.

43.3. Management:
- IV, monitor, and pulse oximeter.
- You may order appropriate diagnostic studies now or after the history and secondary survey.

43.4. History:
- Allergies: None.
- Medications: None.
- PMH: Migraine headaches controlled by acetaminophen and ibuprofen.
- Last meal: 6 hours ago.
- Events: 3 days ago, she experienced an explosive headache lasting 1 hour with vomiting and photophobia. The intensity decreased but the headache remained. No complaint of fever, chills, or vomiting. This headache is worse than her usual migraines. No history of trauma.
- Family: Noncontributory.
- Records: None.
- Immune: Up to date.
- EMTs: Noncontributory.
- Narcotics: No illicit drug use.
- Doctor: No doctor.
- Social history: No alcohol or tobacco use.

43.5. Secondary Survey:
- General: Continues to complain of a headache, with VS unchanged.
- Skin: Normal.
- HEENT: Small round hemorrhages seen near the optic nerve.
- Neck: Mild nuchal rigidity.
- Chest: Normal.
- Lungs: Normal.
- Heart: Normal.
- Abdomen: Normal.
- Perineum/genital: Normal.
- Rectal: Normal.
- Back: Normal.
- Extremities: Normal.
- Neuro: Alert to person, place, but not time. CN II to XII intact, bilateral Babinskis present.

43.6. Management:
- Appropriate laboratory studies and x-rays can be ordered now.
- Allow candidate to send the patient to CT scan.
- Treat the headache.

While the patient is in CT scan, the nurse tells you that another patient is in room #2.

Patient #2 (Hand Laceration)

Examiner

This patient presents with a human bite to the second metacarpal-phalangeal joint of the right hand. Do not tell the candidate it was a result of hitting someone's tooth, unless specifically asked. This patient requires admission but is resistant, have the candidate talk him in to it. He can be completely worked up and dispositioned without interruption. If the candidate takes too long, have the third patient arrive.

43.1. Introduction: (**Patient #2**)

A 21 y/o male presents with a cut to his right hand.

Vital signs: BP 126/72, P 88, R 16, T 100.8°F.

43.2. Primary Survey:
- General: Pleasant 21 y/o, right-handed male sitting upright on the cart, asking for his hand to be "fixed" so he can go.

- Airway: Intact.
- Breathing: Normal.
- Circulation: Normal.
- Disability: Normal.

43.3. History:

- Allergies: Penicillin.
- Medications: None.
- PMH: No significant illnesses or injuries. No past surgeries.
- Last meal: 1 hour ago.
- Events: Patient states he was at a bar, had a "few too many drinks," and cut his hand about 12 hours ago. Only after specifically asking him how he did it, does he say that he punched someone in the mouth.
- Family: Older brother is in the waiting area.
- Records: None.
- Immune: Up to date.
- Narcotics: No illicit drug use.
- Doctor: None.
- Social history: Smokes two packs of cigarette per day, drinks one case of beer per week.

43.4. Secondary Survey:

- General: No change in vital signs.
- Skin: Normal.
- HEENT: Normal.
- Neck: Normal.
- Chest: Normal.
- Lungs: Normal.
- Heart: Normal.
- Abdomen: Normal.
- Perineum/genital: Normal.
- Rectal: Deferred.
- Back: Normal.
- Extremities: A full-thickness laceration over the second MP joint with extension into the joint is present. There is normal sensation, motor function, and capillary refill to that digit. Red streaks are present and moderate swelling to the dorsum of the hand is noted.
- Neuro: Normal.

43.5. Laboratory:

- CBC: WBC 19, Hgb 12.5, Hct 37.5, Plt 240,000.
- Differential: Polys 80, bands 38%, lymphs 15, eos 2, mono 3.
- Chemistries: Na 138, K 4.0, Cl 109, CO_2 32.
- BUN/Cr: 10/0.9.
- Glucose: 90.
- PT/PTT: Normal.
- Blood cultures: Pending.
- Wound culture: Pending.
- U/A: Normal.
- Drug screen: Negative.
- ETOH: 80.

43.6. X-rays:

- Right hand: No fracture or foreign body.

43.7. Management:

- IV.
- Irrigate wound.

- Start antibiotics.
- Consult a hand surgeon.
- Convince the patient to be admitted.

The nurse informs you the patient in room 3 is not breathing well.

Patient #3 (32 y/o Male with a Bee Sting)

Examiner

This patient was stung by a bee and is in acute respiratory distress. Regardless of the treatment rendered, the patient deteriorates requiring airway management and pressor support. The candidate will be unable to intubate, thereby requiring a cricothyrotomy. Once the airway is established and appropriate therapy is given, the patient will stabilize. A family member arrives after the primary survey and initial management.

43.1. Introduction:

A 32 y/o male presents via ambulance in respiratory distress with a rash.

Vital signs: BP 80/P, P 124, R 40, T 98.8°F, Wt 80 kg.

43.2. Primary Survey:

- General: A 32 y/o male in acute respiratory distress.
- Airway: Significant oral angioedema, patient continually grabs his throat, drooling.
- Breathing: Diminished breath sounds in both bases with wheezing in all fields.
- Circulation: Capillary refill >4 seconds, peripheral pulses are weak and thready.
- Disability: GCS 15, PERRLA
- Exposure: Medic alert tag indicates allergic to bee.
- Finger: Deferred.

43.3. Management:

- IV.
- Monitor.
- Albuterol 2.5 mg per nebulizer.
- Epinephrine 0.3 mL (1:1,000) subcutaneously × 3, 15 minutes apart.
- 1 L bolus of 0.9% NS.
- Solumedrol 125 mg IV.
- Benadryl 50 mg IV.
- Consider an H_2 blocker IV.
- Tetanus prophylaxis.

43.4. Primary Survey (recheck)

- Patient is still in respiratory distress, requires rapid sequence intubation. Endotracheal intubation is unsuccessful, requiring a cricothyrotomy. Have the candidate describe the procedure.

43.5. History:

The patient is unable to give a history, the EMTs are gone, but the patient's wife is in the waiting room.

- Allergies: Bee stings (last bee sting caused a mild case of wheezing and a rash) and sulfa.
- Medications: None.
- PMH: No illnesses or injuries. No surgeries.
- Last meal: Unknown.
- Events: Wife states her husband was working in the garden when she heard him call to her. When she arrived he was lying on the ground, unable to speak, in respiratory distress.
- Family: Noncontributory.
- Records: None.
- Immune: Last tetanus 15 years ago.
- EMTs: Gone.

- Narcotics: None.
- Doctor: None.
- Social history: No alcohol or tobacco use.

43.6. Secondary Survey:
- General: Patient is paralyzed, being ventilated.
- Skin: Raised wheels diffusely distributed.
- HEENT: Clear rhinorrhea, eye lid edema, chemosis, tongue, and uvular swelling.
- Neck: Urticaria.
- Chest: Urticaria.
- Lungs: Wheezing present but louder than before.
- Heart: Rapid rate, no murmur.
- Abdomen: Normal.
- Perineum/genital: Normal.
- Rectal: Normal.
- Back: Urticaria
- Extremities: After fluid bolus capillary refill is <2 seconds, pulses equal and stronger.
- Neuro: Patient paralyzed.

43.7. Laboratory:
- CBC: WBC 21, Hgb 15, Hct 45, Plt 300,000.
- Differential: Polys 65, bands 8, lymphs 10, eos 20, mono 5.
- Chemistries: Na 138, K 4.5, Cl 112, CO_2 24.
- BUN/Cr: 9/1.0.
- Glucose: 138.
- Ca/Mg: Normal.
- LFTs: Normal.
- Amylase/Lipase: Normal.
- PT/PTT: Normal.
- Cardiac enzymes: Normal.
- ABG: pH 7.45, pO_2 360, pCO_2 27, HCO_3 25.
- U/A: Normal.

43.8. X-rays:
- CXR: No pulmonary edema, cric tube in place.

43.9. Special Tests:
- ECG: Sinus tachycardia.

43.10. Management:
- Admit to the ICU.

Patient #1 returns from the CT scan with the headache still present and vital signs and neurologic status unchanged.

Patient #1

43.1. Laboratory:
- CBC: WBC 14, Hgb 13.2, Hct 39.6, Plt 185,000.
- Chemistries: Na 125, K 3.8, Cl 108, CO_2 24.
- BUN/Cr: 15/1.0.
- Glucose: 140.
- Ca/Mg: Normal.
- LFTs: Normal.
- Amylase/Lipase: Normal.
- PT/PTT: Normal.
- Cardiac enzymes: Normal.

- ABG: pH 7.48, pO_2 98, pCO_2 27, HCO_3 23 (room air).
- Blood cultures: Pending.
- U/A: Normal.
- Drug screen: Negative.
- ETOH: Negative.

43.2. X-rays:

- CXR: Normal.
- CT head: Normal.

43.3. Special Tests:

- ECG: Nonspecific ST-T-wave abnormalities.
- CSF results: Opening pressure 200, protein 600, glucose normal, RBCs 100,000, WBCs 500, Appearance xanthochromia, Gram stain negative, culture pending.

43.4. Management:

- Consult neurosurgery.
- Call the radiologist to set up CT or MR angiography.
- Elevate the head of the bed to 30 degrees.
- Start esmolol, nicardipine, or nitroprusside drip to lower the BP (SBP <150 or DBP <90 mmHg or within 5% of baseline).
- Give phenytoin (15–20 mg/kg loading dose), for seizure prophylaxis.
- Use antiemetic, if vomiting continues.
- Give nimodipine 60 mg po to decrease the risk of cerebral vasospasm.
- Admit to the ICU.
- Perform an LP when the CT scan is negative.
- Decrease the diastolic blood pressure below 100 mm Hg.

43.5. Pearls (**Patient #1**)

❍ **When does xanthochromia first appear in the cerebral spinal fluid?**

Six hours after the initial hemorrhage.

❍ **What is the cause of hyponatremia seen in some patients with a subarachnoid hemorrhage?**

Inappropriate secretion of antidiuretic hormone or excessive release of natriuretic peptides.

❍ **What are the CNS complications commonly seen in patients surviving an initial subarachnoid hemorrhage?**

Rebleeding, vasospasm, and an acute hydrocephalus.

Patient #2 (Human Bite)

43.1. Critical Actions:

- Admit.
- Consult a hand surgeon.
- Start IV antibiotics.
- Do not suture the wound.
- Irrigate wound.

43.2. Pearls (**Patient #2**)

❍ **What are the indications for admission in a patient with a human bite?**

Lymphangitis, symptoms of systemic infection, suspected joint, tendon, or bone infection, and patients that are immunocompromised or have vascular insufficiency.

❍ **What are the most common bacteria found in infected human bite wounds?**

Staphylococcus aureus and streptococcus species.

Patient #3 (Anaphylactic Shock)

43.1. Critical Actions:
- Epinephrine.
- Early airway when the medical therapy doesn't work.
- Describe how to perform a cricothyrotomy.
- Steroids.
- Fluid bolus to correct hypotension.
- ICU admission.
- Tetanus prophylaxis.

43.2. Pearls (Patient #3)

❍ **What is the most common cause of life-threatening anaphylaxis?**

Penicillin.

❍ **What is the most common cause of death from anaphylaxis?**

Laryngeal edema resulting in upper airway obstruction.

CASE 44 (80 y/o Male with Abdominal Pain)

Examiner

This is a difficult case but the patient has many risk factors for mesenteric ischemia/occlusion. Have the candidate call and talk with the surgeon. The surgeon will be resistant to seeing the patient because of the equivocal CT angiogram results. He/She is requesting a formal angiogram. The candidate must convince the surgeon to see the patient quickly based on the risk factors, laboratory findings, and ECG. The surgeon will eventually accept the consult. Continue to point out how much pain the patient has despite the paucity of physical findings.

44.1. Introduction:

An 80 y/o male presents via ambulance from a retirement home, with a complaint of abdominal pain.

Vital signs: BP 100/70, P 92 (irregular only if asked), R 26, T 100.6°F, Wt 76 kg.

44.2. Primary Survey:
- General: Slender, cachectic appearing male, pale, diaphoretic, sitting upright holding his abdomen, in severe pain.
- Airway: Intact.
- Breathing: Normal.
- Circulation: Capillary refill >2 seconds, weak peripheral pulses.
- Disability: Normal.
- Exposure: Medic alert tag stating "Heart disease."
- Finger: Deferred to secondary survey.

44.3. Management:
- IV, O_2, monitor, and pulse oximeter.
- IV pain medication.
- CT angiogram of abdomen and pelvis.
- Cardiac monitor.
- Order appropriate laboratory studies and x-rays.

44.4. History:
- Allergies: None.
- Medications: Furosemide 40 mg bid.
  - Digoxin 0.125 mg qd.
  - Glipizide 5 mg qd.

  - Nitroglycerine SL prn chest pain.
  - Aspirin 160 mg qd.
  - Mylanta 30 cc ac $^+$ hs.
- PMH: Cardiac angioplasty 1996.
  - Carotid endarterectomy 1997.
  - NIDDM.
  - Myocardial infarction 1990, 1994.
- Last meal: 1 hour ago.
- Events: This 80 y/o patient began complaining of pain shortly after eating breakfast. The pain is crampy, diffused, nonradiating, and increasing in intensity. The patient complains of nausea, no vomiting, diarrhea, fever, chills, or urinary complaints. Last bowel movement was 10 hours ago and it was normal. A 20 lb weight loss has been noted over the past 4 months.
- Family: Father, mother, and brother all died from heart disease.
- Records: None.
- Immune: "Flu" shot this year.
- EMTs: Left department.
- Doctor: Dr. Internist.
- Social history: Retired accountant, smokes half pack of cigarette per day for 40 years, quit 15 years ago. No alcohol use.

44.5. Secondary Survey:
- General: Patient appears very uncomfortable complaining of increasing pain.
- Skin: Pale, moist, no rash, or petechiae.
- HEENT: Arcus senilis, EOM-I PERRLA.
- Neck: Normal.
- Chest: Normal.
- Lungs: Normal.
- Heart: Irregular rhythm, loud III/VI systolic ejection murmur, laterally displaced PMI.
- Abdomen: Soft, mild, and diffused tenderness to palpation. No rebound or guarding. Bowel sounds are present but diminished. No pulsatile mass or organomegaly.
- Perineum/genital: Normal.
- Rectal: Slightly enlarged, firm prostate, brown stool, hemoccult positive.
- Back: Normal.
- Extremities: Femoral pulses are strong but peripheral pulses are weak in the lower extremities. Pretibial edema, no calf tenderness, negative Homan's sign.
- Neuro: Intact.

44.6. Laboratory:
- CBC: WBC 14.2, Hgb 16.6, Hct 50, Plt 240,000.
- Differential: Polys 68, bands 29%, lymphs 18, eos 1, mono 0.
- Chemistries: Na 150, K 4.0, Cl 112, CO_2 15.
- BUN/Cr: 60/2.5.
- Glucose: 201.
- Ca/Mg: 10/2.1.
- LFTs: Normal.
- Amylase/Lipase: 150/15.
- PT/PTT: 13.5/36.
- Cardiac enzymes: Normal.
- ABG: pH 7.10 pO_2 94, pCO_2 40, HCO_3 13.
- Blood cultures: Pending.
- Digoxin: 1.7 (0.8–2.1).
- Phosphorus 7.0 (3–4.5).

- Type & Cross: Pending.
- U/A: Ketones 2+, all other values are negative.

44.7. X-rays:
- CXR: Normal.
- Abdominal series: Ileus.

44.8. Special Tests:
- ECG: Atrial fibrillation.
- Aortic and mesenteric CT angiography: Vasoconstriction in the superior mesenteric artery and bowel edema.

44.9. Management:
- Consult a surgeon.
- NS bolus.
- IV pain medication.

44.10. Critical Actions:
- Pain medication.
- Recognize the diagnosis from the presence of all the risk factors.
- Consult and convince surgery to see patient.
- Obtain a CT angiogram.
- NS fluid bolus.
- Administer triple antibiotics.

44.11. Pearls

❍ **What are the risk factors for mesenteric ischemia?**

Advanced age, advanced cardiovascular disease, a history of thromboembolic events, concurrent medication with digoxin and a diuretic, and atrial fibrillation.

❍ **What are the plain radiographic findings seen in mesenteric ischemia?**

Thumb-printing of the intestinal mucosa, gas in the intestinal wall, gas in the portal venous system, and an ileus pattern. In the majority of cases, the films will be normal or have nonspecific findings.

❍ **What is the gold standard test for diagnosing mesenteric ischemia/infarct?**

Mesenteric angiography.

CASE 45 (Child with Knee Swelling)

Examiner

A 12 y/o girl presents after a fall with an acute pain to the right knee and severe swelling. She has a known history of hemophilia C. The case should demonstrate the candidate's ability to treat hemophilia as well as evaluate a severe knee injury and patellar dislocation.

45.1. Introduction:

A 12 y/o girl is brought to the ED by her mother with a complaint of severe right knee

Vital signs: BP 110/80, P 80, R 20, T 98.6°F, Wt 42 kg.

45.2. Primary Survey:
- General impression: Child in severe pain with very swollen right knee.
- Airway: Normal.
- Breathing: Normal.
- Circulation: Normal.
- Disability: Normal.
- Exposure: No signs of trauma other than right knee, hemophilia medic alert tag.
- Finger: Not indicated.

45.3. Management:
- Start IV.
- Administer appropriate IV pain medicine (avoid an NSAID or aspirin)
- Order CBC, Factor XIII and XI levels, von Willebrand factor level, PT, PTT, and thrombin time.
- Order x-ray of R knee.
- Order ice packs to the right knee.
- Order fresh frozen plasma 15 to 20 mL/kg IV loading dose.
- Consider tranexamic acid.

45.4. History:
- Allergies: None.
- Medications: None.
- PMH: No significant illnesses or major injuries.
- Last meal: 2 hours ago.
- Events: A 12 y/o girl is brought to the ED by her mother with a complaint of severe right knee pain after she fell down the steps 3 hours ago. The mother indicates the child has hemophilia C. No LOC or other complaints of pain.
- Family: Mother is present to answer the questions. Family history is not applicable as the child is adopted.
- Records: None.
- Immune: Up to date.
- Doctor: Dr. Hematologist. Available for consult.

45.5. Secondary Survey:
- General: Awake and alert in severe pain.
- Skin: Normal.
- HEENT: Normal.
- Neck: Supple, no nodes.
- Chest: Normal.
- Lungs: Clear to auscultation.
- Heart: Normal.
- Abdomen: Normal.
- Perineum/GU: Normal.
- Rectal: Not indicated.
- Back: Normal.
- Extremities: Normal and equal pulses. Right knee severe swelling and pain with any attempt at movement.
- Neuro: Normal.

45.6. Laboratory:
- CBC: Normal.
- Chemistry: Normal.
- BUN/Cr: Normal.
- Glucose: Normal.
- PT: Normal, PTT moderately elevated, thrombin time normal.
- U/A: Normal.
- Factor levels: Pending.

45.7. X-rays:
- Knee: Right patella dislocated.

45.8. Critical Actions:
- Appropriate early pain relief.
- Administer FFP.
- Relocate dislocated patella and immobilize knee.
- Consult a hematologist.
- Consider DDAVP and epsilon-aminocaproic acid (amicar).
- Admit.

45.9. Pearls:

❍ **What concerns do you have with FFP administration?**

Volume overloading, hypersensitivity reactions, and transmission of infection from plasma products.

❍ **Why should you double check the current treatment recommendations before administering FFP?**

In Europe, Factor XI concentrates are available. Soon they should be available in the United States.

CASE 46 (Female with Vomiting and Diarrhea)

Examiner

A 34 y/o female presents with a lithium overdose. As part of the workup, the candidate should order a lithium level, however, this test should be slow to return and the laboratory should call and indicate the lithium level will have to be sent to another institution because of an equipment problem. The neuro examination, laboratory studies, EKG, and history of tetracycline and ibuprofen use (increase lithium levels), and dehydrated state should alert the candidate of the diagnosis. Therapy should be started in the ED.

46.1. Introduction:

A 34 y/o female presents from home anxious, pale in obvious discomfort.

Vital signs: BP 100/70, P 110, R 20, T 99.0°F, pulse ox 94% RA, Wt 60 kg.

46.2. Primary Survey:

- General: The patient is a slim female actively vomiting, anxious, pale, and in obvious discomfort. She is a very poor historian, however, her husband, with prompting, reports a history of confusion and a seizure and symptoms getting worse over the last 3 days. With further questioning, he provides a history of running a 10 K race 5 days ago and taking Ibuprofen for a muscle pull. She also takes tetracycline for her acne.
- Airway: Intact.
- Breathing: Slightly increased rate.
- Circulation: Rapid pulse.
- Disability: Negative.
- Exposure: No obvious injuries.
- Finger: Normal rectal, heme negative.

46.3. Management:

- Determine that patient is at risk for lithium toxicity.
- Start IV with NS bolus.
- Place on O_2, pulse oximeter, and cardiac monitor.
- Perform frequent VS.
- Order screening laboratory studies, lithium level, ECG, and possibly head CT scan.

46.4. History:

- Allergies: None.
- Medications: Lithium, ibuprofen, and tetracycline, unknown dose. The husband thinks she take her lithium several times a day and that "slow release" lithium was tried in the past and did not work.
- PMH: Well-controlled manic-depression.
- Last meal: Last night.
- Events: A 34 y/o female presents with nausea, vomiting, diarrhea, weakness, and confusion. She has a tremor and had a first time seizure witnessed by her husband. A detailed history taken from her husband reveals that she has a history of manic-depression and takes lithium. He does not think that she is taking more than her usual dose. She is also taking tetracycline for acne and ibuprofen for pain after running. The symptoms started 3 days ago but have gotten worse. She ran a 10 K race 4 days ago.
- Family: Husband is present for the information. Parents died from cancer in their seventies.

- Records: Available upon request.
- Immune: Up to date.
- Narcotics: No illicit drug use.
- Doctor: Consultants are available.
- Social history: No alcohol or tobacco use. Lives with her husband. She is a psychologist.

46.5. Secondary Survey:

- General: Continues to be anxious, uncomfortable, vomiting, and had multiple episodes of diarrhea.
- Skin: Pale, dry.
- HEENT: Mucous membranes dry.
- Neck: Normal.
- Chest: Nontender.
- Lungs: Clear.
- Heart: Tachycardic and regular.
- Abdomen: Bowel sounds are normal, no pain to palpation.
- Perineum/GU: Normal.
- Rectal: Normal.
- Back: No CVA tenderness.
- Extremity: Slow capillary refill, pulses are equal.
- Neuro: Severe tremor, muscle fasciculations and symmetrical weakness, choreoathetosis, hyperreflexia, clonus, and confusion.

46.6. Laboratory:

- CBC: Normal.
- Chemistry: Na 124, K 3.5, Cl 98, CO_2 20.
- BUN/Cr: 28/1.5.
- Glucose: Normal.
- Ca/Mg: Normal.
- LFTs: Normal.
- Amylase/Lipase: Normal.
- Cardiac enzymes: Normal.
- U/A: Normal.
- Stool: Hemoccult negative.
- Lithium: Results back after full workup and admit to the ICU. 4.4 mEq/L.

46.7. X-rays:

- Chest x-ray: Normal.
- CT head: Normal.

46.8. Special Tests:

- ECG: Depressed ST-segments, T-wave inversion and prolonged QT interval.

46.9. Critical Actions:

- Elicit a history from husband of taking lithium.
- Give a normal saline bolus, keeping the urine output at 1 to 2 mL/kg/h.
- Admit to the ICU.
- Arrange hemodialysis for chronic lithium toxicity.
- Consult nephrology and internal medicine.
- Do not give activated charcoal.

46.10. Pearls:

❍ **What electrolyte and EKG findings are associated with lithium toxicity?**

Lithium toxicity may cause a decrease in the anion gap. Both Na^+ and K^+ may be low. Chronic lithium toxicity is associated with depressed ST-segments and T-wave inversion. In acute toxicity you see T wave inversions, complete heart block, and a prolonged QT interval.

❍ **When should dialysis be used in lithium toxicity?**

Guidelines for hemodialysis are controversial in patients with an acute intoxication, but it is generally recommended for high lithium levels (>4 mEq/L) despite minor symptoms, serious CNS and/or cardiovascular abnormalities. Consider dialysis in patients with chronic toxicity and serum lithium concentrations higher than 4 mEq/L and in unstable chronic patients with lithium levels higher than 2.5 mEq/L.

CASE 47 (44 y/o Male with a Cough)

Examiner

This case tests the candidate's ability to recognize anthrax infection as well as activate reasonable exposure precautions. The patient is a psychotic microbiologist who arrives with respiratory distress, advanced active disease, and initially no reported history of exposure. As the case develops, he has physical findings highly suggestive of anthrax and the substance is on his clothes. Shortly after the emergency physician questions the patient about possible exposure to something at work, the patient bolts from the treatment room and in the course of being tackled by security in the waiting room, dumps a plastic sac containing white powder into the air. He has exposed nine individuals in the waiting room, the triage nurse, the patient care nurse, two security officers, and the candidate.

After the incident, the candidate must suspect the diagnosis, confront the patient, treat the patient, treat the exposure within the department, and contact the appropriate physicians, hazmat team and law enforcement agency to assist with management of the patient and exposure, and CDC.

47.1. Introduction:

A 44 y/o male presents with fever, nonproductive cough, malaise, shortness of breath, and vomiting. Patient is very evasive but admits to symptoms getting worse over the last few days. Patient denies tobacco use or a history of asthma. He says, he is a microbiologist, knows what he has, and requests Ciprofloxacin®.

Vital signs: BP 120/80, P 100, R 24, T 102.2°F.

47.2. Primary Survey:

- General: 44 y/o male, who appears in moderate respiratory distress.
- Airway: Intact.
- Breathing: Tachypneic with retractions.
- Circulation: Capillary refill 4 seconds.
- Disability: Pupils normal.
- Exposure: Patient has all his clothes on and did not put on the hospital gown provided.

47.3. Management:

- Initiate IV rehydration with NS.
- Order appropriate laboratory studies, including blood and urine cultures, and chest x-ray.
- Place on O_2, cardiac monitor, and pulse oximeter.

47.4. History:

- Allergies: None.
- Medications: None.
- PMH: None.
- Last meal: 24 hours ago.
- Events: A 44 y/o male presents with fever, nonproductive cough, malaise, shortness of breath, and vomiting. Patient is very evasive but admits to symptoms getting worse over the last few days. He says, he is a microbiologist, knows what he has, and requests Ciprofloxacin®.
- Family: None.
- Records: None.
- Immune: Up to date.

- Doctor: None.
- Social: Anxious, admits to being fired from job teaching microbiology at a local college.

47.5. Secondary Survey:

- General: Anxious and hyper alert.
- Skin: Normal.
- HEENT: Sclera nonicteric, PERRL, oral mucosa dry, pharynx normal, TMs normal.
- Neck: Supple, no meningeal signs.
- Chest: Nontender to palpation.
- Lungs: Crackles with basilar consolidation.
- Heart: Tachy, cardic no murmur.
- Abdomen: Nontender, no masses, no organomegaly.
- Perineum/GU: Normal.
- Rectal: Hemoccult negative.
- Back: Normal.
- Extremities: Capillary refill >3 seconds.
- Neuro: No focal deficits, normal DTRs.
- Lymphatic: Multiple sites of shotty lymph nodes.

47.6. Laboratory:

- CBC: WBC 14, Hgb 14.1, Hct 43, Plt 225,000.
- Chemistry: Na 132, K 4.0, Cl 80, CO_2 13.
- BUN/Cr: 26/0.9.
- Glucose: 130.
- Ca/Mg: Normal.
- LFTs: Normal.
- PT/PTT: Normal.
- Pulse Ox: 91%.
- ABG: pH 7.27, pO_2 93, pCO_2 30, HCO_3 14.
- Cultures: Blood/urine/ pending.
- Gram stain: Gram-positive rods.
- U/A: RBC 0–2, WBC 0–2, ketones 2+, specific gravity 1.025.

47.7. X-rays:

- CXR: Wide mediastinum with paratracheal and hilar fullness and bibasilar pleural effusions.

47.8. Critical Actions:

- Start fluid bolus therapy with 0.9 NS or LR.
- Restrain patient or appropriate security in ED.
- Admit to the ICU in isolation with security detail.
- Start IV ciprofloxin 400 mg q12 hours.
- Consult infectious disease and internal medicine physicians.
- Call hazmat emergency and close down emergency department and waiting room for decontamination.
- All exposed should be hosed down and should scrub with soap and water.
- All exposed should be started on ciprofloxin 500 mg bid for 60 days.
- Call CDC to report high-probability exposure and obtain access to vaccine.
- Give the anthrax vaccine.
- Call local authorities.

47.9. Pearls:

❍ **What is the key laboratory finding in patients with anthrax?**

Gram-positive rods.

❍ **What are the expected chest x-ray findings in inhalational anthrax?**

Prominent mediastinum with hilar adenopathy and pleural effusions.

CASE 48 (8 y/o with a Neck Injury)

Examiner

An 8 y/o male presents with impending airway obstruction. He has sustained a serious neck injury. Paramedics arrive in the ED and indicate they have attempted to intubate the patient but have been unable to do so with three attempts. O_2 saturation has been dropping and on arrival is 85%. The paramedic screams they are having increasing difficulty bagging the patient as they wheel the patient into the trauma room.

When the candidate enters the room, the nurse says the patient is worse and the saturation has dropped to 85%. The patient is cyanotic and limp. Any attempt at intubation fails. The candidate should perform a needle cricothyroidotomy, appropriate x-rays, and ENT consultation. A cricothyroidotomy is not recommended in patients younger than 12 years and should the candidate attempt this, the patient should develop severe hemorrhage, inability to access the airway, and the patient should expire.

48.1. Introduction:

An 8 y/o male is brought to the ED by paramedics in severe respiratory distress.

Vital signs: BP 90/60, P 130, R 30, T 98.6, pulse ox 85% by bag-valve-mask, Wt 30 kg.

The paramedics attempted to intubate three times but have been unsuccessful. O_2 saturation has been dropping and on arrival is 85%. The paramedic screams they are having increasing difficulty bagging the patient.

48.2. Primary Survey:

- General: An 8 y/o in severe respiratory distress with stridor and shallow, rapid respirations.
- Airway: Nearly impossible to bag.
- Breathing: Rapid.
- Circulation: Tachycardic.
- Disability: Unresponsive.
- Exposure: Large red mark in anterior neck, with extensive soft tissue swelling, and subcutaneous air. No c-collar has been placed on the patient.

48.3. Management:

- IV, O_2, pulse oximeter, monitor.
- Give IV sedation
- Ask the paramedics to maintain in-line traction and stabilize the neck.
- Attempt immediate intubation (which fails).
- Perform a needle cricothyrotomy (ask the candidate to describe the procedure in detail).
- Place on 100% O_2 with intermittent jet insuflation and have the assistant hold the catheter in place at all times.
- Order CT neck
- CT c-spine.
- CXR.
- Call anesthesiology and ENT immediate surgery.

48.4. History:

- Allergies: Unknown.
- Medication: Unknown.
- PMH: Unknown.
- Last meal: 1 hour ago.
- Events: Paramedics state he was riding his bicycle and according to his sister, struck his neck on a wire stretched across a bridge. No other information is available
- Family: Unknown, cannot reach mother, 9 y/o sister is crying and cannot be calmed.
- Records: None.
- Immune: Unknown.
- Doctor: Dr. Pediatrician.
- Social: Unknown.

48.5. Secondary Survey:

- General: Improved after placement of needle cricothyrotomy.
- Skin: Normal.
- HEENT: Normal.
- Neck: Red deep line across anterior neck with extensive soft tissue swelling.
- Chest: Normal.
- Lungs: Good breath sounds with insufflation.
- Heart: Normal.
- Abdomen: Normal.
- Perineum/GU: Normal.
- Rectal: Not indicated.
- Back: Normal.
- Extremities: Normal.
- Neuro: Normal.

48.6. Laboratory:

- CBC: Normal.
- Chemistry: Normal.
- BUN/Cr: Normal
- Glucose: Normal.
- PT/PTT: Normal.
- U/A: Normal.

48.7. X-rays:

- CT neck: Extensive soft tissue swelling with fracture of hyoid bone.
- CXR: Normal.
- CT c-spine: Normal.

48.8. Critical Actions:

- Attempt oral intubation.
- Perform needle cricothyrotomy.
- C-spine precautions until cleared.
- Immediate consult of anesthesiology and ENT.
- Attempt to contact parents but send patient to OR even though parents cannot be reached.

48.9. Pearls:

❍ **What is the minimum recommended age for surgical cricothyrotomy?**

12 years.

❍ **Why is a needle cricothyrotomy indicated in children younger than 12 years?**

There is a high incidence of late airway complications such as subglottic stenosis.

CASE 49 (Triple)

Patient #1 (Abdominal Pain in a Postoperative Female)

Examiner

This patient is 1 week post-op from a Roux-en-Y gastric bypass. She has an anastomotic leak and is in early sepsis. She had an uneventful operation and was recovering at home when she started having abdominal pain. It is important to recognize the potential deadly complications of bariatric surgery and the subsequent workup and treatment.

Once the patient is stabilized and the workup is underway, she may go to CT with a nurse. While the patient is in CT, Cases 2 and 3 may be started and completed. Eventually the patient comes back from CT with a diagnosis of an anastomotic leak and surgery is immediately consulted.

49.1. Introduction: (**Patient #1**)

A 35 y/o morbidly obese female is lying on the cart restless, pale, and in a moderate degree of pain.

Vital signs: BP 90/65, P 110, R 24, T 100.9°F, Wt 172.7 kg (382 lb).

49.2. Primary Survey:

- General: Pale and restless.
- Airway: Intact.
- Breathing: Tachypneic.
- Circulation: Rapid weak pulses.
- Disability: None.
- Exposure: Healing laparoscopy incisions.
- Finger: Hemoccult negative stool.

49.3. Management:

- CBC, BMP, PT/PTT/INR, UA, Lipase, LFTs, Lactate, T&S, beta-HCG, CT abd/pelvis with IV contrast only. Unable to tolerate po contrast.
- 1 L NS bolus.
- Abdominal x-rays and CXR.
- Morphine for pain.
- Antiemetic for N/V.

49.4. History:

- Allergies: None.
- Medications: Colace 100 mg bid, oxycodone 10 mg q 4 hours, fluoxetine 20 mg qd, metformin 500 mg bid.
- PMH: Obesity, HTN, diabetes, depression.
- Last meal: Drank water 3 hours ago.
- Events: A 35 y/o obese female started having diffuse abdominal pain 16 hours ago. Pain is sharp, 8/10, and radiating to the back. She has a fever, N/V, weakness, fatigue, and constipation. Her postoperative period was uneventful and she went home 2 days after surgery.
- Family: Husband is at the bedside.
- Records: Easy to obtain.
- Immune: Up to date.
- EMTs: N/A.
- Narcotics: Oxycodone.
- Doctor: Dr. Roux surgery. Dr. Wenckebach internal medicine.
- Social history: Lives at home with husband and three children.

49.5. Secondary Survey:

- General: Unchanged unless pain medication and fluids are given.
- Skin: Warm, dry, no rash.
- HEENT: Mucous membranes dry.
- Neck: Supple.
- Chest: Normal.
- Lungs: Clear.
- Heart: Tachycardic, regular rhythm.
- Abdomen: Obese, diffusely tender, decreased bowel sounds.
- Perineum/GU: Normal.
- Rectal: Hemoccult negative.
- Back: Normal.
- Extremities: Normal.
- Neuro: Normal.

At this point the nurse asks you to see a patient that is in severe pain.

Patient #2 (Female with Severe Flank Pain)

Examiner

This patient has an obstructing kidney stone that must be diagnosed and appropriately managed in the ED. Even though she present with signs and symptoms of pyelonephritis, a simple admission and antibiotics are not enough. The ureteral stone must be found on CT or the patient will have a bad outcome in the hospital. She wants no "special" tests because of having no insurance. You must spend the time it takes to talk her into having a CT. You must also order the CT without contrast or the collecting system and stone will be obscured. Once the ureteral stone is found, consult urology and interventional radiology for a possible percutaneous nephrostomy tube.

49.1. Introduction: (**Patient #2**)

A 52 y/o female presents with right flank and abdominal pain, fever, and n/v for 1 day. She thinks it is related to her dinner last night or she is getting another "kidney infection."

Vital signs: BP 130/85, P 110, R 24, T 101.3°F, Wt 98 kg (215.6 lb).

49.2. Primary Survey:

- General: Moderately obese female in mild distress due to pain. She appears uncomfortable and has vomited in the ED.
- Airway: Normal.
- Breathing: Tachypnea.
- Circulation: Rapid full pulses, good capillary refill.
- Disability: Normal.
- Exposure: No abnormalities.

49.3. Management:

- IV, pulse oximeter, and monitor.
- Give pain medication IV.
- Give an antiemetic IV.
- Give a 500 mL to 1 L NS IV bolus.
- Give acetaminophen or ibuprofen po for fever.
- Draw blood for labs, UA with culture, CT abd/pelvis without IV/po contrast, consider a US of gallbladder and/or kidney.

49.4. History:

- Allergies: Penicillin.
- Medications: Metformin 500 mg po bid.
- PMH: Diabetes, pyelonephritis × 3, hysterectomy.
- Last meal: 10 hours ago.
- Events: Patient presents with right flank and abdominal pain for the past 24 hours. She has had many bouts of pyelonephritis in the past and states this feels the same. She has had a fever, n/v, diffuse abdominal pain, dysuria, increasing frequency and urgency.
- Family: DM and cancer.
- Records: None.
- Immune: Up to date.
- EMTs: None.
- Narcotics: None.
- Doctor: Dr. Renin
- Social history: Nonsmoker, nondrinker.

49.5. Secondary Survey:

- General: If given fluids, pain medication, and an antiemetic patient appears in no distress.
- Skin: Pale and dry.

- HEENT: Normal.
- Neck: Normal.
- Chest: Normal.
- Lungs: Normal.
- Heart: Normal.
- Abdomen: Hypoactive bowel sounds, some RUQ tenderness to palpation, no rebound or guarding.
- Perineum/GU: Normal.
- Rectal: Normal.
- Back: Significant right CVA tenderness.
- Extremities: Normal.
- Neuro: Normal.

At this point, the nurse states CT is ready for patient #2, and that another patient is in room 3. If candidate asks about patient #1 states that she is on her way back to the ED from radiology.

Patient #3 (Male with Diarrhea)

Examiner

This is a case of bacterial diarrhea and moderate dehydration. It is important to treat symptoms, replace the low potassium, and hydrate the patient. If he feels better, he may be discharged home with close follow up. Start on antibiotics after it is determined there are WBCs in the stool smear.

49.1. Introduction: (**Patient #3**)

A 33 y/o male presents with bloody diarrhea times 3 days.

Vital signs: BP 100/70, P 105, R 14, T 99.5°F (37.5°C), Wt 86 kg.

49.2. Primary Survey:

- General: Patient appears comfortable lying on cart.
- Airway: Normal.
- Breathing: Normal.
- Circulation: Tachycardic.
- Disability: None.
- Exposure: Normal.

49.3. Management:

- 1 to 2 large IVs.
- Bolus 1 to 2 L NR or LR.
- Order CBC, BMP, stool for O&P, WBCs, gram stain, and culture.

49.4. History:

- Allergies: Sulfa causes a rash.
- Medications: None.
- PMH: None.
- Last meal: 2 days ago
- Events: Started having crampy abdominal pain followed by multiple bouts of watery diarrhea about 2 days ago. He noted each BM was bloody starting today. Associated symptoms include abdominal cramping, fever, malaise, and anorexia. No complaints of n/v, recent antibiotic use, or hematuria. Patient lives with wife, and has had no sick contacts.
- Family: None.
- Records: None.
- Immune: Up to date.
- EMTs: None.

- Narcotics: None.
- Doctor: None.
- Social history: Nonsmoker, nondrinker.

49.5. Secondary Survey:
- General: Alert, nontoxic appearing, comfortable on cart.
- Skin: Decreased skin turgor, warm, no rash.
- HEENT: Normal.
- Neck: Normal.
- Chest: Normal.
- Lungs: Normal.
- Heart: Tachycardic rate, normal rhythm.
- Abdomen: Nontender, hyperactive bowel sounds.
- Perineum/GU: Normal.
- Rectal: Nontender, blood on glove, hemoccult positive.
- Back: Normal.
- Extremities: Normal.
- Lymph: No nodes.
- Neuro: Normal.

49.6. Laboratory:
- CBC: WBC 10.5, Hgb 12, Hct 36, Plt 270.
- Differential: Pending.
- Chemistry: Na 135, K 2.9, Cl 102, CO_2 21.
- BUN/Cr: 14/1.0.
- Glucose: 100.
- U/A: Normal.
- Stool: + WBCs, negative for O&P. Culture and Gram stain pending.

49.7. Critical Actions:
- IV hydration.
- Start on antibiotics for bacterial diarrhea.
- Treat the Low potassium.

Patient # 1 (Abdominal Pain in a Postoperative Female)

49.6. Laboratory:
- CBC: WBC 18,000, Hgb 11.5, Hct 35, Plt 385.
- Differential: Pending.
- Chemistry: Na 131, K 3.0, Cl 98, CO_2 18.
- BUN/Cr: 30/1.0.
- Glucose: 330.
- Ca/Mg: Pending.
- LFTs: Pending.
- Amylase/Lipase: Pending.
- Lactate: Pending.
- PT/PTT/INR: Pending.
- Blood cultures: Pending.
- U/A: Spec G 1.036, 2 + ketones. Otherwise normal.

49.7. X-rays:
- CXR: Normal.
- Abdominal x-ray: No visible abnormality due to body habitus and a poor quality film.

- CT abd/pelvis: Free fluid and air in peritoneal cavity.
- Barium enema: Diagnostic and therapeutic for intussusception.

49.8. Special Tests:
- ECG: None.

49.9. Critical Actions:
- Give an IV fluid bolus.
- Obtain a surgical consult.
- Order a CT abd/pelvis.
- Admit for surgical or endoscopic repair.
- Start appropriate antibiotics.

Patient #2

49.6. Laboratory:
- CBC: WBC 17, Hgb 14.1, Hct 37.8, Plt 190,000.
- Differential: Segs 55%, lymphs 38%, mono 5%, eos 1%, bands 15%.
- Chemistry: Na 139, K 4.2, Cl 104, CO_2 24.
- BUN/Cr: 15/1.3.
- Glucose: 130.
- Ca/Mg: Pending.
- LFTs: Pending.
- Amylase/Lipase: Pending.
- PT/PTT/INR: 12/28/1.0.
- Cardiac enzymes: Not indicated.
- ABG: Not indicated.
- Blood cultures: Pending.
- U/A: WBC's 100 hpf, RBC's 25–50 hpf, + bacteria, + nitrite.
- Urine culture pending.
- CT abd/pelvis: 1 cm stone proximal right ureter with significant hydronephrosis and perinephric fat stranding.

49.7. X-rays:
- KUB: 1 cm calcification right upper quadrant.
- CXR: Normal

49.8. Special Tests:
- US RUQ: Normal gallbladder, mild right hydronephrosis.
- CT abd/pelvis: 1 cm stone proximal right ureter with significant hydronephrosis and perinephric fat stranding.

49.9. Critical Actions:
- Diagnose the presents of an obstructing stone and early sepsis.
- Keep the patient NPO
- Urgent urology consult.
- Admit
- Start appropriate antibiotics.

49.10. Pearls: **(Patients# 1–3)**

❍ **What are the potential complications seen in the first postoperative month, from bariatric surgery?**

Anastomotic leak, obstruction, dumping syndrome, gastric necrosis, wound infection, GI bleed, and postcibal syndrome.

❍ **What is the most common late complication from gastric bypass?**

Stomal stenosis.

❍ **What is the purpose of ordering a KUB in a patient with renal colic, diagnosed by CT?**

The KUB provides valuable information for follow-up and can be repeated at a later date to track the progress. This prevents having to repeat a CT scan.

❍ **Is it true that a negative KUB and UA rules out the presence of a kidney stone?**

This is false. UA may be negative for blood in 15% to 25% of cases, while 10% of stones will not be seen on KUB.

❍ **What are two significant hematologic complications from infection with *Escherichia coli* 0157:H7?**

TTP and hemolytic-uremic syndrome.

References

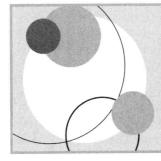

1. *Advanced Cardiac Life Support.* Dallas: American Heart Association; 2011.
2. American College of Surgeons. Committee on Trauma. *Advanced Trauma Life Support.* 9th ed. Chicago, IL: American College of Surgeons; 2012.
3. American Board of Emergency Medicine. *Examination Information for Candidates, Oral Certification.* 2014.
4. Anderson JE. *Grant's Atlas of Anatomy.* 8th ed. Baltimore, MD: Williams & Wilkins; 1983.
5. Bakerman S. *ABCs of Interpretive Laboratory Data.* 5th ed. Greenville: Interpretive Laboratory Data, Inc.; 2014.
6. Beers M, Porter R. *The Merck Manual.* 18th ed. Rahway: Merck Sharp & Dohme Research Laboratories; 2006.
7. Blok B, Cheung D, Platts-Mills T. *First Aid for the Emergency Medicine Boards.* 2nd ed. New York, NY: McGraw-Hill; 2012.
8. Bork K. *Diagnosis and Treatment of Common Skin Diseases.* 2nd ed. Philadelphia, PA: W.B. Saunders Company; 1999.
9. Christos SS. *Mnemonics & Pearls for Residents, Medical Students, Nurses, and Pre-Hospital Personnel.* Presence Resurrection Medical Center Emergency Department. Chicago, IL; 2012.
10. Dambro MR. *Griffith's 5 Minute Clinical Consult 2005.* Williams & Wilkins; 2004.
11. DeGowin EL. *Bedside Diagnostic Examination.* 8th ed. New York, NY: McGraw-Hill; 2004.
12. Wolff K. *Fitzpatrick's Color Atlas and Synopsis of Clinical Dermatology.* 5th ed. New York, NY: McGraw-Hill; 2005.
13. Gossman W. *Emergency Medicine.* eMedicine.com Inc.; 2006.
14. Harris JH. *The Radiology of Emergency Medicine.* 4th ed. Baltimore, MD: Lippincott, Williams & Wilkins; 2000.
15. Harrison TR. *Principles of Internal Medicine.* 18th ed. New York, NY: McGraw-Hill; 2011.
16. Harwood-Nuss A. *The Clinical Practice of Emergency Medicine.* 5th ed. Philadelphia, PA: Lippincott Williams & Wilkins Company; 2009.
17. Hoppenfeld S. *Physical Examination of the Spine and Extremities.* Norwalk: Appleton-Century-Crofts; 1976.
18. Howes D. *First Aid for the Emergency Medicine Oral Boards.* 1st ed. New York, NY: McGraw-Hill; 2010.
19. Kazzi Z, Shih R. *AAEM Resident & Student Association Toxicology Handbook.* 2nd ed. 2011.
20. Marriott HJL. *Practical Electrocardiography.* 10th ed. Baltimore, MD: Lippincott, Williams & Wilkins; 2001.
21. Moore KL. *Clinically Oriented Anatomy.* 4th ed. Baltimore, MD: Lippincott, Williams & Wilkins; 1999.
22. Yasuhara O. *Emergency Medicine Oral Board Review Illustrated.* 1st ed. Cambridge University Press; 2009. PEPID EM Platinum Suite 15.2, Chicago: 2014.
23. Perkins ES. *An Atlas of Diseases of the Eye.* 3rd ed. London: Churchill Livingstone; 1986.
24. Thomson PDR Staff. *Physicians' Desk Reference.* 59th ed. Oradell: Medical Economics Company Inc.; 2005.
25. Plantz SH. *Emergency Medicine PreTest, Self-Assessment and Review.* McGraw-Hill; 1990.
26. Plantz SH. *Emergency Medicine.* Baltimore, MD: Lippincott, Williams & Wilkins; 1998.
27. Plantz SH. *Emergency Medicine.* eMedicine.com, Inc.; 2005.
28. Plantz SH. *Emergency Medicine Pearls of Wisdom.* 6th ed. McGraw-Hill; 2005.
29. Robbins SL. *Pathologic Basis of Disease.* 7th ed. Philadelphia, PA: WB Saunders Company; 2004.
30. Roberts JR, Hedges JR. *Clinical Procedures in Emergency Medicine.* 5th ed. Philadelphia, PA: W.B. Saunders Company; 2009.
31. Rosen P. *Emergency Medicine Concepts and Clinical Practice.* 8th ed. Saunders; 2013.

32. Simon RR. *Emergency Orthopedics The Extremities.* 4th ed. Norwalk: Appleton & Lange; 2001.
33. Simon R. *Emergency Procedures and Techniques.* 4th ed. Baltimore, MD: Lippincott, Williams and Wilkins; 2001.
34. Simon R. *Clinical Neurology.* 7th ed. McGraw-Hill; 2009.
35. Slaby F. *Radiographic Anatomy.* New York, NY: John Wiley & Sons; 1990.
36. Squire LF. *Fundamentals of Radiology.* 5th ed. Cambridge: Harvard University Press; 1997.
37. Stedman TL. *Illustrated Stedman's Medical Dictionary.* 27th ed. Baltimore, MD: Williams & Wilkins; 2000.
38. American Society for Surgery of the Hand. *The Hand Primary Care of Common Problems.* 2nd ed. London: Churchill Livingstone; 1990.
39. Tintinalli JE. *Emergency Medicine: A Comprehensive Study Guide.* 7th ed. New York, NY: McGraw-Hill; 2010. UpToDate, Waltham, MA. Accessed from November 2014 to January 2015.
40. Weinberg S. *Color Atlas of Pediatric Dermatology.* 3rd ed. New York, NY: McGraw-Hill; 1997.

INDEX

U

V

W